Thyroid Eye Disease

Thyroid Eye Disease

Third Edition

Devron H. Char, M.D.
Professor of Ophthalmology and Radiation Oncology,
University of California, San Francisco, School of Medicine
and San Francisco General Hospital

Butterworth–Heinemann
Boston   Oxford   Johannesburg   Melbourne   New Delhi   Singapore

Every effort has been made to ensure that the drug dosage schedules within this text are accurate and conform to standards accepted at time of publication. However, as treatment recommendations vary in the light of continuing research and clinical experience, the reader is advised to verify drug dosage schedules herein with information found on product information sheets. This is especially true in cases of new or infrequently used drugs.

∞ Recognizing the importance of preserving what has been written, Butterworth–Heinemann prints its books on acid-free paper whenever possible.

Library of Congress Cataloging-in-Publication Data

Char, Devron H., 1945-
    Thyroid eye disease / Devron H. Char. -- 3rd ed.
        p.   cm.
    Includes bibliographical references and index.
    ISBN 0-7506-9893-4
    1. Thyroid eye disease.   I. Title.
    [DNLM: 1. Eye Diseases--etiology. 2. Thyroid Diseases--complications.   WW 140 C469t 1997]
    RE715.T48C43   1997
    617.7--dc21
    DNLM/DLC
    for Library of Congress   96-50467
                                                                                   CIP

British Library Cataloguing-in-Publication Data
A catalogue record for this book is available from the British Library.

The publisher offers special discounts on bulk orders of this book.
For information, please contact:

Manager of Special Sales
Butterworth–Heinemann
313 Washington Street
Newton, MA 02158-1626
Tel: 617-928-2500
Fax: 617-928-2620

For information on all B-H medical publications available, contact our World Wide Web home page at: http://www.bh.com/med

10 9 8 7 6 5 4 3 2 1

Printed in the United States of America

To Dr. Valerie Charlton and Danton Char, without whom life
would be far less fun and less exciting
and
To my friend Bill Coblentz, a man whose everyday actions make
an adumbration of the classic line in act I, scene 2 of *Henry VI Part 2*

Contents

Preface

Writing a third edition of a book is an interesting experience for the author. Among his or her considerations are how fast basic pathophysiologic concepts have changed, what errors need correction from the previous editions, and what modifications in patient management have been made since the second edition.

I have tried to continue the format and scope of the first two editions to produce a short, readable monograph and lucidly discuss basic disease mechanisms as well as patient management. In a few areas, new experimental data have increased our understanding of the pathophysiology of thyroid eye disease, and that material has been included in this edition. Molecular biology techniques have also begun to increase our understanding of disease pathophysiology. Clinical trials based on those findings and gene therapy approaches are just being organized.

Some treatment issues have become better clarified with more experience. Many more surgeons, including myself, have had greater experience with orbital decompression, which has led to alterations in surgical technique. Finally, new drugs have been tried in the treatment of severe thyroid orbitopathy; their role in our therapeutic armamentarium is discussed.

It has become more difficult to exhaustively review the large body of literature of over 2,500 papers spanning almost 200 years. Whereas in previous editions I have tried to be all-inclusive, the exponentially expanding literature makes that impossible. Libraries continue to parse their journal subscriptions, and a myriad of journals are not in Medline. I have limited the references principally to those in which there are primary data, papers that promulgate a major theory, or those that lucidly address the point discussed. I am sure that some papers that have made important contributions to our understanding have not been cited, and I apologize in advance for those omissions.

In writing this book I very much appreciate the advice and assistance of my editor, O.E.E. Anderson, and the people at Butterworth–Heinemann. Peg Coakley has graciously word-processed versions of this manuscript. As always, Mike Narahara has produced excellent photographs. I am indebted to Doctors Crowell Beard, Creig Hoyt, Art Jampolsky, Alan Scott, Andrew Murr, Basil Rappoport, and Frank Greenspan, who read portions of the manuscript and made valuable suggestions. Walter Denn and Joan Weddell have produced wonderful drawings that improve the lucidity of the text. Dr. William Dillon has kindly allowed me to use CT and MRI scans from our institution. They have all added much positive input; I take sole responsibility for the errors. I invite readers to contact me with questions.

Devron H. Char, M.D.
Department of Ophthalmology
University of California, San Francisco, Medical Center
10 Kirkham Street, Box 0730
San Francisco, CA 94143-0730
(415) 334-2792
email: char-tumori@worldnet.ATT.net

1

Introduction

The association between eye disease and hyperthyroidism has been recognized for more than 200 years. Parry[1] first described diffuse toxic goiter and proptosis in 1786. In 1835 Graves[2] described a female patient: "It was now observed that the eyes assumed a singular appearance, for the eyeballs were apparently enlarged, so that when she slept or tried to shut her eyes, the eyelids were incapable of closing. When the eyes were open, the white sclerotic could be seen, to a breadth of several lines around the cornea." Perhaps Brain[3] made the most telling statement about thyroid ophthalmopathy when he wrote: "There is an exception to every statement that can be made."

There are more than 40 theories to account for the development of eye changes in hyperthyroidism since von Basedow[4] hypothesized that the orbital contents were probably hypertrophied ("strumous hypertrophy"). The disproved hypotheses for thyroid ophthalmopathy include cervical sympathetic stimulation, laxity of the extraocular muscles, orbital venous congestion, contraction of the nonstriated orbital muscles, and the presence of a simple pituitary factor.[5–14]

Many terms and classifications have been advocated by various clinicians to describe thyroid eye findings (Table 1-1), including malignant exophthalmos, infiltrative ophthalmopathy, endocrine exophthalmos, and thyroid ophthalmopathy.[15–19] More than 30 eponyms for various eye signs of thyroid ophthalmopathy exist (see Chapter 4).

This book is written for medical practitioners who manage patients with thyroid-related eye problems. Thyroid eye disease literature, even excluding those publications addressing nonophthalmic aspects of Graves' disease, is voluminous. Approximately 2,500 manuscripts have been published that discuss thyroid ophthalmopathy since its first clinical description in 1786. The etiology, pathophysiology, diagnosis, and treatment of hyperthyroidism and its associated ophthalmopathy remain an enigma to many physicians who must evaluate and treat patients with these conditions. In some areas, researchers and clinicians have improved our understanding of these disease processes; laboratory tests including sensitive thyroid-stimulating hormone (TSH) assays and orbital scanning procedures have increased diagnostic accuracy and demonstrated the mechanism of thyroid optic neuropathy (see Chapter 6). In other areas, historical theories, unsupported by controlled clinical trials, still influence the management of thyroid ophthalmopathy. As discussed in

Table 1-1. Thyroid and Euthyroid Ophthalmopathy: Descriptive Terms

Thyrotoxic exophthalmos
Progressive exophthalmos
Malignant exophthalmos
Exophthalmic ophthalmoplegia
Thyrotropic exophthalmos
Hyperophthalmopathic form of Graves' disease
Edematous exophthalmos of endocrine origin
Infiltrative ophthalmopathy
Endocrine exophthalmos
Exophthalmic goiter
Thyrotropic exophthalmos
Postoperative exophthalmos

Chapter 7, the effect of various hyperthyroidism therapies (surgery, drugs, and radioactive iodine) on thyroid eye disease is still unclear.

Major issues remain unresolved in thyroid ophthalmopathy. These include the following:

1. What is the relationship between autoimmune thyroid disease and eye findings? Are these components of the same disease, or are they separate but closely related?
2. What are the inciting factors for the pathogenesis of thyroid eye disease?
3. What is the putative shared thyroid-orbital antigen?
4. Why do some patients with hyperthyroidism develop clinical eye changes while other patients do not?
5. What is the relationship between the course of treated systemic thyroid disease and thyroid ophthalmopathy?
6. Why do a small minority (usually < 5%) of thyroid ophthalmopathy patients develop serious ocular sequelae while most do not?
7. What mechanisms are responsible for asymmetric thyroid eye disease with either unilateral or predominant inferior rectus muscle involvement?
8. What is the role of the thyroid in the development of euthyroid ophthalmopathy?

This book stresses the diagnosis and management of thyroid eye disease and offers ophthalmologists a thorough overview of the associated eye changes. There are some excellent reviews of components of thyroid ophthalmopathy, but a single author's experience with these diverse areas has been lacking.[20–33] The purpose of this book is to consolidate current ideas of pathogenesis, diagnosis, and management. Chapter 2 is an overview of current concepts regarding thyroid regulation and the pathophysiology of Graves' disease. Chapter 3 discusses the use of nonocular tests in establishing the diagnosis of thyroid ophthalmopathy. Chapter 4 covers the eye signs and symptoms and thyroid orbitopathy classification systems. Chapter 5 discusses differential diagnosis, ocular tests, and orbital studies useful in diagnostic evaluation. Chapter 6 discusses current concepts of pathogenesis and pathophysiology. Chapter 7 outlines the natural history of thyroid eye disease including development of major complications such as restrictive myopathy, exposure, optic neuropathy, and the effect of systemic therapy on ocular disease. The remainder of the book suggests rational approaches to the management of thyroid eye disease. An overview of treatment is presented, and medical, radiation, and surgical approaches to therapy are outlined. A surgical atlas covers most of the procedures that I find useful in the management of thyroid ophthalmopathy.

REFERENCES

1. Parry CH. Enlargement of thyroid gland in connection with enlargement or palpitation of the heart. Collections from unpublished writings of late Caleb Hillier Parry (Vol 2). London: Underwoods, 1825;111.
2. Graves RJ. Newly observed affection of the thyroid gland in females. London Med Surg J 1835;7:516.
3. Brain R. Discussion of endocrine exophthalmos. Proc R Soc Med 1952;45:237.
4. Von Basedow CA. Exophthalmos durch hypertrophie des cellgewebes in der augenhöhle. Wochenschr Ges Heilk 1840;6:197, 220.
5. Cooper WW. On protrusion of the eyes in connection with anemia, palpitation and goitre. Lancet 1849;1:551.
6. Dobyns BM. Present concepts of pathologic physiology of exophthalmos. J Clin Endocrinol Metab 1950;10:1202.
7. Askanasy M. Pathologische-Anatomische beitraege zur kenntnis des morbus basedowii, insbesonders ueber die dabei auftretende muskelerkrankung. Dtsch Arch Klin Med 1898;61:118.
8. Sattler H. Ueber den sogenannten landstroemischen muskel und seine bedeutung fur den exophthalmus bei morbus basedowii. Ber Versamml Ophthalmol Ges Heidelberg 1911;37:181.
9. Mulvany JH. Exophthalmos of hyperthyroidism (part I). Am J Ophthalmol 1944;27:589.
10. Aran FA. De la nature et du traitement de l'affection connue sous le nom de goitre exophtalmique, cachexia exophtalmique, maladie de basedow. Bull Acad Med 1860–1861;26:122.
11. Marine D. Studies on pathological physiology of exophthalmos of Graves' disease. Ann Intern Med 1938;12:443.
12. Bernard C. Leçons sur la Physiologie et la Pathologie due Système Nerveux (Vol 2). Paris: J B Ballière et Fils, 1858;499.
13. Loeb J, Friedman H. Exophthalmos produced by injections of acid extract of anterior pituitary gland of cattle. Proc Soc Exp Biol Med 1932;29:648.
14. Smelser GK. A comparative study of experimental and clinical exophthalmos. Am J Ophthalmol 1937;20:1189.
15. Brain WR. Exophthalmic ophthalmoplegia. Trans Ophthalmol Soc UK 1937;57:107.
16. Jensen VA. Malignant exophthalmos after strumectomy. Acta Ophthalmol 1940;18:1.
17. Thomas HM Jr, Woods AC. Progressive exophthalmos following thyroidectomy. Bull Johns Hopkins Hosp 1936;59:9.
18. Warner F. Ophthalmoplegia externa, complicating case of Graves' disease. Br Med J 1882;ii:843.
19. Werner SC. Ocular Manifestations. In SC Werner, S Ingbar (eds), The Thyroid. New York: Harper & Row, 1971;528.
20. McGill DA, Asper SP Jr. Endocrine exophthalmos. A review and a report on autoantibody studies. N Engl J Med 1962;267:188.
21. Woods AC. The ocular changes of primary diffuse toxic goitre; review. Medicine 1946;25:113.
22. Havard CWH. Endocrine exophthalmos. Br J Med 1972;1:1360.
23. Gorman CA. The presentation and management of endocrine ophthalmopathy. J Clin Endocrinol Metab 1978;7:67.
24. Kriss JP, Konishi J, Herman M. Studies on the pathogenesis of Graves' ophthalmopathy (with some related observations regarding therapy). Recent Prog Horm Res 1975;31:533.
25. DeSanto LW. The total rehabilitation of Graves' ophthalmopathy. Laryngoscope 1980;90:1652.
26. Sergott RC, Glaser JS. Graves' ophthalmopathy: a clinical and immunologic review. Surv Ophthalmol 1981;26:1.
27. Jacobson DH, Gorman CA. Endocrine ophthalmopathy: current ideas concerning etiology, pathogenesis and treatment. Endocr Rev 1984;5:200.

28. Kriss JP, McDougall IR, Donaldson SS. Graves' Ophthalmopathy. In DT Krieger, CW Bordin (eds), Therapy in Endocrinology. Philadelphia: Decker, 1983.

29. Mullin BR. Dysthyroid exophthalmos. In A Garner, GK Klintworth (eds), Pathobiology of Ocular Disease: A Dynamic Approach. New York: Dekker, 1983;1077.

30. Cordes FC. Endocrine exophthalmos: Evaluation of present knowledge. Am J Ophthalmol 1954;38:1.

31. Gorman CA, Waller RR, Dyer JA (eds). The Eye and Orbit in Thyroid Disease. New York: Raven, 1984.

32. Weetman AP. Extrathyroidal complications of Graves' disease. QJM 1993;86:473.

33. Burch HB, Wartofsky L. Graves' ophthalmopathy: current concepts regarding pathogenesis and management. Endocr Rev 1993;14:747.

2

Normal Thyroid Gland and Mechanisms of Hyperthyroidism

NORMAL ANATOMY AND PHYSIOLOGY

The thyroid gland weighs approximately 20 g; its upper isthmus margin can be palpated just below the cricoid cartilage. The gland has a rich vascular and lymphatic supply. Kriss and coworkers have demonstrated, using radionuclide tracer techniques, that the lymphatic drainage from the thyroid gland and the orbit is probably into the cervical lymph node chain.[1]

The thyroid gland is composed primarily of acini, or follicles—closely packed saccules invested with a rich capillary network. The clear proteinaceous colloid they contain constitutes the thyroid's major mass. Iodination and the initial phase of hormone secretion occur at or near the apical microvilli of follicular cells located in the colloid.[2] Thyroglobulin, a protein that is the major component of the colloid, is the matrix in which thyroid hormones are formed and stored.

A hypothalamic-anterior pituitary-thyroid complex, modulated by a negative feedback loop, regulates thyroid function (Figure 2-1).[3,4] The cerebral cortex may also play a role, by regulating hypothalamic secretion of the thyrotropin-releasing hormone (TRH). TRH, a tripeptide synthesized in the supraoptic and paraventricular nuclei of the hypothalamus, is stored in the median eminence and reaches its target organ through the hypophyseal portal venous circulation. In the anterior pituitary it is specifically bound to thyrotroph and lactotroph cells and stimulates adenylate cyclase.

TRH promotes the release and synthesis of the thyroid-stimulating hormone (TSH) thyrotropin by bonding with thyrotroph cells in the anteromedial portion of the adenohypophysis. This action is inhibited mainly by unbound (free) triiodothyronine (T_3) and thyroxine (T_4) hormones, which diminish the number of available TRH receptors on pituitary thyrotrophs. Although TRH and thyroid hormones are the major components of the homeostatic control mechanism for TSH release, somatostatin, dopamine, steroids, iodide, and other compounds can modulate this servocontrol circuit.

The glycoprotein TSH is composed of alpha and beta subunits.[5] Many of its effects on the thyroid gland are mediated by cyclic adenosine monophosphate (cAMP). There is a TSH receptor (TSHr) on the membrane of follicular cells. Stimulation of this receptor by autoantibodies is the cause of hyperthyroidism in the pathophysiol-

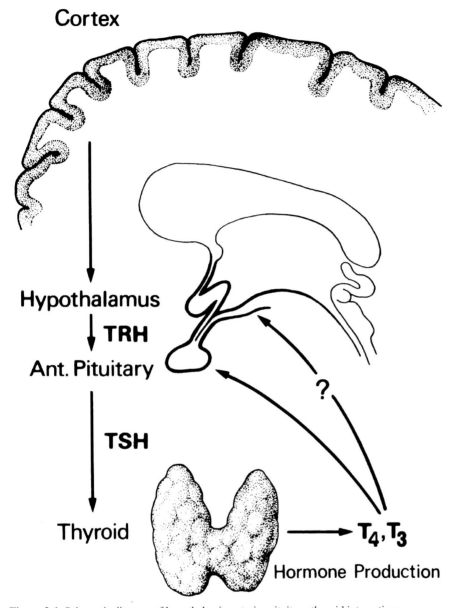

Figure 2-1. Schematic diagram of hypothalamic-anterior pituitary-thyroid interactions.

ogy of Graves' disease.[6] The thyrotropin receptor has been cloned.[7] It is a hepta-helical receptor that can stimulate G proteins.[8] The anti-TSHr antibodies appear to be secreted mainly by clonally restricted B cells in the thyroid gland.[9] As discussed in Chapter 3, the availability of newer, more sensitive TSH assays have revolutionized the evaluation of thyroid eye disease patients. In addition to the exogenous anterior pituitary influence, the thyroid gland also has some autoregulatory capacity.

Table 2-1. Thyroxin-Binding Alpha Globulin (TBG) Alteration

1. Increases TBG levels
   a. Genetic predisposition
   b. Pregnancy
   c. Neonatal period
   d. Drugs: estrogens, birth control pills, perphenazine, etc.
   e. Liver disease: biliary cirrhosis, hepatitis
2. Decreases TBG levels
   a. Genetic predisposition
   b. Steroids
   c. Systemic illness
   d. Nephrotic syndrome
   e. Acromegaly

Hormone formation in the thyroid gland occurs in three steps: active iodide transportation into the thyroid, iodide oxidation and iodination with tyrosyl residues to form inactive iodotyrosines, and coupling of iodotyrosines to form T_3 and T_4. Release of hormones from the thyroid gland is also an active process requiring thyroglobulin hydrolysis and release of iodothyronines (T_3 and T_4) before exit into the lymphatic and systemic circulations.

Almost all thyroid hormone is released as T_4; peripheral conversion by deiodination of that hormone produces more than 80% of the body's T_3.[10] T_4 is highly bound to two serum proteins, thyroxin-binding globulin (TBG) and thyroxin-binding prealbumin (TBPA).[11] T_3 binds mainly to TBG. Both T_3 and T_4 are minimally bound to plasma albumin (<5%). Numerous conditions alter TBG concentrations (Table 2-1). While these conditions do not affect the amount of hormone that enters the cell, they can artifactitously alter the laboratory assessment of T_3 and T_4 levels. Some systemic illnesses, pregnancy, and drugs can also alter hormone secretion and the peripheral conversion of T_4 to T_3.[12]

A summary of abbreviations and synonyms is given in Table 2-2.

MANIFESTATIONS OF HYPERTHYROIDISM

Thyrotoxicosis can result from overproduction of hormone by the thyroid (true hyperthyroidism), from inflammation-induced glandular hormone leakage, from oral ingestion of excess thyroid hormone, or (rarely) as a result of extrathyroidal hormonal production.[12] Hyperthyroidism due to Graves' disease (termed von Basedow's disease in Europe) most commonly presents in the third or fourth decade of life with a female to male ratio between 4 to 1 and 7 to 1.[13,14] In the United States the disease's incidence is estimated to be 0.4%.[15]

Other causes of thyrotoxicosis not associated with ophthalmopathy include toxic multinodular goiter, toxic adenoma, inappropriate thyroid stimulation (tumors, molar pregnancy, hypothalamic-pituitary abnormalities, etc.), thyrotoxicosis factitia, and diffuse micronodular goiter.[16] Only in Graves' disease is there a statistically significant increased prevalence of eye disorders, although eye findings occur in approximately 3% of Hashimoto's disease patients and occasionally in individuals with primary hypothyroidism, thyroid cancer, and those with a history of other forms of

Table 2-2. Abbreviations and Synonyms

AMP	Adenosine monophosphate
cAMP	Cyclic adenosine monophosphate
DQ/DR	HLA-class II antigens
FRTL	Rat thyroid cell line used in TSI assay
HLA	Human leukocyte antigen
IL	Interleukin
LAI	Leukocyte adherence inhibition
LATS	Long-acting thyroid stimulator
LPA	LATS protector activity
MHC	Major histocompatibility complex
MIF	Migration-inhibiting factor
RT_3	Resin T_3
T_3	Triiodothyronine
T_4	Tetraiodothyronine (thyroxine)
TBA	Thyroxin-binding albumin
TBG	Thyroxin-binding globulin
TBII	Thyrotropin-binding inhibitory immunoglobulin
TBPA	Thyroxin-binding prealbumin
TPO	Thyroid peroxidase
TRAb	Thyrotropin receptor antibody
TRH	Thyrotropin-releasing hormone
TSH	Thyroid-stimulating hormone (thyrotropin)
TSHr	Thyrotropin receptor
TSI	Thyroid-stimulating immunoglobulin

thyroid inflammation.[16–24] Hancock and colleagues reviewed 1,787 Hodgkin's disease patients treated with chemotherapy, radiation, or both; approximately 10% had some thyroid abnormalities.[23] Most of these patients had their thyroid in the radiation field. Of the 30 patients who developed Graves' disease after Hodgkin's disease therapy, 21 had eye changes (Figure 2-2).[23]

Graves' disease, or diffuse toxic goiter, is actually a constellation of disorders including diffuse primary thyroid hyperplasia and thyrotoxicosis that is one of a number of conditions associated with elevated levels of thyroid hormones. It is often accompanied by ophthalmopathy and occasionally by an infiltrative dermopathy. Fatourechi and coworkers noted that dermopathy was present in less than 4% of all Graves' disease patients but was present in 15% of those with orbitopathy.[25] Almost all dermopathy patients have ocular findings, and 30% require orbital decompression.[25] Rarely, hyperthyroid patients develop thyroid acropathy, which encompasses endocrine exophthalmos, pretibial myxedema, and peripheral clubbing.

While eye signs and symptoms can be present at the time of diagnosis in 20–40% of Graves' disease patients, less than 20% of hyperthyroid patients initially present to their physician because of ocular manifestations without a history of hyperthyroidism.[26–35] Most hyperthyroid patients seek medical care because of the systemic signs and symptoms of thyrotoxicosis—gradually occurring nervousness, irritability, emotional lability, fatigue, weight loss, abnormal heat sensitivity, increased sweating, palpitations, and weakness. In individual cases, different elements of this symptom complex may predominate. Occasionally patients seek help because of abnormal thyroid tests, hormones, or after thyrotoxic exacerbation of other systemic illnesses

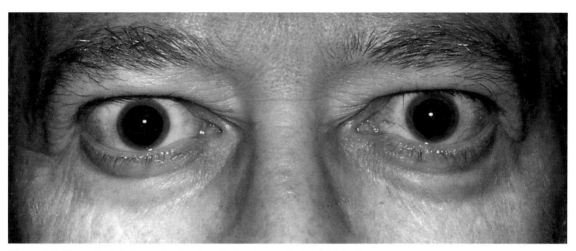

Figure 2-2. Graves' ophthalmopathy developed after therapy for Hodgkin's disease.

such as cardiac disease, or with acute thyroid storm. The frequency of signs and symptoms in 247 thyrotoxic patients is shown in Table 2-3.[36]

In all forms of true hyperthyroidism there are increased levels of circulating T_3 and T_4; the serum T_3 is usually increased proportionately more than the T_4 concentration, leading to an abnormally elevated T_3/T_4 ratio. In as many as 10% of hyperthyroid patients, only T_3 levels are elevated (T_3 toxicosis). A significant number of patients referred to ophthalmologists for the diagnosis of proptosis have thyroid ophthalmopathy with normal or borderline elevated T_3 and T_4 levels.[33,35,37,38] In almost all forms of hyperthyroidism, TSH secretion is suppressed; direct measurement of several techniques shows it to be very low.[39] As discussed in Chapter 3, these newer TSH assays are at least an order of magnitude more sensitive than older ones. In these situations, the thyroid gland functions independently of the pituitary-hypophyseal axis.

An enlarged thyroid gland (goiter) and bilateral exophthalmos are the most characteristic signs of Graves' disease, present in approximately one-third of patients at the time of diagnosis.[40-42] As shown in Figure 2-3, occasionally the cause of proptosis can be missed if the neck is not palpated (this patient was referred with a unilateral orbital tumor and the correct diagnosis was initially missed because an

Table 2-3. Signs and Symptoms in Thyrotoxicosis Patients

% of Cases	Symptoms	Signs
85–100	Nervousness, sweating, heat insensitivity, palpitation, fatigue, weight loss	Tachycardia, goiter, skin changes, tremor
70–85	Tachycardia, dyspnea, weakness	Thyroid bruit, eye signs
30–65	Increased appetite, eye symptoms, leg swelling, increased bowel movements	

Source: Modified from RH Williams. Thiouracil treatment of thyrotoxicosis: the results of prolonged treatment. J Clin Endocrinol 1946;6:1.

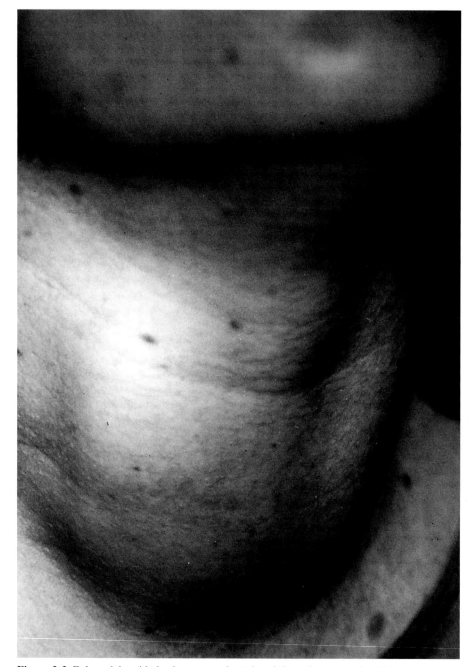

Figure 2-3. Enlarged thyroid gland was not palpated, and the patient was referred for management of a unilateral orbital tumor.

enlarged thyroid was not recognized). The thyroid gland is usually diffusely enlarged in hyperthyroid patients; however, many patients examined first because of eye findings have a normal gland, depending on the evolution of the thyroid gland pathology.[30,33,43] When there is diffuse enlargement of the gland, a thrill may often be palpable and a bruit audible over the thyroid. Patients usually have a tremor, tachycardia, and warm, moist skin; appear flushed due to increased cutaneous blood flow, and display nervous behavior. Often there are other integumentary changes including loss, brittleness, or increased fineness of hair, soft nails, increased skin pigmentation, and vitiligo.

PATHOGENESIS OF HYPERTHYROIDISM

A number of clinical and research observations document the autoimmune nature of Graves' disease; however, neither the initiating events nor the precise immunopathology is well delineated.[44–48] Probably a local insult or perturbation in the thyroid gland is responsible for the initiation of the autoimmune process, but a number of areas require elucidation. As discussed below, a viral infection, as with a retrovirus or other insults, increases class II histocompatibility antigen expression (human leukocyte antigen [HLA]-D) on thyrocytes and alters the local immunologic milieu.[49–51] It is uncertain whether Graves' disease is secondary to an abnormality in systemic immune regulation or results from a local perturbation of immune cells in the thyroid gland. Graves' disease, Hashimoto's thyroiditis, and primary thyroid atrophy are all different autoimmune thyroid diseases.[47] Some patients with Graves' disease have thymic hyperplasia, lymphadenopathy, or splenomegaly,[46,48] as well as other concurrent autoimmune diseases including pernicious anemia, myasthenia gravis, idiopathic adrenal atrophy, polymyalgia rheumatica, diabetes mellitus, autoimmune vitiligo, idiopathic thrombocytopenia purpura, and rheumatoid arthritis.[47,48,52]

Graves' disease and Hashimoto's thyroiditis share a number of features; some Graves' disease patients later develop Hashimoto's thyroiditis. Patients with Graves' disease or Hashimoto's thyroiditis have lymphocytic infiltration of the thyroid gland, and HLA disease associations have been observed in both entities.[52–58] The nature of these HLA disease associations is unclear. There is a different association with different racial groups.[52–59] More recent work suggests that autoimmune thyroid disease is more closely associated with the HLA-DQ locus, -DQA1*0501.[60,61]

Families with histories of both Graves' and Hashimoto's thyroiditis have been described. The conditions have been diagnosed in identical twins and even histologically in the same thyroid gland.[44,62–66] In identical twins, the concordance rate of 30–70% suggests that nonhereditary factors are also necessary for disease development.[64,65] A positive family history of thyroid disease is found in approximately 30% of cases.

Graves' disease and Hashimoto's thyroiditis are closely related. However, they are separate entities based on disparity in some HLA disease associations; marked differences in many disease manifestations, including the prevalence of ophthalmopathy, individual associations with other diseases, and different patterns of immunologic reactivity toward thyroid antigens.[46,50,56,67,68]

Initial immunologic studies used humoral techniques, since the requisite methodology for antibody investigations was characterized earlier than that for cell-mediated studies.[69] Early studies by Rose and Witebsky and by Adams and Purves established that an experimental model of thyroiditis was possible, and that some Graves' patients had a long-acting immunoglobulin that stimulated the thyroid gland.[6] A number of other thyroid-associated antibodies were described, but some have little importance in the disease process.[46,69–73] In 1956 Roitt et al. were the first to demonstrate antibodies toward thyroglobulin in patients with hyperthyroidism.[74] Before Roitt, some investigators hypothesized that thyroglobulin was a sequestered antigen and that its systemic exposure and subsequent antibody formation led to the development of autoimmune thyroiditis.[75] A large body of data makes this concept untenable.[76] Thyroglobulin has been revealed, using radioimmunoassays, in circulation in utero, in neonates, and in adults.[77] Moreover, although in rare instances of viral subacute thyroiditis an immunologic reactivity toward thyroid antigens including thyroglobulin can develop, neither Graves' disease nor Hashimoto's syndrome routinely follows.[73]

In 1956, Adams and Purvis described a long-acting thyroid stimulator (LATS), which was later identified as an immunoglobulin.[78] Unlike TSH, which reaches peak effectiveness in 2 hours, LATS is biologically active for up to 16 hours.[69] This substance is present in the serum of approximately 40–60% of patients with untreated hyperthyroidism, although most authorities believe that it does not correlate with disease severity, course, or ophthalmopathy.[26,69–73,79–81]

Contemporary TSHr antibody research is in flux. Antibodies can stimulate or inhibit receptor function as well as block it. As described earlier, the TSHr has been cloned, the extracellular protein of the molecule is quite antigenic, and it can stimulate G proteins.[6] Locally produced antibody directed against the TSHr is responsible for the hyperthyroidism in Graves' disease.[68,82–84] Many different antibodies that bind to TSHrs on thyroid cells have been described; some thyrotropin receptor antibodies (TRAbs) stimulate the thyroid while others do not.[57,68,69] Even the nomenclature for these antibodies is changing, although their general functions are more firmly codified.[39,85] TRAbs compete for the TSHr and stimulate the production of adenyl cyclase through the cyclic adenosine monophosphate (cAMP) system. They also increase radioactive iodine uptake and colloid droplet formation in the thyroid. TRAb describes human serum immunoglobulins that stimulate the release of radioactive iodine from primed guinea pig or murine thyroid cells, or that increase thyroid cellular cAMP in fresh or tissue culture human thyroid cells or an immortalized rat thyroid line (FRTL5 cells).[86] Assays for thyroid-stimulating immunoglobulins (TSIs) biologically active with human thyroid were previously difficult to perform, inaccurate, and costly. As discussed in Chapter 3, some of these TRAb/TSI assays are now commercially available using a number of different techniques. A common approach has been to use aliquots of cryopreserved primary human thyroid cell cultures, which appear to offer efficient, accurate, and reproducible TSI measurements.[39,86,87] Other reported TRAbs do not appear to be biologically active with human thyroid tissue, including TSH-displacing antibody and TSH-binding inhibitory immunoglobulin (TBII), among others. Antibodies demonstrated with the above testing techniques are termed *thyrotropin receptor antibodies*.[56,82,88] Molecular analysis of these various classes of TSHr antibodies should clarify the nature of these immunoglobulins that appear to be hypermutable.[88a]

Some of these antibodies can initiate thyroid glandular hypertrophy, increase vascularity, and cause hormone secretion by activation of cell membrane adenyl cyclase.[56,83] Some investigators have observed correlations between these thyroid-stimulating antibodies and nonsuppressibility of thyroid function. In treated hyperthyroid patients, correlations between antithyrotropin receptor antibody persistence and an increased likelihood of disease recurrence has also been noted. However, other investigators have not concurred.[56,71,79,89–93] Some discrepancies probably relate to the method used to measure the antibodies. In a meta-analysis of 18 publications between 1975 and 1991, the absence of TSHr antibodies after drug therapy was correlated with a 65% lower chance of relapse of hyperthyroidism.[94]

As previously mentioned, causes of autonomous production of these TSHr antibodies are unknown. Increased evidence supports the concept that these antibodies are responsible for hyperthyroidism in Graves' disease.[6,68,93] A clonal intrathyroid

B cell population is at least partially responsible for their development.[9] Probably more than one clone of B cells is activated since, while a preponderance of these antibodies have lambda-light chains, some have kappa-light chains and therefore appear to be polyclonal.[95,96] More data are needed since there are many epitopes on the TSH molecule; possibly a clonal expansion is responsible for the pathogenic antibody, but current techniques also measure other immunoglobulins. Once TRAb production results in hyperthyroidism, altered thyroid function may help perpetuate the immune system abnormalities, since both hyperthyroidism and TSH have many effects on immunologic function.[97,98]

In Graves' disease and Hashimoto's thyroiditis, antithyroid peroxidase (anti-TPO, formerly termed antimicrosomal) and antithyroglobulin antibodies, directed toward other antigens on or in thyroid cells, have diagnostic value (see Chapter 3).[56] Anti-TPO microsomal antibodies fix complement- and lyse-cultured thyroid cells in vitro. Their importance in the pathophysiology of thyroid disease has not been demonstrated. Demonstration of their reactive site led to the nomenclature change from antimicrosomal to anti-TPO antibodies.[99] Different investigators have tried to demonstrate abnormal thyroid antigens in patients with various thyroid diseases, but no novel antigens characteristic of either Graves' disease or Hashimoto's thyroiditis have been described.[100]

The nature and importance of immunologic homeostatic mechanisms for the control of both normal and abnormal immune responses have been investigated extensively in animals and humans. Cellular and humoral feedback loops have been demonstrated, and suppressor cells and anti-idiotypic antibodies have been identified (Figure 2-4). Suppressor cells of various lineages can nonspecifically and specifically dampen, amplify, and modulate cellular immune responses.[76,101] The lack of autoreactivity in normal individuals is probably due to T cell tolerance either by an antigen alone or indirectly by suppressor cells. There is no demonstrable B cell tolerance to several antigens, including thyroglobulin.[76,102] Autoreactivity does not occur in many organ systems, probably because there is no effective autoantigen presentation. Cells require HLA-DR antigen on their surface to effectively present an antigen to lymphocytes. Antigen-presenting cells such as macrophages have class I antigens (HLA-A, -B, -C) and class II antigens (HLA-DR) in contrast to other nucleated cells that lack class II antigens and cannot effectively present antigens to immunologically competent cells.

Several factors, including local viral infection and various inflammatory cells, stimulate interferon production, which is the best known inducer of HLA-DR antigen expression.[103] When a cell expresses DR antigen, immunocompetent T cells can usually recognize both DR and extrinsic antigens. In the presence of various interleukins (ILs), this leads to lymphocyte activation and division.

Our understanding of the immunogenetics of Graves' hyperthyroidism is limited. Under certain conditions, normal thyroid epithelium in culture can express DR antigens.[103,104] Several workers have shown that interferon-gamma can induce class II expression on thyrocytes.[50,105,106] Thyroid glands from Hashimoto's and Graves' disease patients routinely have DR antigen expression and may act as ancillary antigen-presenting cells. The data supporting this latter point are not certain since these class II positive thyrocytes are unable to stimulate T cells.[50] In a small number of thyroid gland studies, DR antigen expression preceded lymphocyte invasion of the thyroid or glandular damage, but there was no correlation between the number of activated T cells in the thyroid and the level of DR expression.[107] The fact that an antithyroid drug such as methimazole seems to reduce DR ex-

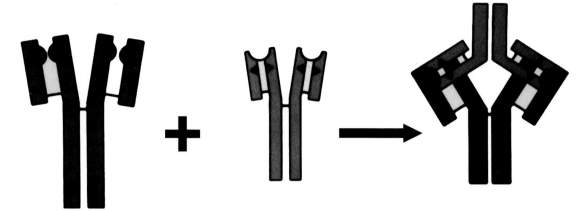

Figure 2-4. Schematic representation of an anti-idiotypic antibody.

pression on thyrocytes as well as diminish TSHr's antibodies also have made it difficult to interpret some studies.[108,109]

Jerne and others have developed network theories and demonstrated the importance of idiotypic and anti-idiotypic antibodies for feedback control of immunologic processes.[101,110] These antibodies recognize antigen-binding sites, or idiotypes, of other host antibodies and control the production and persistence of humoral responses. Anti-idiotypic antibodies against antithyroglobulin antibodies have been reported in some humans.[111] Anti-idiotypic antibodies can substitute for antigens and stimulate the immune system to produce an antibody with the idiotype and/or antigen-binding specificity of the antibody against which it had originally been generated. Zanetti et al. have induced autoantibodies to thyroglobulin in mice immunized with purified anti-idiotypic antibody directed against a monoclonal antibody that bears the recurrent idiotype of the mouse immune response to thyroglobulin.[112] The anti-idiotype to the antibody directed against this self-antigen appeared sufficient to activate autoimmunity in the mouse's system. This suggests that the autoimmune response is partially dependent on perturbation of the immune system by the anti-idiotypic antibody, and that these antibodies may be involved in the termination of natural tolerance to self-antigens. This mechanism could play a role in the maintenance of chronic autoimmune thyroid disease. The above mentioned investigations led to the concept of an intricate, finely tuned, homeostatic control system to amplify and suppress normal and abnormal cellular and humoral immune reactions. In normal individuals, some lymphocytes and antibodies are directed toward the different tissue antigens, but with their reactivity rigidly controlled to avoid the development of autoimmune disease. In Graves' disease a number of investigators have demonstrated anti-idiotypic antibodies; however, their reactivity is relatively weak and it is uncertain whether they play a role in the pathophysiology of the disease.[113–115] There is a great deal of controversy surrounding immunoregulation of thyroid disease.[68,116,117] Some investigators believe T-suppressor cells are important in normal thyroid regulation, but others do not.[68]

Similarly, as previously discussed, the role of immunogenetic abnormalities in the pathogenesis of Graves' disease is unclear. Close amino acid sequence homology does not always imply a near identical immune response as demonstrated in thyroid antigen studies.[118,119]

Immunogenetic abnormalities have also been postulated to have an important role in the pathogenesis of Graves' disease. Some investigators demonstrated that patients with Graves' disease have an altered incidence of HLA-B8, -Bw35, -Cw3, HLA-DR3, and -DQA1* 0501.[52–55,58,60,61] B8 and DR3 HLA antigens have been observed more frequently in patients with various types of autoimmune disease.[76] The level of association between Graves' disease and various HLA haplotypes suggest that the linkage is relatively weak and probably reflects an association with another genetic factor in proximity to the histocompatibility loci.[51]

The nature of the HLA disease association is uncertain; at least five mechanisms have been identified as possibly operative in Graves' disease and other autoimmune processes.[101] In congenic animals, which differ only in a small portion of the major histocompatibility complex (MHC), minor histocompatibility alteration produces a marked difference in immunologic responsiveness. Similarly, in humans, HLA antigens may code for immunogenetic behavior patterns. Thus, patients having a given set of HLA haplotypes may be at a higher risk of developing Graves' disease because of a genetic abnormality affecting immunologic control of cellular or humoral immunity. Certain HLA antigens may also serve as receptors for viral antigens, and bacterial or viral antigens might sufficiently mimic HLA antigens on a molecular level to cause autoimmune disease. Amino acid sequence studies have demonstrated close homology between some common HLA antigens and viral, bacterial, or fungal antigens.[118] It is possible that this close but incomplete homology might result in a breakdown of immunologic tolerance. It is also possible that HLA disease associations occur because certain HLA antigens are in linkage disequilibrium with the relevant non-HLA genetic loci responsible for disease development. The relative ease of induction of class II antigens on thyroid cells may also upregulate the system and produce a lower threshold for autoimmune disease.[51]

In a few diseases, including anterior uveitis associated with ankylosing spondylitis or Vogt-Koyanagi-Harada syndrome, more than 95% of patients are of a given HLA type.[84] There is a much lower, although significant, percentage of Graves' disease patients with a given HLA haplotype, and there is marked ethnic diversity. It is likely that other factors not related to HLA may also be important in thyroid disease development. It is conceivable the HLA type partially controls the immunogenetic propensity for disease severity. While this has not been well documented in systemic thyroid disease, it is speculated, and one group of investigators observed that the severity of ophthalmopathy correlates with the presence or absence of HLA-Bw35.[55,56,76]

Early studies that used different rosette assays to demonstrate a generalized alteration of T cell numbers in patients with active thyroid disease were probably spurious.[47,56,120–122] More recent investigations demonstrate that some hyperthyroid patients have increased levels of IL-2 in the serum.[123] There is controversy about alteration of T-suppressor cells in these patients.[68,124–126] When normal T cells are mixed with T cells from patients with either Graves' disease or Hashimoto's thyroiditis and incubated with thyroid antigens, migration inhibition is suppressed.[127,128] If normal cells are treated with either low-dose radiation or mitomycin C to abrogate the T-suppressor cell response, there is no suppression. While some investigators have observed circulating immune complexes in both Graves' disease and Hashimoto's thyroiditis, others have not, and a correlation with disease status or prognosis has not been documented.[47,56,72,124,129–133] Immune complexes with thyroglobulin have been noted on extraocular muscle membranes, however, and may play a role in the ophthalmopathy (see Chapter 6).[134–138]

Investigators have also used classic cell-mediated immunologic assays of migration-inhibiting factor (MIF) and leukocyte adherence inhibition (LAI) to demonstrate that patients with Graves' disease have cellular reactivity toward various thyroid and orbital antigens (see Chapter 6).[135–139] The importance of this cellular reactivity in disease pathophysiology has not been established. Almost all studies have been performed with nonspecific blood lymphocytes, not those specifically reactive with thyroid or orbital antigens, so enumeration of T cell or B cell subsets probably has little meaning to thyroid disease. Akamizu and colleagues have produced a T cell line reactive with the TSHr.[139]

Volpe and others hypothesize that an alteration, not in the number of suppressor cells but in organ-specific T-suppressor cells, is probably responsible for the development and maintenance of autoimmune thyroid diseases.[6,68,102,127,140] It is difficult to demonstrate an alteration in such a small minority of T-suppressor cells. Nevertheless, alterations in T-suppressor cells directed toward the thyroid could occur as part of the normal aging process, they could be secondary to hyperthyroidism (which is itself immunosuppressive), or they could be due to other unknown factors.[102] If such an alteration in immunologic homeostatic control mechanisms exists, it requires elucidation. The concept is partially supported, however, by observations that some antithyroid drugs appear to exert their effect on the disease partially by altering immunologic reactivity towards thyroid cells.[50,68,108,140,141]

CONCLUSION

The thyroid gland is a semiautonomous endocrine organ with hypothalamic-pituitary feedback control. In Graves' disease, thyrotropin receptor antibodies bind to the thyroid cells' TSHrs and stimulate glandular activity independent of neuroendocrine control mechanisms.

Immunologic factors are important in the pathogenesis of hyperthyroidism, but the inciting event or events in the development of Graves' disease remain unclear. As discussed, it is likely that an alteration results in a perturbation of normal humoral and/or cellular immunologic control mechanisms with an abnormal immunologic reactivity toward thyroid-related antigens. Consequently, thyroid-stimulating antibodies are produced and increase the secretion of thyroid hormones without the mediating control of TRH or TSH. Lymphocytes, immunoglobulins, and lymphokines directed against thyroid tissue antigens then lead to immunologic destruction of thyroid tissue. A schematic representation of possible immune mechanisms for Graves' disease is shown in Figure 2-5.

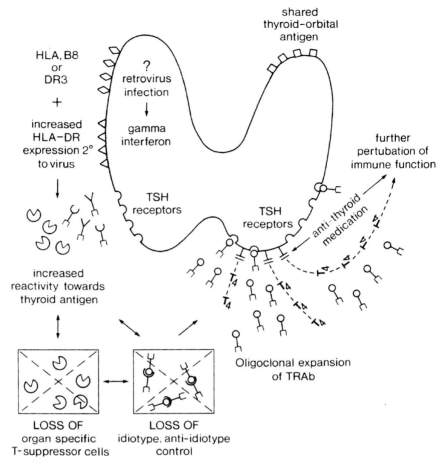

Figure 2-5. Schematic representation of immune mechanisms in Graves' disease.

REFERENCES

1. Kriss JP. Radioisotopic thyroid lymphography in patients with Graves' disease. J Clin Endocrinol Metab 1970;31:315.

2. Fawcett DW, Long JA, Jones AL. The ultrastructure of endocrine glands. Recent Prog Horm Res 1969;25:315.

3. Florsheim WH. Control of Thyrotropin Secretion. In E Knobil, WH Sawyer (eds), Handbook of Physiology (Vol 4) Section VII Endocrinology, the Pituitary Gland and Its Neuroendocrine Control. Washington: American Physiological Society, 1974;449.

4. Reichlin S. Neuroendocrine Control. In SC Werner, SH Ingbar (eds), The Thyroid. Hagerstown, MD: Harper & Row, 1978.

5. Pierce JG. Pituitary Thyrotropin: Chemistry. In SC Werner, SH Ingbar (eds), The Thyroid. Hagerstown, MD: Harper & Row, 1978.

6. Volpe R. Autoimmune thyroid disease—a perspective. Mol Biol Med 1986;3:25.

7. Parmentier M, Libert F, Maenhaut C, et al. Molecular cloning of the thyrotropin receptor. Science 1989;246:1620.

8. Laugwitz KL, Allgeier A, Offermanns S, et al. The human thyrotropin receptor: a heptahelical receptor capable of stimulating members of all four G protein families. Proc Natl Acad Sci U S A 1996;93:116.

9. Weetman AP, et al. Thyroid-stimulating antibody activity between different immunoglobulin G subclasses. J Clin Invest 1990;86:723.

10. Cavalieri RR, Rapoport B. Impaired peripheral conversion of thyroxine to triiodothyronine. Annu Rev Med 1977;28:57.

11. Levey, GS, Klein I. Disorders of the Thyroid. In JH Stein (ed), Internal Medicine: Diagnosis and Therapy. Norwalk, CT: Appleton & Lange, 1993.

12. Oppenheimer JH. Thyroid Hormone Action at the Molecular Level. In SC Werner, SH Ingbar, LE Braverman, RD Utiger (eds), Thyroid: A Fundamental and Clinical Text (6th ed). Philadelphia: Lippincott, 1991;46.

13. Von Basedow CA. Exophthalmos durch hypertrophie des zellgewebes in der augenhöhle. Wochenschr F D Ges Heilk 1840;6:197, 220.

14. Cordes FC. Endocrine exophthalmos: an evaluation of present knowledge; Fourth Estelle Doheney Eye Lecture. Am J Ophthalmol 1954;38:1.

15. McDougall, IR. Thyroid Disease in Clinical Practice. New York: Oxford University Press, 1992.

16. Schleusener H, Joseph K, Mahlsted J, et al. Differences between immunogenic toxic diffuse goiter (Graves' disease) and goiter with disseminated autonomy: preliminary results. J Mol Med 1980;3:129.

17. Fox RA, Schwartz TB. Infiltrative ophthalmopathy and primary hypothyroidism. Ann Intern Med 1967;67:377.

18. Wasnich RD, Grumet FC, Payne RO, Kriss JP. Graves' ophthalmopathy following external neck irradiation for nonthyroidal neoplastic disease. J Clin Endocrinol Metab 1973;37:703.

19. Wyse EP, McConahey WM, Woolner LB, et al. Ophthalmopathy without hyperthyroidism in patients with histologic Hashimoto's thyroiditis. J Clin Endocrinol Metab 1968;28:1623.

20. Brownlie BEW, Newton OAG, Singh SP. Ophthalmopathy associated with primary hypothyroidism. Acta Endocrinol (Copenh) 1979;79:691.

21. Leiter L, Seidlin SM, Marinelli LD, Maumann EJ. Adenocarcinoma of the thyroid with hyperthyroidism and functional metastases. J Clin Endocrinol Metab 1946;6:247.

22. Bartley GB, Fatourechi V, Kadramas EF, et al. The chronology of Graves' ophthalmopathy in an incidence cohort. Am J Ophthalmol 1996;121:426.

23. Hancock SL, Cox RS, McDougall IR. Thyroid diseases after treatment of Hodgkin's disease. N Engl J Med 1991;325:599.

24. Jacobson DR, Fleming BJ. Case report: Graves' disease with ophthalmopathy following radiotherapy for Hodgkin's disease. Am J Med Sci 1984;288:217.

25. Fatourechi V, Pajouhi M, Fransway AF. Dermopathy of Graves' disease (pretibial myxedema). Medicine 1994;73:1.

26. Havard CWH. Endocrine exophthalmos. Br J Med 1972;1:360.

27. Grove AS Jr. Evaluation of exophthalmos. N Engl J Med 1975;292:1005.

28. Werner SC. Euthyroid patients with early eye signs of Graves' disease; their responses to L-triiodothyronine and thyrotropin. Am J Med 1955;18:608.

29. Mornex R, Fournier G, Berthezene F. Ophthalmic Graves' disease. Mod Probl Ophthalmol 1975;14:426.

30. Hall R, Kirkham K, Doniach D, El Kabir D. Ophthalmic Graves' disease. Lancet 1970;1:375.

31. Ivy HK. Medical approach to ophthalmopathy of Graves' disease. Mayo Clin Proc 1972;47:980.

32. Franco PS, Hershman JM, Haigler ED Jr, Pittman JA Jr. Response to thyrotropin-releasing hormone compared with thyroid suppression tests in euthyroid Graves' disease. Metabolism 1973;22:1357.

33. Solomon DH, Chopra IJ, Chopra U, Smith FJ. Identification of subgroups of euthyroid Graves' ophthalmopathy. N Engl J Med 1977;296:181.

34. Tamai H, Nakagawa T, Ohsako N, et al. Changes in thyroid functions in patients with euthyroid Graves' disease. J Clin Endocrinol Metab 1980;50:108.

35. Teng CS, Yeo PPB. Ophthalmic Graves' disease: natural history and detailed thyroid function studies. Br Med J 1977;1:273.

36. Williams RH. Thiouracil treatment of thyrotoxicosis: the results of prolonged treatment. J Clin Endocrinol 1946;6:1.

37. Schimmel M, Utiger RD. Thyroidal and peripheral production of thyroid hormones: review of recent findings and their clinical implications. Ann Intern Med 1977;87:760.

38. Lawton NF, Fells P, Lloyd GAS. Medical Investigation of Dysthyroid Eye Disease. In W Junk (ed), Third International Symposium on Orbital Disorders Headed by Orbital Center Amsterdam. The Hague: BV Publishers, 1978;343.

39. Singer PS, Cooper DS, Levy EG, et al. Treatment guidelines for patients with hyperthyroidism and hypothyroidism. JAMA 1995;273:808.

40. Holloway TB, Fry WE, Wentworth HA. Ocular signs in 100 unselected cases of goiter. JAMA 1929;92:35.

41. Woods AC. The ocular changes of primary diffuse toxic goitre; review. Medicine (Baltimore) 1946;25:113.

42. Jones DIR, Munro DS, Wilson GM. Observations on the course of exophthalmos after ^{131}I therapy. Proc R Soc Med 1969;62:15.

43. Kasagi K, Hidaka A, Misaki T, et al. Scintigraphic findings of the thyroid in euthyroid ophthalmic Graves' disease. J Nucl Med 1994;35:811.

44. Kriss JP, Pleshakov V, Rosenblum AL, et al. Studies on the pathogenesis of the ophthalmopathy of Graves' disease. J Clin Endocrinol Metab 1967;27:582.

45. Sergott RC, Glaser JS. Graves' ophthalmopathy. A clinical and immunologic review. Surv Ophthalmol 1981 ;26:1.

46. Volpe R, Farid NR, Von Westarp C. The pathogenesis of Graves' disease and Hashimoto's thyroiditis. Clin Endocrinol (Oxf) 1974;3:239.

47. Kidd A, Okita N, Row VV, Volpe R. Immunologic aspects of Graves' and Hashimoto's diseases. Metabolism 1980;29:80.

48. Warthin AS. The constitutional entity of exophthalmic goiter and so-called toxic adenoma. Ann Intern Med 1928;2:553.

49. Ciampolillo A, Mirakian R, Schultz T, et al. Retrovirus-like sequences in Graves' disease: implications for human autoimmunity. Lancet 1989;1:1096.

50. Weetman A. The potential immunological role of the thyroid cell in autoimmune thyroid disease. Thyroid 1994;4:493.

51. Sosperda M, Obiols G, Santamaria Babi LF, et al. Hyperinducibility of HLA class II expression of thyroid follicular cells from Graves' Disease. J Immunol 1995;154:4213.

52. Hall R. Immunological aspects of thyroid function. N Engl J Med 1962;266:1204.

53. Bech K, Lumholtz B, Nerup J, et al. HLA antigens in Graves' disease. Acta Endocrinol (Copenh) 1977;86:510.

54. Farid NR, Sampson L, Noel EP, et al. A study of human leukocyte D locus related antigens in Graves' disease. J Clin Invest 1979;63:108.

55. Sergott RC, Felberg NT, Savino PJ, et al. Association of HLA antigen Bw35 with severe Graves' ophthalmopathy. Invest Ophthalmol Vis Sci 1983;24:124.

56. Strakosch CR, Wenzel BE, Row VV, Volpe R. Immunology of autoimmune thyroid diseases. N Engl J Med 1982;307:1499.

57. Farid NR, Bear JC. The human major histocompatibility complex and endocrine disease. Endocr Rev 1981;2:50.

58. Scherthaner G, Ludwig H, Mayr WR, Hofer R. Genetic heterogeneity in thyrotoxicosis patients with and without endocrine ophthalmopathy. Diabet Metab 1977;3:189.

59. Dong R-P, Kimura A, Okubo R, et al. HLA-A DPB1 loci confer susceptibility to Graves' disease. Hum Immunol 1992;35:165.

60. Badenhoop K, Schwartz G, Walfish PG, et al. Susceptibility to thyroid autoimmune disease: molecular analysis of HLA region genes identifies new markers for goitrous Hashimoto's thyroiditis. J Clin Endocrinol Metab 1990;71:1131.

61. Yaganawa T, Mangklabruks A, Chang YB, et al. Human histocompatibility antigen-DQAI*0501 allele associated with genetic susceptibility to Graves' disease in a Caucasian population. J Clin Endocrinol Metab 1993;76:1569.

62. Vail D. Exophthalmos. Postgrad Med 1949;5:439.

63. Chertow BS, Fidler WJ, Fariss BL. Graves' disease and Hashimoto's thyroiditis in monozygous twins. Acta Endocrinol (Copenh) 1973;72:18.

64. Skillern PG. Genetics of Graves' disease. Mayo Clin Proc 1972;47:848.

65. Friedman JM, Fialkow PJ. The genetics of Graves' disease. J Clin Endocrinol Metab 1978;7:47.

66. Fatourechi V, McConahey WM, Woolner LB. Hyperthyroidism associated with histologic Hashimoto's thyroiditis. Mayo Clin Proc 1971;46:682.

67. Brown J, Solomon DH, Beall GN, et al. Autoimmune thyroid diseases—Graves' and Hashimoto's. Ann Intern Med 1978;88:379.

68. Volpe R. Immunoregulation in autoimmune thyroid disease. Thyroid 1994;4:373.

69. McKenzie JM, Zakarija M. LATS in Graves' disease. Recent Prog Hormone Res 1977;33:29.

70. Lipman LM, Green DE, Snyder NJ, et al. Relationship of long-acting thyroid stimulator to the clinical features and course of Graves' disease. Am J Med 1967;43:486.

71. Mukhtar ED, Smith BR, Pyle GA, et al. Relation of thyroid-stimulating immunoglobulins to thyroid function and effects of surgery, radioiodine and antithyroid drugs. Lancet 1975;1:713.

72. Kriss JP, Konishi J, Herman MM. Studies on the pathogenesis of Graves' ophthalmopathy (with some related observations regarding therapy). Recent Prog Horm Res 1975;31:533.

73. Volpe R. The pathogenesis of Graves' disease: an overview. J Clin Endocrinol Metab 1978;7:3.

74. Roitt IM, Doniach D, Campbell PN, Hudson RV. Autoantibodies in Hashimoto's disease (lymphadenoid goitre). Lancet 1956;2:820.

75. Owen CA, Jr. A review of "auto-immunization" in Hashimoto's disease. J Clin Endocrinol Metab 1958;18:1015.

76. Theofilopoulos AN, Dixon FJ. Autoimmune diseases: immunopathology and etiopathogenesis. Am J Pathol 1982;108:321.

77. Roitt IM, Torrigiani G. Identification and estimation of undergraded thyroglobulin in human serum. Endocrinology 1967;81:421.

78. Adams DD, Purvis HD. Abnormal response in assay of thyrotrophin. Proc Univ Otago Med Sch 1956;34:11.

79. Kendall-Taylor P. LATS and human-specific thyroid stimulator; their relation to Graves' disease. J Clin Endocrinol Metab 1975;4:319.

80. Adams DD, Kennedy TH, Stewart RDH. Correlation between long-acting thyroid stimulator protector level and thyroid ^{131}I uptake in thyrotoxicosis. Br Med J 1974;2:199.

81. Wall JR, Odgers R, Hetzel BS. Immunological studies of the eye changes of thyrotoxicosis. Aust N Z J Med 1973;3:162.

82. Smith BR, Hall R. The Interaction of Graves' Immunoglobulins with TSH Receptor. In JR Stockigt, S Nagataki (eds), Thyroid Research VIII. Proceedings of the Eighth International Thyroid Congress. Oxford, England: Pergamon, 1980;715.

83. Volpe R. The immunoregulatory disturbance in autoimmune thyroid disease. Autoimmunity 1988;2:55.

84. Clague R, Mukhtar ED, Pyle GA, et al. Thyroid stimulating immunoglobulins and the control of thyroid function. J Clin Endocrinol Metab 1976;43:550.

85. Davies TF. Thyroid-stimulating hormone receptor antibodies—the calm after the calm? Mayo Clin Proc 1988;63:736.

86. Gupta MK. Recent advances in laboratory tests for autoantibodies to thyrotropin receptor protein in Graves' disease. Clin Lab Med 1988;8:303.

87. Rapoport B, Greenspan FS, Filetti S, Pepitone M. Clinical experience with a human thyroid cell bioassay for thyroid-stimulating immunoglobulin. J Clin Endocrinol Metab 1984;58:332.

88. Onaya T, Kotani M, Yamada T, Ochi Y. New in vitro tests to detect thyroid stimulator in sera from hyperthyroid patients by measuring colloid droplet formation and cyclic AMP in human thyroid slices. J Clin Endocrinol Metab 1973;36:859.

88a. Akamizu T, Matsuda F, Okuda J, et al. Molecular analysis of stimulatory anti-thyrotropin receptor antibodies (TSAbs) involved in Graves' disease. J Immunol 1996;157:3148.

89. Zakarija M, McKenzie JM, Banovac K. Clinical significance of assay of thyroid-stimulating antibody in Graves' disease. Ann Intern Med 1980;93:28.

90. Fenzi G, Hashizume K, Roudebush CP, DeGroot LJ. Changes in thyroid-stimulating immunoglobulins during antithyroid therapy. J Clin Endocrinol Metab 1979;48:572.

91. McGregor AM, Rees Smith B, Hall R, et al. Prediction of relapse in hyperthyroid Graves' disease. Lancet 1980;1:1101.

92. Teng CS, Yeung RTT, Khoo RKK, Alagaratnam TT. A prospective study of the changes in thyrotropin binding inhibitory immunoglobulins in Graves' disease treated by subtotal thyroidectomy or radioactive iodine. J Clin Endocrinol Metab 1980;50:1005.

93. Zakarija M, Garcia A, McKenzie JM. Studies on multiple thyroid cell membrane—directed antibodies in Graves' disease. J Clin Invest 1985;76:1885.

94. Feldt-Rasmussen U, Schleusener H, Carayon P. Meta-analysis evaluation of the impact of thyrotropin receptor antibodies on long term remission after medical therapy of Graves' disease. J Clin Endocrinol Metab 1994;78.

95. Williams RC Jr, Marshall NJ, Kilpatrick K, et al. Kappa/lambda immunoglobulin distribution in Graves' thyroid-stimulating antibodies. J Clin Invest 1988;82:1306.

96. Knight J, Laing P, Knight A, et al. Thyroid-stimulating autoantibodies usually contain only gamma-light chains: evidence for the "forbidden clone" theory. J Clin Endocrinol Metab 1986;62:342.

97. Kruger TE, Smith LR, Harbour DV, Blalock JE. Thyrotropin: an endogenous regulator of the in vitro immuno response. J Immunol 1989;142:744.

98. Stein-Streilein J, Zakarija M, Papic M, McKenzie JM. Hyperthyroxinemic mice have reduced natural killer cell activity. Evidence for a defective trigger mechanism. J Immunol 1987;139:2502.

99. Pratt DE. Thyroid antibodies. Immunol Allerg Clin North Am 1994;14:835.

100. Von Westar C, Knox AJS, Row VV, Volpe R. Comparison of thyroid antigens by the experimental production of precipitating antibodies to human thyroid fractions and the identification of an antibody which competes with long-acting thyroid stimulator (LATS) for thyroid binding. Acta Endocrinol (Copenh) 1977;84:759.

101. Autoimmunity. In A Coutinho, MD Kazatchkine (eds), A Physiology and Disease. New York: Wiley-Liss, 1994.

102. Mignog OD, Efroy K, Brazillet MP, et al. Distinctive modulation by IL-4, IL-10 of the effect or function of murine thyroglobulin-primed cells in "transfer-experimental autoimmune thyroiditis." Cell Immunol 1995;162:171.

103. Pujol-Borrell R, Hanafusa T, Chiovato L, Bottazzo GF. Lectin induced expression of DR antigen on human cultured follicular thyroid cells. Nature 1983;304:71.

104. Pujol-Borrell R, Hanafusa T, Doniach D. Expression of HLA antigens and their relation to thyroid microsomal antigen on microvilli of human thyroid monolayers. Ann Endocrinol (Paris) 1982;43:58A.

105. Jannson R, Karlsson A, Forsum U. Intrathyroidal HLA-DR expression and T lymphocyte phenotypes in Graves' thyrotoxicosis, Hashimoto's thyroiditis and nodular colloid goitre. Clin Exp Immunol 1984;58:264.

106. Aichinger G, Fill H, Wick G. In situ immune complexes, lymphocyte subpopulations, and HLA-DR positive epithelial cells in Hashimoto's thyroiditis. Lab Invest 1985;52:132.

107. Bottazzo GF, Pujol-Borrell R, Hanafusa T, Feldmann M. Role of aberrant HLA-DR expression and antigen presentation in induction of endocrine autoimmunity. Lancet 1983;2:1115.

108. Volpe R. Immunoregulation in autoimmune thyroid disease. N Engl J Med 1987;316:44.

109. Bohlmann BJ. Hyperthyroidism. Ann Intern Med 1995;122:393.

110. Jerne NK. Towards a network theory of the immune system. Ann Immunol (Paris) 1974;125:373.

111. Zouali M, Fine JM, Eyquem A. Human monoclonal IgG 1 with anti-idiotypic activity against anti-human thyroglobulin autoantibody. J Immunol 1984;133:190.

112. Zanetti M, Rogers J, Katz DH. Induction of autoantibodies to thyroglobulin by anti-idiotypic antibodies. J Immunol 1984;133:240.

113. Bach J-F. Antireceptor or antihormone autoimmunity and its relationship with the idiotype network. Adv Nephrol 1987;16:251.

114. Paschke R, Teuber J, Schwedes U, Usadel KH. Is remission of Graves' disease regulated by anti-idiotypic antibodies? Acta Endocrinol 1987 (Suppl);281:99.

115. Raines KB, Baker JR, Lukes YG, et al. Antithyrotropin antibody in the sera of Graves' disease patients. J Clin Endocrinol Metab 1985;61:217.

116. Kolsch E. T suppressor lymphocytes and aspects of immunological tolerance. Res Immunol 1989;140:286, discussion 339.

117. Nabozny GH, Flynn JC, Kong YCM. Synergism between mouse thyroglobulin and vaccination-induced suppressor mechanisms in murine experimental autoimmune thyroiditis. Cell Immunol 1991;136:340.

118. Goldstone MBA. Molecular mimicry in autoimmune disease. Cell 1987;50:819.

119. Quaratino S, Thorpe CJ, Travers PJ, Londei M. Similar antigenic surfaces, rather than sequence homology, dictate T-cell epitope molecular mimicry. Proc Natl Acad Sci U S A 1995;92:10398.

120. Sergott RC, Felberg NT, Savino PJ, et al. E-rosette formation in Graves' ophthalmopathy. Invest Ophthalmol Vis Sci 1979;18:1245.

121. Wybran J, Fudunberg HH. Thymus-derived rosette-forming cells in various human disease states: cancer, lymphoma, bacterial and viral infections and other diseases. J Clin Invest 1973;52:1026.

122. Wall JR, Gray B, Greenwood DM. Total and "activated" peripheral blood T lymphocytes in patients with thyroid disorders. Acta Endocrinol (Copenh) 1977;85:753.

123. Prummel MF, Wiersinga WM, Van der Gaag R, et al. Soluble IL-2 receptor levels in patients with Graves' ophthalmopathy. Clin Exp Immunol 1992;88:405.

124. Bene M-C, Derennes V, Faure G, et al. Graves' disease: in situ localization of lymphoid T-cell subpopulations. Clin Exp Immunol 1983;52:311.

125. Canonica GW, Bagnasco M, Moretta L, et al. Human T-lymphocyte subpopulations in Hashimoto's disease. J Clin Endocrinol Metab 1981;52:553.

126. Sridama V, Pacini F, DeGroot LJ. Decreased suppressor T-lymphocytes in autoimmune thyroid diseases detected by monoclonal antibodies. J Clin Endocrinol Metab 1982;54:316.

127. Aoki N, Pinnamaneni KM, De Groot LJ. Studies on suppressor cell function in thyroid disease. J Clin Endocrinol Metab 1979;48:803.

128. Okita N, Row VV, Volpe R. Suppressor T-lymphocyte deficiency in Graves' disease and Hashimoto's thyroiditis. J Clin Endocrinol Metab 1981;52:528.

129. Calder EA, Penhale WJ, Barnes E, Irvine WJ. Evidence for circulating immune complexes in thyroid disease. Br Med J 1974;2:30.

130. Takeda Y, Kriss JP. Radiometric measurement of thyroglobulin-antithyroglobulin immune complex in human serum. J Clin Endocrinol Metab 1977;44:46.

131. Konishi J, Herman MM, Kriss JP. Binding of thyroglobulin and thyroglobulin-antithyroglobulin immune complex to extraocular muscle membrane. Endocrinology 1974;95:434.

132. Brohee D, Derennes V, Bonnyns M. Circulating immune complexes in thyroid disease [abstract]. Ann Endocrinol (Paris) 1978;39:20A.

133. Wall JR, Strakosch CR, Fang SL, et al. Thyroid-binding antibodies and other immunological abnormalities in patients with Graves' ophthalmopathy: effect of treatment with cyclophosphamide. Clin Endocrinol 1979;10:79.

134. Wall JR, Walters BAJ, Grant C. Leukocyte adherence inhibition in response to human orbital and lacrimal extracts in patients with Graves' ophthalmopathy. J Endocrinol Invest 1979;2:375.

135. Mullin BR, Levinson RE, Friedman A, et al. Delayed hypersensitivity in Graves' disease and exophthalmos: identification of thyroglobulin in normal orbital muscle. Endocrinology 1977;100:351.

136. Munro RE, Lamki L, Row VV, Volpe R. Cell-mediated immunity in the exophthalmos of Graves' disease as demonstrated by the migration inhibition factor (MIF) test. J Clin Endocrinol Metab 1973;37:286.

137. Robinson RG, Guttler RB, Rea TH, Nicoloff JT. Delayed hypersensitivity in Graves' disease. J Clin Endocrinol Metab 1974;38:322.

138. Lamki L, Row VV, Volpe R. Cell-mediated immunity in Graves' disease and in Hashimoto's thyroiditis as shown by the demonstration of migration inhibition factor (MIF). J Clin Endocrinol Metab 1973;36:358.

139. Akamizu T, Kohn LD, Mori T. Molecular studies on thyrotropin (TSH) receptor and anti-TSH receptor antibodies. Endocr J 1995;42:617.

140. Volpe R. Auto-immunity in the endocrine system. Monogr Endocrinol 1981;20:19.

141. Klein I, Becker DV, Levey GS. Treatment of hyperthyroid disease. Ann Intern Med 1994;121:281.

3

Systemic Diagnostic Tests for Thyroid Ophthalmopathy and Euthyroid Ophthalmopathy

Correct diagnosis of patients with classic thyrotoxicosis symptoms is relatively easy. Bilateral exophthalmos in association with an enlarged thyroid gland is virtually pathognomonic for Graves' disease. Thyroid eye disease commonly occurs in association with Graves' disease hyperthyroidism, but it develops in less than 3% of Hashimoto's thyroiditis patients and very rarely with primary hypothyroidism.[1–4] As discussed in Chapter 2, a significant number of patients treated with radiation of their neck or thyroid for Hodgkin's disease develop Graves' ophthalmopathy.[5]

On the other hand, diagnosis of patients with bilateral or unilateral exophthalmos, without obvious systemic signs or abnormal laboratory findings of thyroid disease, is difficult. This chapter's discussion of systemic tests is not all-inclusive. It is limited to those assays useful to the nonendocrinologist evaluating patients suspected of having thyroid ophthalmopathy. Laboratory evaluation of these patients has been revolutionized by the widespread availability of newer assays. Tables 3-1 and 3-2 highlight changes during the last several years.

Five laboratory test categories have been used to evaluate thyroid function. Double-label sandwich assays allow sensitive serum thyrotropin or thyroid-stimulating hormone (TSH) measurement, and commercial tests to detect serum thyrotropin receptor antibodies (TRAbs) are available. Thyroid hormones (triiodothyronine [T_3] and thyroxine [T_4]) predominantly bound to serum carriers can be measured; historic assays (basal metabolism rate, etc.) can determine the impact of thyroid hormones on tissue. In rare instances, alterations of thyroid gland regulation can be studied with older assays (thyroid suppression test and thyrotropin-releasing hormone [TRH] test). Other miscellaneous assays (antibodies, scans, biopsies, etc.) can also be performed.

As discussed in Chapter 2, increasing evidence indicates that the final common pathway of hyperthyroidism in Graves' disease is through autoimmune, antireceptor antibodies. These immunoglobulins bind the thyrotropin receptor (TSHr) to the thyrocyte and stimulate production of thyroid hormones. Virtually all patients with Graves' disease have these antibodies at some time.

Most thyroid eye disease patients have evidence of systemic hyperthyroidism when they initially present with orbital disease, but in approximately 50% of thyroid eye patients initially referred to an ophthalmic consultant with proptosis of unknown etiology, that is not the case. Graves' ophthalmopathy can present before,

Table 3-1. Historic List of Classic Sequential Studies Used to Evaluate Patients with Suspected Thyroid Orbitopathy: Sequential Laboratory Approach Circa 1985

1. Serum T_4
2. Serum T_3
3. Resin T_3 uptake test
4. Calculated free T_4 index and free T_3 index
5. Thyrotropin receptor antibodies
6. Antithyroid antibodies
7. TRH test
8. Thyroid (T_3 or Werner) suppression test

T_4 = thyroxine; T_3 − triiodothyronine; TRH = thyrotropin-releasing hormone.

Table 3-2. Current Sequential Laboratory Approach for the Diagnosis of Thyroid Ophthalmopathy

1. Serum thyrotropin
2. Calculated free T_4 index
3. Thyroid-stimulating immunoglobulin (TSI)
4. Antithyroid antibodies
5. Serum T_3

T_4 = thyroxine; T_3 = triiodothyronine.

during, or after the hyperthyroid state has become manifest. The goals of laboratory studies are to demonstrate systemic hyperthyroidism or altered immune response to thyroid-related antigens, or both.

Advances in laboratory techniques have altered the evaluation protocol of patients with possible thyroid eye disease. An historical laboratory flow sheet from the 1985 edition of this book lists sequential laboratory tests to evaluate patients suspected of having thyroid-related eye disease (see Table 3-1). It has since been discovered that only 50% of ophthalmopathy patients without a history of hyperthyroidism have elevated serum T_3 or T_4 levels. The widespread availability, rapid assays, and improved sensitivity of serum TSH assays have completely altered the evaluation of patients with possible thyroid disease. Historically, TSH could only be detected in normal or hypothyroid patients—radioimmunoassay measurements of serum TSH took 5–7 days to perform. Newer techniques have improved the sensitivity of the TSH assay tenfold with results available in 2–5 hours.[6] This change in test sensitivity and measurement ease, coupled with the fact that a twofold change in serum T_4 results in approximately a fiftyfold change in serum TSH, are the reasons that the TSH assay has supplanted thyroid hormone studies as the initial test to detect either covert or overt hyperthyroidism.[7,8]

Sensitive serum TSH measurements are performed using a sandwich technique. Two monoclonal antibodies are directed toward different epitopes (antigen-binding sites) on the thyrotropin molecule.[6] One of the antibodies functions as a component of a separation system, often linked to solid beads, and the other monoclonal antibody is attached to a signal system. The latter monoclonal-signal ligand can be radioactive, chemiluminescent, or enzymatic, and the TSH measurement assay is termed immunoradiometric, immunoenzymometric, or immunochemiluminometric assay depending on the signal system used.[7-9] There is no evidence to demonstrate clinical superiority of any of these different TSH measurement systems.[7] Normal serum levels of TSH vary in different laboratories but are usually between 0.35–6.7 μU/ml—hyperthyroid patients have serum levels less than 0.1 μU/ml. Reproducibility in different laboratories and with different techniques has been excellent.[10,11]

In 1985, Caldwell and coworkers reported on the sensitivity of serum TSH results in 285 patients referred to a thyroid clinic. They observed that a detectable and normal serum TSH obviates the need for thyroid hormone assays to screen for hyperthyroidism.[8,12] There is no clear delineation between normal and abnormal TSH levels. Serum TSH concentrations are very low or unmeasurable with active thyrotoxicosis.[13] These newer, sensitive TSH assays are quite useful as screening tests for hyperthyroidism for three reasons.[14] One, as discussed above, they are very sensitive—a small alteration in serum T_4 produces a larger change in serum TSH and subclinical disease is detectable earlier with serum TSH than with conventional hormone studies.[15] Two, they are less affected by nonthyroidal illnesses than most conventional T_3 or T_4 assays.[8] Three, they are not affected by alteration in thyroid-binding proteins.

The serum TSH assay has become widely available and is an excellent initial screening test to evaluate proptotic patients who may have thyroid orbitopathy. Its sensitivity has resulted in the elimination of either the TRH assay or Werner T_3 suppression test in the ophthalmic evaluation of most of these patients.[12] While serum TSH measurements are very useful, a few false-positive findings have been demonstrated. Diagnostically inaccurate serum TSH values can occur in patients who are receiving thyroid, dopamine, or steroids; who are in the first trimester of pregnancy; who have hypopituitarism; who are acutely ill; who are hospitalized with psychiatric diseases; or who are elderly.[7,8,16-20]

In some patients with a marginally altered serum TSH without clinical signs of hyperthyroidism, other assays are needed.[21] Free T_3 or free T_4 levels are raised more than bound forms of these hormones in hyperthyroidism.[12,22] Discussion of these hormonal assays follows.

A summary of abbreviations and synonyms is given in Table 2-2.

SERUM THYROXINE AND TRIIDOTHYRONINE ASSAYS

Ninety percent of hyperthyroid patients display elevated serum T_3 or T_4 levels, but as many as 10% of Graves' disease patients experience T_3 elevation only (T_3 toxicosis). In this latter group, T_4 can be normal or borderline.[21,23,24] In some studies of Graves' ophthalmopathy, a significant proportion of patients fit into this latter group.[25]

Historically, numerous techniques have been used to measure serum levels of thyroid hormones, but their results were affected by iodine ingestion and numerous other artifacts.[26] Currently most thyroid hormone analyses are obtained through radioimmunoassays, which are not influenced by iodine ingestion. The range of normal values in each laboratory varies—for most laboratories, the normal range for total (bound and unbound) plasma T_4 is 5–12 μg/dl; the T_3 range is 80–180 mg/dl.

Standard laboratory T_3 and T_4 assays measure the total amount of hormone in the blood, more than 99% of which is bound to plasma-binding proteins (see Chapter 2). The patient's actual metabolic state is more closely related to free thyroid hormone concentrations, which are difficult to measure directly. Elevations of either T_3 or T_4 hormones are not necessarily diagnostic of thyrotoxicosis. As shown in Table 2-1, a number of factors can alter the serum concentration of thyroxin-binding globulin (TBG) and other serum proteins binding T_3 and T_4. Consequently, any abnormalities that alter the concentration of TBG, thyroxin-binding prealbumin (TBPA), or albumin will change the level of T_3 or T_4, modifying the results of standard laboratory evaluations.[8,20,21] In circumstances such as pregnancy, the use of certain medicines, or systemic illness in which an abnormality of TBG or TBPA may be expected, the serum concentration of circulating, unbound, free T_3 or T_4 should be assessed to detect hyperthyroidism. Assays that directly measure free T_3 or T_4 levels are available but not very reliable, and free thyroid hormone concentrations are more commonly measured indirectly.

TESTS TO ASSESS HORMONE BINDING TO SERUM PROTEINS

The free T_4 index is proportional to the free thyroxine concentration. Measurement of resin T_3 uptake and its derivative, the free T_4 (thyroxine) index, is useful in a number of situations. The determination of the free T_4 index is relatively simple, yet the historic term for one of its components has led to confusion.

Plasma binding is measured using the T_3-resin (RT_3) uptake test. This test is based on the principle that the amount of an aliquot of either radioactive T_3 or T_4 recovered on a uniform resin after incubation with a patient's serum is inversely proportional to the relative saturation of plasma protein binding. In hyperthyroidism, plasma T_4 is elevated, there is a high degree of TBG saturation, and the RT_3 uptake is elevated. In contrast, when TBG levels are elevated without hyperthyroidism, there is a low degree of TBG saturation and a low RT_3 uptake.

The product of this binding index (T_3 uptake) and the plasma T_4 equals the free T_4 index. In hyperthyroidism, usually both the plasma T_4 level and RT_3 uptake are elevated and their product exceeds the upper limit of the free T_4 index. In a patient on oral contraceptives, with increased TBG, there is an elevated plasma T_4 level with a low RT_3 uptake and a normal free T_4 index. The calculated free T_4 index is more useful clinically than the free T_4 level, which is an expensive test.[27]

ANTIBODIES IN THYROID DISEASE

As discussed in Chapter 2, long-acting thyroid stimulator (LATS) was one of the first abnormal immunoglobulins described in thyroid disease.[28,29] It is found in approximately 60% of patients with active Graves' disease.[30–38] This antibody is of historic interest only; it does not correlate with disease status or prognosis. A few reports have noted a correlation between LATS and ophthalmopathy; however, most have not.[30–38] In some studies, antibodies towards the TSH receptor are the most common abnormal immunoglobulin in thyroid eye disease patients and are found in more than 85% of such cases.[39]

In a tertiary referral center, a significant number of patients with proptosis who eventually are diagnosed as having thyroid orbitopathy are not clinically hyperthyroid. Often they do not have elevated serum thyroid hormone levels nor suppressed serum TSH. Some of these patients have had spontaneous resolution of the hyperthyroid state on the basis of autoimmune thyroid gland damage, while others have yet to develop clinical hyperthyroidism (euthyroid ophthalmopathy) at the time of presentation with eye findings.

TRAbs, discussed in Chapter 2, are directed against the TSHr. They carry a variety of labels depending on the type of assays used to demonstrate their presence and their function (stimulate or inhibit receptor or block receptor).[8,39,40] Almost all patients with systemic hyperthyroidism have these antibodies detected at one point in their disease course. Standard nomenclature includes TRAb, thyroxin-binding albumin (TBA), LATS protector antibody, thyroid-stimulating immunoglobulin (TSI), and TSH-binding inhibitory immunoglobulin (TBII).[33,40–47] Techniques used to measure these antibodies include preventing LATS inactivation by human thyroid extracts (LATS-protector activity or LPA), stimulation of colloid droplet formation, enhancement of cyclic adenosine monophosphate (cAMP) formation in human thyroid slices, increased cAMP in a primary of human thyroid cells, displacement of labeled thyrotropin in a radioreceptor assay using human thyroid membranes, and promotion of the release of radioiodine from primed murine thyroids.[20,21,42,43,48]

TRAbs, measured in primary human thyroid cultures, cryopreserved thyroid cells, or an immortalized rat thyroid cell line are present in more than 90% of active Graves' disease and Hashimoto's thyroiditis patients.[39,49–52] They compete with TSH binding to thyroid cells and increase the secretion of T_4. TRAbs are present in approximately 40–95% of thyroid eye disease patients even without other evidence of autoimmune thyroid disease and are one of the most useful antibody tests to diagnose a patient suspected of having thyroid-related eye disease.[39,40,44,53–57] In most cases, these antibodies correlate with response to systemic thyroid therapy, disappearing in remission and returning when there is a recurrence.[40,49,58–60] Measurement of these antibodies is especially useful in patients with normal serum TSH levels.[8,54–59]

Four types of other antithyroid antibodies have been demonstrated—an antithyroglobulin antibody, an antibody directed against a component of thyroid microsomes (thyroid peroxidase, TPO), an anticolloidal immunoglobulin distinct from thyroglobulin, and an antibody reactive with a nuclear component of thyroid cells.[39,61,62] All except the antinuclear antibody are organ-specific. Only the antithyroglobulin and anti-TPO antibodies are useful diagnostically. Molecular characterization of these antibodies will increase our understanding of their development and importance.[62a]

The anti-TPO, formerly termed antimicrosomal antibody, is found more often in thyroid disease patients and has a higher titer and lower incidence of false-positives than antithyroglobulin antibodies. In a patient with a suppressed serum TSH and a normal free T_4, anti-TPO antibody studies are useful—if antibodies are present patients are more likely to develop clinical disease, while if absent, it is less likely for clinical hyperthyroidism to become manifest.[7,8,63] Positive antithyroglobulin antibody titers are present in 10–20% of healthy elderly women. Anti-TPO antibody titers are present in up to 90% of Hashimoto's and 80% of Graves' disease patients, whereas antithyroglobulin antibody levels are positive in only 55% of Hashimoto's and 25% of Graves' disease patients (and in 10% of disease-free subjects). In vitro assays of these substances are widely available, relatively inexpensive, and convenient to perform.[39,61,62,64] Classic antithyroid antibodies (antithyroglobulin and anti-TPO antibodies) are also useful in that they rarely disappear during the disease course and have some prognostic implications.[65] We generally obtain these studies either simultaneously with or after TSHr antibody assays. Other immunologic tests may be useful in atypical patients—some of these assays are research tools but in one study all euthyroid orbitopathy patients were positive in at least one assay.[66]

The ophthalmologist presented with a patient whose chief complaint is proptosis is in a different position than an endocrinologist examining a patient with the systemic stigmata of Graves' disease. While approximately 95% of patients with thyrotoxicosis have a suppressed TSH and an elevated free T_4 index, 10–25% of patients who present to the ophthalmologist with proptosis and are eventually diagnosed as having thyroid-related eye disease do not display the systemic signs or the thyroid hormone alterations characteristic of classical Graves' disease.

A number of other assays are used in rare circumstances by the endocrinologist. I have briefly listed some of these assays, and have described some of the data that has been generated with them on Graves' and euthyroid ophthalmopathy. As discussed in the next section, the latter diagnosis is often difficult to make. The use of TSHr antibodies, antithyroid antibodies, and serum TSH are more sensitive in the diagnosis of euthyroid ophthalmopathy than older assays such as T_3 suppression and serum TRH.[56] Still, about 10% of euthyroid ophthalmopathy patients are not definitely diagnosed with these tests.

RADIOACTIVE IODINE UPTAKE TEST

The radioactive iodine uptake (RAIU) test, which measures the rate of synthesis and release of thyroid hormones, is usually performed with ^{123}I since it has a shorter half-life (12–13 hours) and a lower radiation dose to patients' thyroid than ^{131}I. Twenty-four hours after the oral ingestion of radioactive iodine (RAI), two gamma scintillation counts are obtained—one over the thyroid gland and another background count over the thigh. Percentage of RAIU by the thyroid is calculated using the following formula:

$$\% \text{ RAIU} = 100 \times \frac{\text{Thyroid counts} - \text{thigh counts}}{\text{dose of RAI}}$$

At 24 hours, the normal range is between 5–30%. This average RAIU has decreased over the past 30 years because of increased amounts of iodine in the environment, medications, and diet.

Unlike current serum tests for thyroid hormones, RAIU results are altered by iodine-containing substances. Moreover, RAIU is not used for routine diagnosis of hyperthyroidism. Other more convenient in vitro assays are quite accurate. The RAIU is usually elevated in Graves' disease but can also be above normal in other conditions. The RAIU test is useful as a component of the T_3 suppression test, in distinguishing different forms of hyperthyroidism (thyrotoxicosis factitia, thyroiditis with transient hyperthyroidism, and ectopic thyroid production), and in planning radioactive iodine therapy. In one study, the uneven pattern of uptake was a consistent finding in euthyroid orbitopathy.[67]

THYROID SUPPRESSION (TRIIDOTHYRONINE SUPPRESSION OR WERNER) TEST

In normal subjects, 75–100 µg of sodium T_3 (liothyronine) daily for 8–14 days suppresses thyroid gland function. The RAIU values at the end of this period are less than 50% of those obtained just before.[60] It is unclear why a more complete RAIU suppression does not occur in some normal subjects. In hyperthyroidism there is autonomous thyroid gland function and thus no suppression of RAIU values.[60,68] A schema for this test is shown in Table 3-3.

Historically, in patients suspected of having thyroid ophthalmopathy with normal serum T_3 and T_4 levels, negative antibody titers, and no clinical stigmata of Graves'

Table 3-3. Thyroid Suppression Test Protocol

1. Radioactive iodine (^{123}I) uptake (RAIU) test (normal 5–30%)
2. Oral administration of 75–100 mg/day liothyronine for 8–14 days
3. Repeat RAIU
4. Positive test (abnormal suppression) greater than 50% reduction of baseline RAIU

disease,[44,53,62,69–71] a thyroid suppression test was useful. A normal Werner suppression test almost eliminated the diagnosis of hyperthyroidism, while an abnormal thyroid suppression test was observed (see Table 3-3) in 40–80% of patients with active ophthalmopathy, even with otherwise normal thyroid function.

Abnormal response was consistent with, but not pathognomonic for, hyperthyroidism. Indeed, abnormal suppression may persist for years after thyrotoxicosis has been successfully treated. In patients who are not suppressible, there may be a higher incidence of recurrence.[72]

The thyroid suppression test requires a high degree of patient compliance—T_3 must be taken 8–14 days. The test also carries a risk of morbidity through heart failure for elderly patients or those with cardiac disease. Therefore, the assay is contraindicated in these two groups.

THYROTROPIN-RELEASING HORMONE TEST

The TRH stimulation test entails standardized supraphysiologic excitation of the TSH secretory mechanism of the anterior pituitary thyrotrophic cells. The resultant increase in serum TSH is inversely correlated with basal TSH concentration over a relatively wide range of values.[73] While this assay was useful before the development of sensitive serum TSH studies, the latter test has largely superseded it.

TRH can be administered by any route but is usually given intravenously as a 400-mg bolus. Serum for TSH analyses is drawn just before and 30 minutes after TRH administration. In individuals with normal thyroid function, serum TSH peaks in 20–30 minutes, then declines slowly, reaching baseline (0–8 μU/ml) in 2–3 hours. Concentrations can vary broadly even within a single subject. In healthy subjects, intravenous TRH usually increases the serum TSH level two to eight times baseline. In hyperthyroidism, however, TSH secretion is inhibited and thyrotropin levels do not rise in response to exogenous TRH. Primary hypothyroidism causes an exaggerated response.

The TRH test was clinically useful when there was a suggestion of hyperthyroidism or euthyroid ophthalmopathy with equivocal results from serum T_3 and T_4 tests, serum antibodies, and the free T_4 index. Positive results (subnormal or flat TRH response) were observed in approximately 30–50% of patients with euthyroid ophthalmopathy (see below and Table 3-3).[64,70–81] A subnormal TRH response was not pathognomonic for clinically significant thyrotoxicosis, nor did a negative test exclude the possibility of either Graves' disease or thyroid ophthalmopathy. TRH test results were usually concordant with those of the T_3 suppression test; however, the assay was less cumbersome to perform, did not rely as heavily on patient compliance, and had significantly less potential for morbidity.

In a comparison of TRH and thyroid suppression test results in 57 euthyroid ophthalmopathy patients, Tamai and coworkers noted that both sets of findings were abnormal in 35 patients (61.4%), normal in 15 cases (26%), and incongruent in seven patients (12%).[71]

There are subtle differences between the T_3 suppression test and the TRH test.[77] The suppression test does not indicate how much thyroid hormone is available; rather, it determines whether thyroid function is autonomous (hyperthyroidism) or is being driven by TSH (normal). TRH testing indicates whether the level of available thyroid hormone exceeds physiologic requirements and has therefore induced negative feedback control of TSH secretion.

In normal controls or patients with frank hyperthyroidism, results of both tests were almost always congruent. In some situations, however, the tests contradicted each other. As an example, in treated Graves' disease, an abnormal immunoglobulin may persist, causing continued thyroid stimulation. If there is sufficient loss of thyroid tissue and hormone production is normal or somewhat decreased, the TSH secretory mechanism maintains at least normal activity levels. In this situation, the suppression test would be abnormal while the TRH response would be normal or increased. As discussed under euthyroid ophthalmopathy, diagnostic accuracy may have been minimally increased when both tests are used together with other assays. The reason for discrepant results is sometimes unclear; similarly, the meaning of a supranormal response to TRH is not known.

EUTHYROID OPHTHALMOPATHY (OPHTHALMIC GRAVES' DISEASE)

In the 1940s, Means and Rundle separately described some patients with infiltrative ophthalmopathy without clinical or laboratory signs of thyrotoxicosis.[82,83] This entity was later termed *euthyroid ophthalmopathy* or *ophthalmic Graves' disease*. Some investigators have assigned this diagnosis to patients with mild thyroid enlargement if there are no historic or current signs of hyperthyroidism.[78] Of patients eventually diagnosed as having thyroid exophthalmos, 10–25% fall into this category.[44,53,56,57,66,69,71,79,84] Clinically, the eye findings in this group of patients are identical to those of patients whose ophthalmopathy is associated with Graves' disease. This entity is either becoming more common or is being recognized more frequently. In two Mayo Clinic studies over the past 30 years, the diagnosis has increased from 12% to 20% in patients with presumed thyroid eye disease.[69,84]

The signs and differential diagnosis of thyroid eye disease are discussed in Chapters 4 and 5. Euthyroid ophthalmopathy, which accounts for 10–25% of thyroid-related eye disease, may be the clinician's most difficult diagnostic challenge.

Several studies have attempted to identify correlations between thyroid function and ocular status. Liddle et al. suggested that a combination of Graves' disease and Hashimoto's thyroiditis would account for the euthyroid state in most cases.[85] Solomon et al. demonstrated the heterogeneity of the euthyroid ophthalmopathy patient group, identifying from a number of euthyroid patients some with latent Graves' disease, others with a combination of Graves' and Hashimoto's diseases, and one subgroup that could not be classified.[70] They studied thyroid suppression, LATS, LATS protector, and antithyroid antibody tests in 17 euthyroid ophthalmopathy patients. Two patients had LATS activity, nine (53%) had LATS protector activity (LPA, another measure of LATS effect), 47% had antimicrosomal antibodies, and eight of 16 had abnormal thyroid suppression tests (see Table 3-3). Six patients had LPA and nonsuppressibility consistent with Graves' disease, possibly coexistent with

Hashimoto's thyroiditis. Five patients appeared to have normal thyroid function; three of these had bilateral ocular abnormalities. Six patients had disparity between LPA and T_3 suppression findings and could not be classified. Neither computed tomography nor ultrasound was used in this study, so patients with nonthyroid extraocular myositis could not be excluded.

Teng et al. noted TRAbs in 43% of 56 patients with ophthalmic Graves' disease.[44] There was a 3 to 1 female to male ratio; equal numbers of patients had unilateral and bilateral ocular disease. Forty-five had orbital swelling and 16 had a family history of autoimmunity or thyroid disease. There was no correlation between TSI levels and TRH response or T_3 suppression. They followed many of these patients and noted progressive deterioration in seven; 37 had spontaneous improvement and 12 remained stable. There was no discernible relationship between TSI and changes in ocular status. As in the study by Solomon et al., patients could be divided into three groups: those who had thyrotropin control of thyroid function in the presence of receptor binding by nonstimulating antibodies; those whose thyroid function was controlled by TSI antibodies although hyperthyroidism was prevented by autoimmune destruction of the thyroid gland; and those in which there was TSH control of thyroid function in the absence of any antibodies. In a separate publication, Teng et al. noted that 18 of 46 euthyroid ophthalmopathy patients tested had impaired or absent response to TRH (39%), and 11 of 37 (30%) had normal T_3 suppression tests. Antibody levels in this study did not correlate with eye disease.[53]

In 1970, Hall et al. noted that 18 of 26 euthyroid ophthalmopathy patients (69%) had antithyroid antibodies compared to 10–20% of controls.[78] Fifty percent had abnormal T_3 suppression tests, and one-third had antithyroglobulin antibodies. The researchers concluded the presence of antibodies and nonsuppressibility were the best markers of ophthalmic Graves' disease.

Mornex et al. studied 20 patients and found that T_3 suppression test findings were abnormal in nine (45%) and normal in eleven (55%).[79] TRH test results were abnormal in one case (5%), normal in three (15%), and exaggerated in two cases (10%). These authors concluded that the thyroid suppression test was more reliable, but the two tests should be used together to increase diagnostic accuracy. In their study, the correct diagnosis of thyroid ophthalmopathy was made in eight of nine exophthalmic patients when the tests were used in tandem.

Franco et al. reported on pituitary-thyroid axis tests in 11 euthyroid ophthalmopathy patients. Five patients (45%) were nonsuppressible with T_3; two of these had exaggerated response to TRH, and three had a deficient TRH response.[74] Six patients (55%) were suppressible with T_3; one had a normal and five an exaggerated response to TRH. Neither test correlated with disease activity, course, or exophthalmos. Normal suppression levels were seen in four of six individuals with active ophthalmopathy but were abnormal in three of five patients with inactive ophthalmopathy. Thyroid nonsuppressibility occurred in some patients with an intact pituitary-thyroid reserve. Similar data were generated by Jackson et al.; no false-positive TRH results were observed in their small series.[80]

Three patients in the series reported by Franco et al. and some reported by Teng et al. had repeat T_3 suppression tests on multiple occasions with variable responses. Similar results were observed by Tamai and coworkers. These cases further demonstrate that many euthyroid ophthalmopathy patients do not fit neatly into distinct groups and that their thyroid status changes on long-term follow-up.[53,71,74] Tamai, for instance, noted that nine euthyroid ophthalmopathy patients eventually developed clinical and laboratory evidence of systemic hyperthyroidism.

Table 3-4. Thyroid Suppression and Thyrotropin-Releasing Hormone Tests in Euthyroid Ophthalmopathy*

Series	Abnormal T_3 suppression/patients	Subnormal TSH response
Werner, 1955	10/10	p
Guinet & Descaur, 1962	9/13	p
Hobbs, 1963	15/16	p
Burke, 1967	4/8	p
Bayliss, 1967	11/12	p
Wyse et al. 1968	5/6	p
Bowden & Rose, 1969	15/23	p
Hall et al. 1970	13/26	p
Lawton, 1971	2/2	2/2
Ivy, 1972	31/36	p
Franco et al. 1973	5/11	3/11
Mornex et al. 1975	9/22	1/6
Lawton, 1977	15/31	p
Teng, 1977	11/37	18/46
Solomon et al. 1977	9/17	p
Jackson et al. 1978	5/6	6/6
Zakarija et al. 1980	6/10	p
Tamai et al. 1980	41/57	36/57
Total	196/300 (65%)	87/169 (51%)

T_3 = triiodothyronine; TSH = thyroid-stimulating hormone.
*This tabulation is inclusive for different test protocols; an exaggerated response to thyrotropin-releasing hormone is not included in the data.

Watanabe and colleagues summarized the literature and noted that the TSHr antibody appeared to be the most sensitive assay in euthyroid orbitopathy; however, there was a wide variation in results (an average of 30% in positivity).[56,57] In their study, 12 of 13 euthyroid patients had TSHr antibodies and in followup five developed hyperthyroidism.[56] Using a combination of clinical research studies, Salvi and colleagues showed that all their ophthalmopathy patients had at least one thyroid abnormality demonstrable.[66] In my experience, since management is not altered if the patient is not hyperthyroid, and other diagnoses are excluded, we routinely just obtain TSHr anti-TSHr, anti-TPO, and antithyroglobulin antibodies. If those tests are negative, we manage the patient as we would a thyroid orbitopathy patient who is euthyroid. The obvious caveats are that some of these patients will become hyperthyroid and all require serial thyroid evaluations.

Table 3-4 summarizes a series of published reports concerning T_3 suppression and/or TRH tests. While TRH results usually mirror the T_3 suppression data, there is a 10–30% discrepancy. Many investigators have noted that test results change over time in the same patient.[71]

CONCLUSION

Patients suspected of having thyroid-related ophthalmopathy should have a thorough systemic review and a brief physical examination to ascertain if there are signs and symptoms of Graves' disease. If patients have bilateral ophthalmopathy with thyroid glandular enlargement and hyperthyroid symptoms, no further tests are required to establish the diagnosis of Graves' ophthalmopathy.

The current approach to laboratory evaluation in thyroid eye disease patients who present to an ophthalmologist without a history of systemic thyroid disease is listed in Table 3-2. A serum TSH is obtained, followed by a free T_3 index, free T_4, TSHr antibodies, and standard antithyroid antibodies. Pragmatically, if the first or subsequent tests are positive, other studies are not necessary. With very rare exceptions, serum T_3, TRH, and T_3 suppression tests are no longer needed in the evaluation of patients with possible thyroid-related eye disease.

REFERENCES

1. Fox RA, Schwartz TB. Infiltrative ophthalmopathy and primary hypothyroidism. Ann Intern Med 1967;67:377.
2. Wasnich RD, Grumet FC, Payne RO, Kriss JP. Graves' ophthalmopathy following external neck irradiation for nonthyroidal neoplastic disease. J Clin Endocrinol Metab 1973;37:703.
3. Wyse EP, McConahey WM, Woolner LB, et al. Ophthalmopathy without hyperthyroidism in patients with histologic Hashimoto's thyroiditis. J Clin Endocrinol Metab 1968;28:1623.
4. Brownlie BEW, Newton OAG, Singh SP. Ophthalmopathy associated with primary hypothyroidism. Acta Endocrinol (Copenh) 1975;79:691.
5. Hancock SL, Cox RS, McDougall IR. Thyroid diseases after treatment of Hodgkin's disease. N Engl J Med 1991;325:599.
6. Ridgway EC. Thyrotropin radioimmunoassays: birth, life and demise. Mayo Clin Proc 1988;63:1028.
7. Spencer CA. Clinical utility and cost-effectiveness of sensitive thyrotropin assays in ambulatory and hospitalized patients. Mayo Clin Proc 1988;63:1214.
8. Singer PA, Cooper DS, Levy EG, et al. Treatment guidelines for patients with hyperthyroidism and hypothyroidism. JAMA 1995;273:801.
9. Klee GG, Hay ID. Sensitive thyrotropin assays: analytic and clinical performance criteria. Mayo Clin Proc 1988;63:1123.
10. Hershman JM, Pekary AE, Smith VP, Hershman JD. Evaluation of five high-sensitivity American thyrotropin assays. Mayo Clin Proc 1988;63:1133.
11. Gupta MK. Recent advances in laboratory tests for autoantibodies to thyrotropin receptor protein in Graves' disease. Clin Lab Med 1988;8:303.
12. Caldwell G, Gow SM, Sweeting VM, et al. A new strategy for thyroid function testing. Lancet 1985;1:1117.
13. Wehmann RE, Nisula BC. Radioimmunoassay of human thyrotropin: analytic and clinical developments. CRC Crit Rad Clin Lab Sci 1984;20:243.
14. Toft AD. Use of sensitive immunoradiometric assay for thyrotropin in clinical practice. Mayo Clin Proc 1988;63:1035.
15. Utiger RD. Thyrotropin measurements: past, present, future. Mayo Clin Proc 1988;63:1053.
16. Ehrmann DA, Sarne DH. Serum thyrotropin and the assessment of thyroid status. Ann Intern Med 1989;110:179.
17. Hamblin FS, Dyer SA, Mohr VS, et al. Relationship between thyrotropin and thyroxine changes during recovery from severe hypothyroxinemia of critical illness. J Clin Endocrinol Metab 1986;62:717.
18. Piketty ML, Talbot JN, Askienazy S, Milhaud G. Clinical significance of a low concentration of thyrotropin: five immunometric "kit" assays compared. Clin Chem 1987;33:1237.
19. Spencer C, Eigen A, Hsen D, et al. Specificity of sensitive assays of thyrotropin (TSH) used to screen thyroid disease in hospitalized patients. Clin Chem 1987;33:1391.
20. Klee GG, Hay ID. Biochemical thyroid function testing. Mayo Clin Proc 1994;69:5469.
21. Surks MI, Chopra IJ, Mariash CN, et al. American Thyroid Association guidelines for use of laboratory tests in thyroid disorders. JAMA 1990;263:1529.

22. Midgley JEM, Moon CR, Wilkins TA. Validity of analog free thyroxin immunoassays (part II). Clin Chemistry 1987;33:2145.

23. Hesch RD, Huefner M, Muhlen A von zur, Emrich D. Triiodothyronine levels in patients with euthyroid endocrine exophthalmos and during treatment of thyrotoxicosis. Acta Endocrinol (Copenh) 1974;75:514.

24. Surks MI. Assessment of thyroid function. Ophthalmology 1981;88:476.

25. Lawton NF, Fells P, Lloyd GAS. Medical Investigation of Dysthyroid Eye Disease. In W Junk (ed), Third International Symposium on Orbital Disorders Headed by Orbital Center Amsterdam. The Hague: BV Publishers, 1978;343.

26. McDougall RI. Thyroid Disease in Clinical Practice. New York: Oxford University Press, 1992.

27. Bayer MF, McDougall IR. Radioimmunoassay of free thyroxine in serum: comparison with chemical findings and results of conventional thyroid-function tests. Clin Chem 1980;26:1186.

28. Adams DD, Purvis HD. Abnormal responses in the assay of thyrotropin. Univ Otago Med School Proc 1956;34:11.

29. Kriss JP. Inactivation of long-acting thyroid stimulator (LATS) by anti-kappa and anti-lambda antisera. J Clin Endocrinol Metab 1968;28:1440.

30. Werner SC, Feind CR, Aida M. Graves' disease and total thyroidectomy: progression of severe eye changes and decrease in serum long acting thyroid stimulator after operation. N Engl J Med 1967;276:132.

31. McKenzie JM, McCullagh EP. Observations against a causal relationship between the long-acting thyroid stimulator and ophthalmopathy in Graves' disease. J Clin Endocrinol Metab 1968;28:1177.

32. Wall JR, Odgers R, Hetzel BS. Immunological studies of the eye changes of thyrotoxicosis. Aust N Z J Med 1973;3:162.

33. Wall JR, Strakosch CR, Fang SL, et al. Thyroid-binding antibody and other immunological abnormalities in patients with Graves' ophthalmopathy: effect of treatment with cyclophosphamide. Clin Endocrinol 1979;10:79.

34. Lipman LM, Green DE, Snyder NJ, et al. Relationship of long-acting thyroid stimulator to the clinical features in the course of Graves' disease. Am J Med 1967;43:486.

35. Adams DD, Kennedy TH, Stewart RDH. Correlation between long-acting thyroid stimulator protector level and thyroid ^{131}I uptake in thyrotoxicosis. Br Med J 1974;II:199.

36. Hetzel BS, Mason EK, Wong HK. Studies of serum long-acting thyroid stimulator (LATS) in relation to exophthalmos after therapy for thyrotoxicosis. Aust Ann Med 1968;17:307.

37. Snyder NJ, Green DE, Solomon DH. Glucocorticoid-induced disappearance of long-acting thyroid stimulator in the ophthalmopathy of Graves' disease. J Clin Endocrinol 1964;24:1129.

38. Solomon DH, Green DE, Snyder NJ, Nelson JC. Clinical significance of the long-acting thyroid stimulator of Graves' disease. Clin Res 1964;12:119.

39. McLachlan SM, Bahn R, Rapoport B. Endocrine ophthalmopathy: a re-evaluation of the association with thyroid autoantibodies. Autoimmunity 1992;14:143.

40. Strakosch CR, Wenzel BE, Row VV, Volpe R. Immunology of autoimmune thyroid diseases. N Engl J Med 1982;307:1499.

41. Major PW, Munro DS. Observations on the stimulation of thyroid function in mice by injection of serum from normal subjects and from patients with thyroid disorders. Clin Sci 1962;23:463.

42. Smith BR, Hall R. The Interaction of Graves' Immunoglobulins with TSH Receptor. In JR Stockigt, S Nagataki (eds), Thyroid Research VIII: Proceedings of the Eighth International Thyroid Congress. Oxford, England: Pergamon, 1980;715.

43. Shishiba Y, Shimizu T, Yoshimura S, Shizume K. Direct evidence for human thyroidal stimulation by LATS protector. J Clin Endocrinol Metab 1973;36:517.

44. Teng CS, Smith BR, Clayton B, et al. Thyroid-stimulating immunoglobulins in ophthalmic Graves' disease. Clin Endocrinol (Oxf) 1977;6:207.

45. Claque R, Mukhtar ED, Pyle GA, et al. Thyroid stimulating immunoglobulins and control of thyroid function. J Clin Endocrinol Metab 1976;43:550.

46. Davies TF. Thyroid stimulating hormone receptor antibodies—the calm after the storm. Mayo Clin Proc 1988;63:736.

47. Committee on Nomenclature of the American Thyroid Association. Revised nomenclature for tests of thyroid hormones and thyroid-related proteins in sera. J Clin Endocrinol Metab 1987;64:1089.

48. Onaya T, Kotani M, Yamada T, Ochi Y. New in vitro tests to detect the thyroid stimulator in sera from hyperthyroid patients by measuring colloid droplet formation and cyclic AMP in human thyroid slices. J Clin Endocrinol Metab 1973;36:859.

49. Rapoport B, Greenspan FS, Filetti S, Pepitone M. Clinical experience with a human thyroid cell bioassay for thyroid-stimulating immunoglobulin. J Clin Endocrinol Metab 1984;58:332.

50. Zakarija M, McKenzie JM. The spectrum and significance of autoantibodies reacting with thyrotropin receptor. Endocrinol Metab Clin North Am 1987;16:343.

51. Ollis CA, Tomlinson S, Munro DS. Thyroid stimulating immunoglobulins: measurement and clinical use. Clin Sci 1985;69:113.

52. Jiang N-S, Fairbanks VF, Hay ID. Assay for thyroid stimulating immunoglobulin. Mayo Clin Proc 1986;61:753.

53. Teng CS, Yeo PP. Ophthalmic Graves' disease: natural history on detailed thyroid function studies. Br Med J 1977;1:273.

54. Smith BR, Creagh FM, Hashim FA, et al. TSH receptor antibodies. Mount Sinai J Med 1986;53:53.

55. Spector RH, Carlisle JA. Minimal thyroid ophthalmopathy. Neurology 1987;37:1803.

56. Kashiwai T, Tada H, Asahi K, et al. Significance of thyroid stimulating antibody and long term follow up in patients with euthyroid Graves' disease. Endocr J 1995;42:405.

57. Watanabe M, Iwatani Y, Kashiwai T, et al. Euthyroid Graves' disease showing no thyroid abnormalities except positive thyroid-stimulating antibody (TSAb): two case reports. J Intern Med 1995;238:379.

58. Smith BR, Hall R. Thyroid stimulating immunoglobulins in Graves' disease. Lancet 1974;2:427.

59. Zakarija M, McKenzie JM, Banovac K. Clinical significance of assay of thyroid stimulating antibody in Graves' disease. Ann Intern Med 1980;93:28.

60. Werner SC, Spooner M. New and simple test for hyperthyroidism employing L-triiodothyronine and the 24-hour I-131 uptake method. Bull N Y Acad Med 1955;31:137.

61. Roitt IM, Doniach D, Campbell PN, Hudson RV. Autoantibodies in Hashimoto's disease (lymphadenoid goiter). Lancet 1956;2:820.

62. McGill DA, Asher SR Jr. Endocrine exophthalmos. N Engl J Med 1962;267:133.

62a. Akamizu T, Matsuda F, Okuda J, et al. Molecular analysis of stimulatory anti-thyrotropin receptor antibodies (TSAbs) involved in Graves' disease. J Immunol 1996;157:3148.

63. Hawkins BR, Cheah PS, Dawkins RL, et al. Diagnostic significance of thyroid microsomal antibodies in a randomly selected population. Lancet 1980;2:1057.

64. Wall JR, Henderson J, Strakosch CR, Joyner DM. Graves' ophthalmopathy. Can Med Assoc J 1981;124:855.

65. Scherbaum WA. On the clinical importance of thyroid microsomal and thyroglobulin antibody determination. Acta Endocrinol 1987 (Suppl);281:325.

66. Salvi M, Zhang Z-G, Haegert D, et al. Patients with endocrine ophthalmopathy not associated with overt thyroid disease have multiple thyroid immunological abnormalities. J Clin Endocrinol Metab 1990;70:89.

67. Kasagi K, Hidaka A, Misaki T, et al. Scintigraphic findings of the thyroid in euthyroid ophthalmic Graves' disease. J Nucl Med 1994;35:811.

68. Burke G. The triiodothyronine suppression test. Am J Med 1967;42:600.

69. Ivy HK. Medical approach to ophthalmopathy of Graves' disease. Mayo Clin Proc 1972;47:980.

70. Solomon DH, Chopra IJ, Chopra U, Smith FJ. Identification of subgroups of euthyroid Graves' ophthalmopathy. N Engl J Med 1977;296:181.

71. Tamai H, Nakagawa T, Ohsako N, et al. Changes in thyroid functions in patients with euthyroid Graves' disease. J Clin Endocrinol Metab 1980;50:108.

72. Yamamoto M, Totsuka Y, Kojima I, et al. Outcome of patients with Graves' disease after long-term medical treatment guided by triiodothyronine (T_3) suppression tests. Clin Endocrinol 1983;19:467.

73. Hershman JM. Clinical application of thyrotropin-releasing hormone. N Engl J Med 1974;290:886.

74. Franco PS, Hershman JM, Haigler ED Jr, Pittman JA Jr. Response to thyrotropin-releasing

hormone compared with thyroid suppression tests in euthyroid Graves' disease. Metabolism 1973;22:1357.

75. Clifton-Bligh P, Silverstein GE, Burke G. Unresponsiveness to thyrotropin-releasing hormone (TRH) in untreated Graves' hyperthyroidism and in euthyroid Graves' disease. J Clin Endocrinol Metab 1974;38:531.

76. Bowden AN, Rose FC. Investigation of endocrine exophthalmos. Proc R Soc Med 1969;6:13.

77. Chopra IJ, Chopra U, Orgiazzi J. Abnormalities of hypothalamo-hypophyseal-thyroid axis in patients with Graves' ophthalmopathy. J Clin Endocrinol Metab 1973;37:955.

78. Hall R, Kirkham K, Doniach D, El Kabir D. Ophthalmic Graves' disease: diagnosis and pathogenesis. Lancet 1970;1:375.

79. Mornex R, Fournier G, Berthezne F. Ophthalmic Graves' disease. Mod Probl Ophthalmol 1975;14:426.

80. Jackson WB, Tolis G, Chertman M. The TRH test: its value in the diagnosis of Graves' ophthalmopathy. Can J Ophthalmol 1978;13:10.

81. Lawton NF, Ekins RP, Nabarro JD. Failure of pituitary response to thyrotropin-releasing hormone in euthyroid Graves' disease. Lancet 1971;2:14.

82. Hertz S, Means JH, Williams RH. Graves' disease with dissociation of thyrotoxicosis and ophthalmopathy. West J Surg 1941;49:493.

83. Hales IB, Rundle FF. Ocular changes in Graves' disease: a long-term follow-up study. QJM 1960;29:113.

84. Hamilton RD, Mayberry WE, McConahey WM, Hanson KC. Ophthalmopathy of Graves' disease: a comparison between patients treated surgically and patients treated with radioiodide. Mayo Clin Proc 1967;42:812.

85. Liddle GW, Heyssel RM, McKenzie JM. Graves' disease without hyperthyroidism. Am J Med 1965;39:845.

4

Thyroid Eye Signs and Disease Classification

Normal lid and orbital anatomy is variable. Myopia, race, familial attributes, and systemic and ocular diseases can alter the degree of ocular protrusion and overall lid position. In the normal adult, the upper lid margin is usually midway between the upper edge of the iris-pupillary border and the corneal-scleral limbus.

Since Cohn[1] initially described an instrument in 1867, investigators have used a myriad of exophthalmometers to measure the range of normal ocular protrusion and asymmetry.[2–5] Most devices use the lateral orbital rim as a fixation point since the amount of fat in this location is relatively uniform. Knudtzon[6] studied 362 normal individuals age 15–65 with less than 2.5 diopters of myopia. He observed a Gaussian distribution with a bell-shaped curve. The mean value for ocular protrusion was 17 mm with a standard deviation of 2.08 mm. Ninety-nine percent of normal subjects had exophthalmometer readings between 11.8 and 22.4 mm. In 44% there were no significant differences in bilateral measurements; 19.7% had a difference of less than 0.5 mm, and 33.4% had a difference of less than 1 mm. Only 3% of this normal population had a difference in exophthalmometer readings between their two eyes of greater than 2 mm. Analogous data have been generated by Dreschler and others.[7–9] In contrast, Streeten and coworkers noted that 21% of 308 thyrotoxic patients had exophthalmometry readings greater than 19 mm.[10]

Two commonly used exophthalmometers are shown in Figure 4-1. The choice of an exophthalmometer is not critical. I prefer an instrument that uses both lateral orbital rims for fixation and can detect parallax. Intraobserver variation is considerably decreased if the same device is used for all serial measurements on a patient; the instrument's accuracy on repeat measurements is approximately ±2 mm. Less experienced observers often underestimate exophthalmos.[11] Readings obtained in the supine versus vertical position change but do not differentiate normal from thyroid eye disease subjects.[12] Rarely, pressure on the exophthalmometer can produce damage to the globe.[13]

A few other instruments are available that do not require orbital rim fixation to measure proptosis. The exophthalmometer shown in Figure 4-2 is useful especially if a surgeon elects to remove the lateral rim as part of an orbital decompression operation.

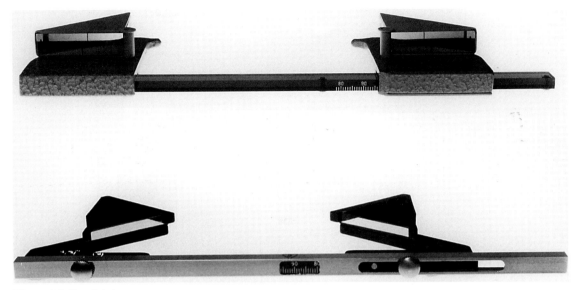

Figure 4-1. Exophthalmometers.

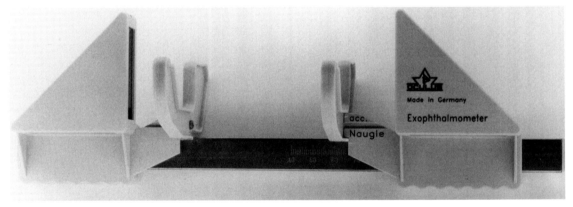

Figure 4-2. Naugle exophthalmometer is useful in cases where the lateral orbital rim has been removed since it uses the cheek and forehead as fixation and reference points.

EYE SIGNS

A number of non–thyroid-related diseases, as well as either endogenous or exogenous sympathetic stimulation, can result in lid retraction.[14–19] Lid retraction is usually diagnosed when the upper or lower eyelid border is at or superior to the corneal limbus, or when the lower lid is 1–2 mm below the inferior limbus. Table 4-1 lists some causes of nonthyroid eyelid retraction. Bartley has summarized an exhaustive list of more than 70 causes of eyelid retraction divided into neurogenic, myogenic, mechanical, and miscellaneous etiologies.[20]

In addition to thyroid ophthalmopathy, systemic diseases, drugs, orbital diseases, and neoplasms of the orbit, brain, and sinus can produce proptosis.[21–23] Most oph-

Table 4-1. Non-Neoplastic Conditions That Can Simulate Early Thyroid Changes of Lid Retraction or Apparent Proptosis

1. Myopia
2. Posterior commissure brain lesions (Parinaud's syndrome)
3. Congenital anomalies
4. Cirrhosis
5. Medication (lithium, steroids, etc.) induced
6. Contralateral ptosis
7. Hydrocephalus
8. Hypokalemic periodic paralysis
9. Cushing's syndrome
10. Chronic obstructive lung disease
11. Uremia
12. Superior vena cava syndrome
13. Sympathomimetic drugs
14. Nerve III lesions
15. Status post lid surgery

thalmologists consider bilateral exophthalmometer readings greater than 22 mm, or a difference between the two eyes of 2 mm or greater, to be suspicious for orbital pathology. Differences of less than 2 mm are questionable since observer error can account for this degree of deviation.

A plethora of thyroid eye signs have been identified since the original description of this disease in 1786.[24] A number of clinicians have described signs that bear their names (Table 4-2).[25–41] A few eponymic signs, such as von Graefe's sign (upper eyelid lag on downgaze, Figure 4-3), and Dalrymple's sign (lid retraction and scleral show, Figure 4-4) are useful, but most are nondiagnostic. The combination of bilateral exophthalmos, lid retraction, stare, and an enlarged thyroid are virtually pathognomonic for endocrine exophthalmos. Some ocular signs are relatively specific for thyroid ophthalmopathy. These include proptosis and lid lag or stare, proptosis plus a restrictive extraocular myopathy (see below), or the presence of isolated enlarged vessels over the insertion of the medial or lateral rectus muscles (Figure 4-5). Conjunctival or periorbital edema (Figures 4-6 and 4-7) is also quite common in thyroid exophthalmos and is occasionally observed in other conditions.

Almost all endocrine exophthalmos patients, even when asymptomatic, have some degree of extraocular muscle involvement demonstrable by abnormal ultrasonography or intraocular pressure (IOP) tests.[42–56] In an ultrasonographic study of 47 patients, 30 of whom had minimal signs of thyroid eye disease (class 0 or 1), 94% had ultrasound evidence of endocrine exophthalmos on the basis of extraocular muscle enlargement; two patients had equivocal changes, and one had normal echographic test findings. Similar data have been generated by other investigators.[44,48,49] The most common extraocular muscles involved in thyroid eye disease, in order of frequency, are the inferior, medial, superior, and lateral recti. The oblique muscles are involved less frequently, and an abnormality of those muscles can be simulated by thyroid involvement of the inferior rectus muscle.[57]

Inferior rectus involvement in thyroid eye disease results in a tethered eye with restricted upward gaze. Increased IOP occurs due to muscle pressure against the eye. This is especially true when the globe is in primary position or attempting a superior duction. Some investigators believe that a 4-mm increase in IOP between inferior

Table 4-2. Eye Signs in Graves' Disease

Name	Signs
Ballet's	Paralysis of one or more extraocular muscles
Boston's	Uneven jerky motion of the upper lid on inferior movement
Cowen's	Extensive hippus of the consensual pupillary light reflex
Dalrymple's	Upper lid retraction
Enroth's	Edema of the lower lid
Gellinek's	Abnormal pigmentation of the upper lid
Gifford's	Difficult eversion of the upper lid
Goffroy's	Absent creases in the forehead on superior gaze
Griffith's	Lower lid lag on upward gaze
Knies'	Uneven pupil dilation in dim light
Kocher's	Spasmatic retraction of the upper lid during fixation
Loewi's	Dilation of the pupil with 1/1,000 epinephrine
Means'	Increased superior scleral show on upgaze
Mobius'	Deficient convergence
Payne/Trousseau's	Dislocation of globe
Pochin's	Reduced amplitude of blinking
Riesman's	Bruit over eyelid
Rosenbach's	Tremor of the gently closed lids
Sainton's	Frontalis contraction after cessation of levator activity
Snellen/Donder's	Bruit over the eye
Suker's	Inability to maintain fixation on extreme lateral gaze
Stellwag's	Incomplete and infrequent blinking
Vigouroux's	Puffiness of the lids
von Graefe's	Upper eyelid lag on downgaze
Wilder's	Jerking of eyes on movement from abduction to adduction

and superior gaze is highly suggestive of a restrictive myopathy. Since the first descriptions of increased IOP by Brailey, Eyre, Wessely, and others, a number of investigators have noted that thyroid eye disease patients have elevated IOP with their eyes in the primary horizontal position.[50–56,58–60] Gamblin et al.[54] observed that all patients with long-standing thyroid exophthalmos had increased IOP; 68% of hyperthyroid patients without measurable proptosis also had an elevated IOP reading in primary position. Others have noted this abnormality less frequently—Allen and coworkers observed this in 22% of their cases.[61] These findings are important for the diagnosis of endocrine eye disease to avoid the false-positive diagnosis of glaucoma in hyperthyroid patients and to demonstrate that, even if patients do not have obvious clinical orbital involvement, a very high percentage of thyroid patients have orbital pathology. Elevated IOP in upgaze is not diagnostic for hyperthyroidism—it was noted in 37% of Hashimoto's patients.[62] When a thyroid ophthalmopathy patient is found to have increased IOP in primary position, the pressure should be rechecked with the eye at an angle of 10–15 degrees below horizontal.

Thyroid ophthalmopathy, like Graves' disease in general, occurs most commonly in females 30–50 years old. Eye findings in association with hyperthyroidism are statistically less common in elderly patients who present with Graves' disease. Nordyke and coworkers observed in a study of 880 patients that eye findings almost disappeared in the seventh and eighth decades.[63] The overall female to male ratio in systemic hyperthyroidism is 4 to 1; however, in thyroid eye disease, the ratio is less, usually documented at approximately 2.5 to 1.[64–66] Bartley and colleagues noted an

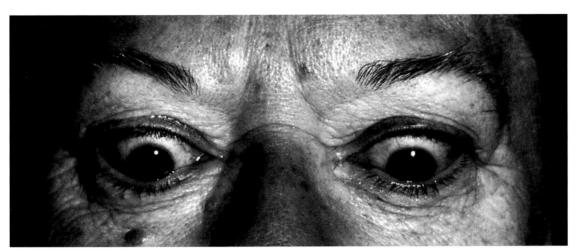

Figure 4-3. Von Graefe's sign of upper eyelid lag on downgaze.

age-adjusted incidence of thyroid orbitopathy for women of 16/100,000/year as compared to 2.9 for men, and there is no change noted over 20 years.[67] Severe exophthalmos develops in older men more commonly than would be expected.[68–76] Thyroid eye disease in children and adolescents is uncommon.[77,78] When ophthalmopathy occurs in children with Graves' disease, eye findings are quite mild.[78–81] Rarely, exophthalmos can transiently develop in the neonatal period secondary to transplacental transfer.[82]

Graves' disease patients usually develop eye symptoms before or simultaneous with noticeable ocular signs. In a study from Amsterdam there was no difference in the systemic disease status between patients who presented with unilateral or bilateral thyroid orbitopathy.[83] Symptoms are usually of gradual or insidious onset. They may include photophobia, tearing, a gritty foreign body sensation, ocular pain, lid edema, diplopia, blurred or decreased visual acuity, and field defects. Rarely, Graves' disease can present as an acute orbititis with an acute, painful proptosis and limitation of eye movements.[84]

The relative frequency of different eye signs in patients with systemic stigmata of hyperthyroidism is shown in Table 4-3. Various clinical studies have shown that approximately 10–70% of Graves' disease patients have clinical eye findings at the time of systemic diagnosis.[85–93] Sloan noted that 115 of 1,500 hyperthyroid patients had eye signs.[94] As previously mentioned, there is computed tomography (CT), magnetic resonance imaging (MRI), or ultrasound evidence for orbital involvement in almost all patients with hyperthyroidism. In a study that was biased toward severe eye disease, Gorman observed that 81% of patients who eventually required orbital decompression developed eye signs within 18 months before or after diagnosis of hyperthyroidism.[94] Approximately 30% of patients with ophthalmopathy and dermopathy required orbital decompression; this is much higher than most other patients with thyroid eye disease.[95]

Clinical evidence of bilateral thyroid eye involvement occurs in 80–90% of cases; unilateral eye findings are present in 10–20% of patients.[21,87,96–99] Among patients referred to an ophthalmologic diagnostic unit, the percentage of unilateral cases can be

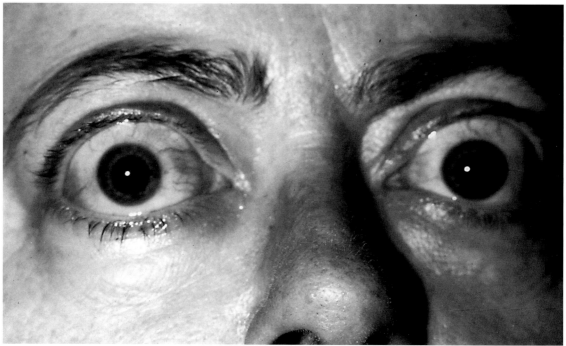

A

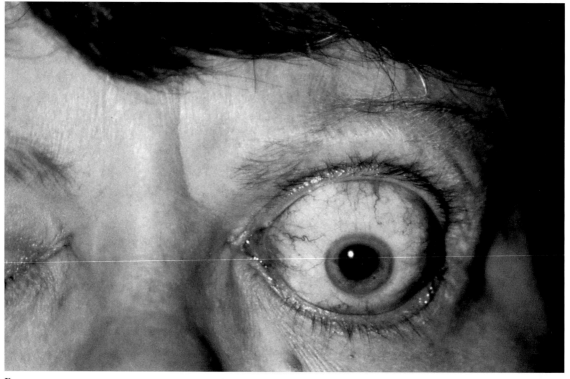

B

Figure 4-4. A. Dalrymple's sign of lid retraction with scleral show. B. Severe retraction and proptosis may produce globe luxation.

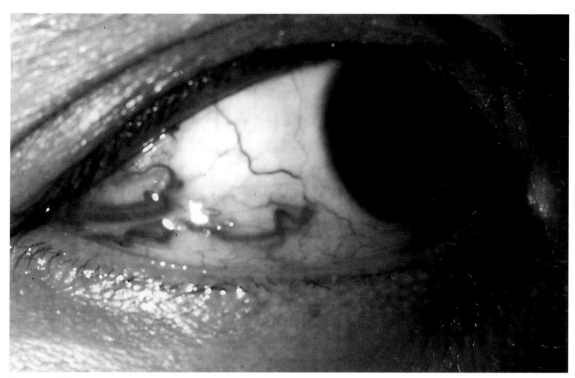

Figure 4-5. Enlarged vessels over the insertion of the medial rectus muscle.

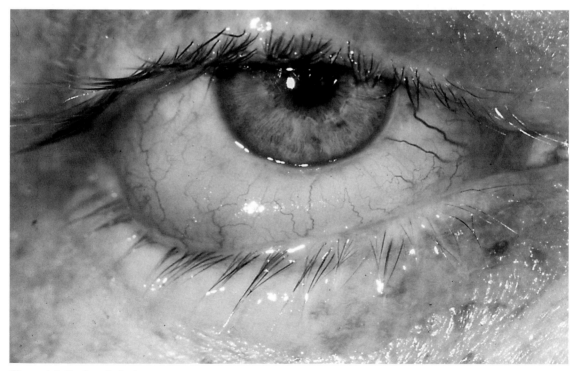

Figure 4-6. Conjunctival edema.

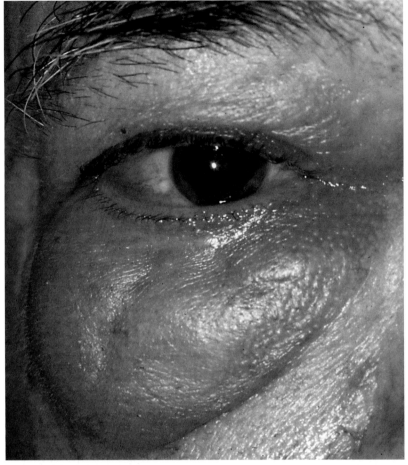

Figure 4-7. Periorbital edema.

Table 4-3. Incidence of Eye Findings in Unselected Graves' Disease Patients

1. Eye lid retraction (Dalrymple's sign), 35–60%
2. Lid lag (von Graefe's sign), 40–50%
3. Increased intraocular pressure, 30%
4. Proptosis, 30%
5. Extreme proptosis, 3–7%
6. Malignant exophthalmos, 2–7%

quite high. In one study, 66% of the patients had apparent unilateral disease.[100,101] In a study of 90 untreated patients with thyroid eye disease referred to a single center, 13 (14%) had unilateral findings.[83] A patient with unilateral inferior rectus involvement is shown in Figure 4-8. As others have noted, many unilateral cases have subtle involvement of the other eye such as increased IOP on upgaze or enlarged extraocular muscles on CT or MRI.[95] Enzmann and colleagues have demonstrated that 50% of patients with unilateral disease had bilateral orbital pathology when evaluated by CT.[102] There are few explanations for unilateral orbital involvement in Graves' disease. Some clinicians have noted more prominent eye findings on the same side as asymmetric thyroid gland swelling,[103] but this thyroid abnormality is rarely observed in patients with unilateral disease. A number of unilateral, presumed thyroid, ophthalmopathy patients have been shown to have CT and ultrasound evidence of unilateral muscle enlargement without demonstrable abnormal thyroid studies.[104]

In unilateral proptosis patients evaluated by an ophthalmologist, the etiology is thyroid ophthalmopathy in 10–30% of cases.[7,21,22,105–109] Thyroid eye disease is the most common cause of both unilateral and bilateral proptosis in adults.[7,21,96,105]

Most patients with thyroid eye disease first present with systemic hyperthyroidism; however, 5–25% seek ophthalmologic evaluation before the discovery of systemic hyperthyroidism[68,69,91,94] (see also the section on euthyroid ophthalmopathy in Chapter 3). Many clinicians since Sattler[110] have noted that eye changes can occur before, simultaneous with, or after the diagnosis of hyperthyroidism.[111,112]

Lid retraction is quite characteristic of thyroid ophthalmopathy; Day noted this finding in 94% of his series of 200 cases.[2,113] As discussed in Chapter 6, there are

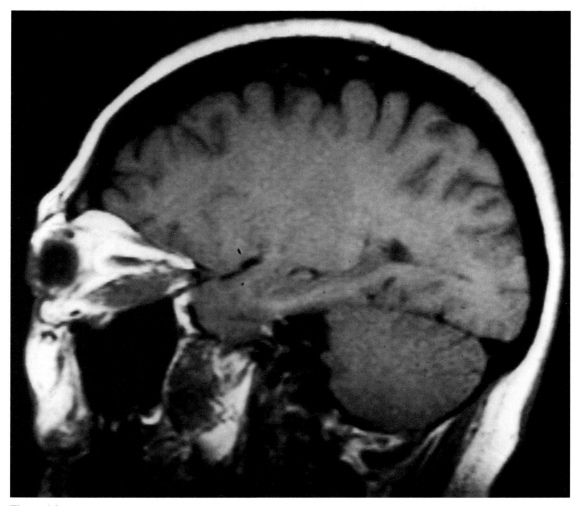

Figure 4-8. Parasagittal T_1-weighted magnetic resonance imaging shows a patient with unilateral inferior rectus involvement.

several mechanisms responsible for eyelid retraction in thyroid orbitopathy.[114–116] In proptosis of nonthyroid origin, patients usually do not have eyelid retraction although exceptions do occur.[20] As an example, Segal et al. noted that 5 (11%) of 44 studied psychiatric patients treated with lithium had findings indistinguishable from thyroid eye disease.[14]

The proptosis associated with thyroid ophthalmopathy is usually relatively symmetric. Drescher and Benedict noted that 58% of thyroid exophthalmos patients had less than 5 mm of orbital asymmetry, 89% less than 7 mm, and no patient more than 10.9 mm.[7] Marked proptosis asymmetry is suggestive of an orbital neoplasm.[8,21,26] Most thyroid ophthalmopathy patients do not have a large degree of exophthalmos. Yamamoto et al. and others have demonstrated that the exophthalmometer readings in the thyroid eye disease population are increased approximately 3 mm versus normal controls.[117–119]

There are no eye signs to predict either the systemic or the ocular course of thyroid disease. Similarly, the ocular findings in thyroid ophthalmopathy, in association with any kind of thyroid disease (hyperthyroidism, Hashimoto's thyroiditis, primary hypothyroidism, thyroid cancer, or euthyroid ophthalmopathy), can be quite similar and cannot be used to differentiate patients[120–125] (see euthyroid section in Chapter 3). Figure 4-9 shows a patient who has had bouts of restrictive myopathy and proptosis after a papillary thyroid carcinoma. Rarely, ophthalmopathy patients who are euthyroid also have myxedema and acropathy.[95,126]

Usually, as described in detail in Chapter 13, thyroid myopathy has a predilection for the inferior and medial recti muscles. Most thyroid myopathy patients have hypotropia, esotropia, or a combination of both. Exotropia is much less common in thyroid eye disease and if present mandates consideration of the possible coexistence of myasthenia gravis.[127] Focal muscle changes are consistent with other causes of myopathy, such as metastases or cystic lesions.[127a]

While corneal changes in the absence of exposure are uncommon in thyroid eye disease, superior limbic keratopathy is associated with thyroid disease. In a summary of 57 superior limbic keratopathy cases, 37 had thyroid dysfunction.[128]

CLASSIFICATION AND GRADING SYSTEMS FOR THYROID EYE DISEASE

Our ability to classify and grade the alterations of thyroid orbitopathy have a number of limitations. In 1969, Werner, as chairman of the American Thyroid Association Ad Hoc Subcommittee on Eye Disease, proposed a classification of ocular changes in thyroid eye disease. This was modified in 1977 to include patients with greater than 23 mm of proptosis into class 3 disease regardless of their symptomatology.[129,130] The abbreviated classification (Table 4-4) has the acronym NO SPECS. The first two categories (classes 0 and 1) have minimal eye findings (NO) (noninfiltrative), and classes 2 through 6 (infiltrative) (SPECS) are associated with more serious eye involvement. As noted in Table 4-5, each class is divided into absent (0), mild (a), moderate (b), or marked (c) involvement. While some patients progress through all disease classes, others do not. The most conspicuous exceptions are the not infrequent optic neuropathy patients (class 6) who may have minimal (< 20 mm exophthalmometry) proptosis.

There is a great deal of overlap between classes 1 and 2. Patients generally present to their endocrinologist (with systemic thyrotoxicosis) or to their ophthalmolo-

Figure 4-9. A. Patient with papillary carcinoma of the thyroid. Histologic review of the thyroid gland demonstrated no evidence of Graves' disease nor inflammation.

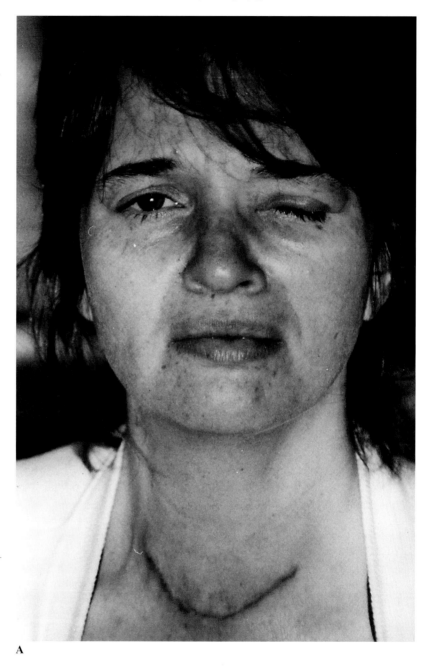

A

gist (with a possible orbital tumor) because of the characteristic startled appearance due to the upper lid retraction. In addition to stare, these patients may have mild lid or periorbital edema. When the patients look downward, there is often upper lid lag (von Graefe's sign). As previously discussed, lid lag is not pathognomonic for thyroid eye disease.[20] In atypical cases, it may be difficult to differentiate a Parinaud's syndrome due to dorsal midbrain pathology from the lid retraction observed in thyroid ophthalmopathy. Lid retraction observed in Parinaud's syndrome is always bilateral without lid lag on downgaze. While there is late vertical gaze impairment,

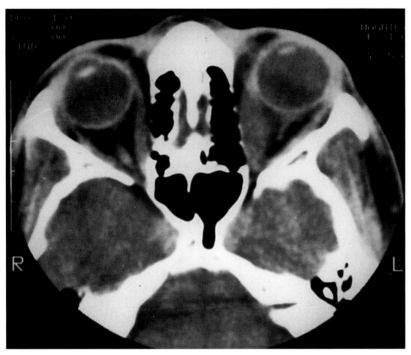

Figure 4-9. *(continued)* B. Axial computed tomography scan.

B

Table 4-4. Abridged (NO SPECS) Classification of Ocular Changes of Graves' Disease

Class	Definition
0	*N*o signs or symptoms
1	*O*nly signs (upper eyelid retraction and stare with or without eyelid lag or proptosis); no symptoms
2	*S*oft-tissue involvement (signs and symptoms)
3	*P*roptosis
4	*E*xtraocular muscle involvement
5	*C*orneal involvement
6	*S*ight loss (optic nerve involvement)

earlier the eyes can be elevated by either a doll's head maneuver or Bell's phenomenon. Patients with Parinaud's syndrome have abnormal pupils (near-light dissociation) and, when they attempt rapid, upward movement using downward optokinetic targets, convergence retraction nystagmus occurs.[131]

Class 3 Graves' ophthalmopathy is defined as at least 23 mm of proptosis. It is extremely unusual for this to occur as an isolated finding; these patients usually have other soft-tissue findings, extraocular muscle involvement, and occasionally decreased vision due to either corneal or optic nerve complications. I routinely perform exophthalmometry with the patient in a standing or sitting position. In a supine position proptosis may be decreased by 2–3 mm. Exophthalmometry

Table 4-5. Detailed Classification of Eye Changes of Graves' Disease

Classes (0–6)	Grades (o, a, b, c)	Ocular signs and symptoms
0	—	No signs or symptoms
1	—	Only signs, no symptoms (signs limited to upper lid retraction and stare, with or without lid lag and proptosis)
—	—	Proptosis associated with class 1 only (specify if difference of 3.0 mm or more between eyes; or progression under observation of 3.0 mm or more, grade o included)
—	o	Absent (20.0 mm or less is normal)
—	a	Minimal (21.0–23.0 mm)
—	b	Moderate (24.0–27.0 mm)
—	c	Marked (28.0 mm or more)
2	—	Soft-tissue involvement (symptoms of excessive lacrimation, sandy sensation, retrobulbar discomfort, and photophobia, but not diplopia; objective signs as follows
—	o	Absent
—	a	Minimal (edema of conjunctivae and lids, conjunctival injection, and fullness of lids, often with orbital fat extrusion palpable lacrimal glands, or swollen extraocular muscle palpable laterally beneath lower lids)
—	b	Moderate (above plus chemosis, lagophthalmos, lid fullness)
—	c	Marked
3	—	Proptosis associated with class 2 through class 6 only (specify if inequality of 3.0 mm or more between eyes, or if progression of 3.0 mm or more under observation)
—	o	Absent (20.0 mm or less)
—	a	Minimal (21.0–23.0 mm)
—	b	Moderate (24.0–27.0 mm)
—	c	Marked (28.0 mm or more)
4	—	Extraocular muscle involvement (usually with diplopia)
—	o	Absent
—	a	Minimal (limitation of motion evident at extremes of gaze in one or more directions)
—	b	Moderate (evident restriction of motion without fixation of position)
—	c	Marked (fixation of position of a globe or globes)
5	—	Corneal involvement (primarily due to lag ophthalmos)
—	o	Absent
—	a	Minimal (stippling of cornea)
—	b	Moderate (ulceration)
—	c	Marked (clouding, necrosis, perforation)
6	—	Sight loss (due to optic nerve involvement)
—	o	Absent
—	a	Minimal (disc pallor or choking, or visual field defect; vision 20/20–20/60)
—	b	Moderate (disc pallor or choking, or visual field defect; vision 20/70–20/200)
—	c	Marked (vision less than 20/200)

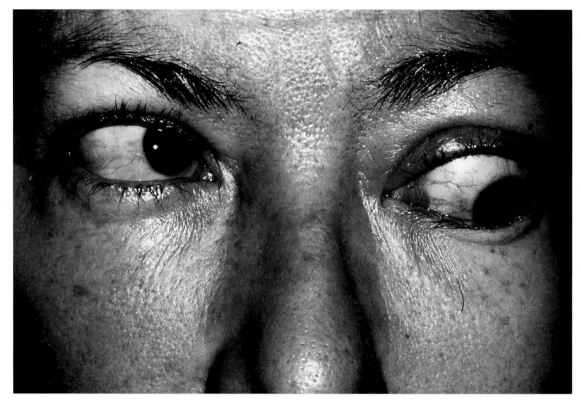

Figure 4-10. Restrictive myopathy. Patient is attempting to look up with inability to elevate the left eye due to inferior rectus fibrosis.

readings may vary by 2 mm when the same patient is measured on different days; however, if asymmetry exists, it should remain unchanged. If the only presenting complaint is proptosis, other causes of orbital disease should be investigated (see below).

Class 4 disease encompasses extraocular muscle involvement. Thyroid eye disease often produces a restrictive myopathy (Figure 4-10). In contrast, the patient shown in Figure 4-11 has idiopathic myositis of the left medial rectus muscle with inability to look into the action of the paretic muscle. As the inferior and medial recti are the most commonly involved in thyroid ophthalmopathy, most patients have problems with vertical and lateral gaze. Initially patients have problems with globe elevation. If extraocular muscle involvement progresses, lateral gaze weakens and eventually a "frozen globe" may occur. Mein and others have noted that eye signs are often worse in the morning.[132] The finding of increased vascularity over the insertion of the medial or lateral recti is fairly typical of thyroid ophthalmopathy; however, this is also occasionally seen with idiopathic orbital myositis (see Figure 4-5).

Class 5 disease involves the cornea. It occurs in patients with enough proptosis to prevent adequate lid closure and causes chronic corneal exposure. These patients usually also have sufficient extraocular muscle involvement to obliterate the protective Bell's phenomenon. It is not uncommon for any patient with more than 23 mm of proptosis to have minimal staining of the inferior cornea on careful slit lamp ex-

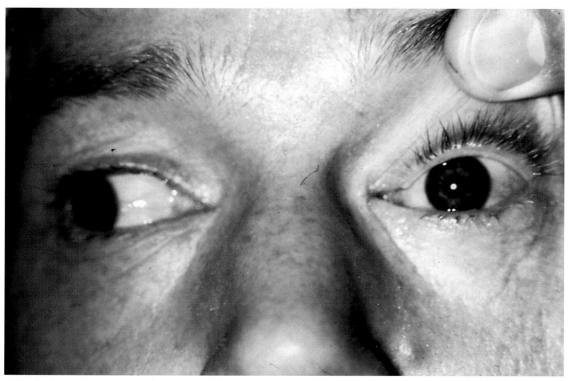

Figure 4-11. Paretic muscle in idiopathic myositis of the left medial rectus muscle. In contrast to thyroid myopathy, in this entity the patient cannot look in the field of action of the muscle.

amination. We usually do not consider a patient to have class 5 disease unless there are symptomatic central corneal exposure problems. The advent of modern treatment options (steroids, radiation, and decompression) have markedly decreased the incidence of corneal complications.

Class 6 patients have visual impairment, usually secondary to optic neuropathy. The incidence of optic neuropathy in thyroid eye disease is 5–10%, but it is a particularly treacherous complication since these patients often do not have marked proptosis (Figure 4-12) and usually do not have evidence of optic nerve changes on fundus examination.[76,133] In Gorman's series of 87 patients with decreased vision, only 12 had papilledema on ophthalmoscopy.[85] In the 18 patients reported by Trobe and colleagues, 50% had normal optic discs.[133] Some investigators have noted only retrobulbar optic nerve changes, a finding that initially led to much confusion regarding the etiology and pathophysiology of this complication.[134,135] Trobe and coworkers noted that the cause of visual impairment was initially misdiagnosed in 15 of 18 cases (83%). A patient with typical fundus changes of thyroid optic neuropathy is shown in Figure 4-13.

Class 6 patients often have minimal to moderate exophthalmos and relatively shallow orbits. The most common presenting complaint is an insidious onset of either visual loss or a visual field defect.[133–138] While visual field changes often are helpful, if they are not performed carefully they can be misleading. Figure 4-14A and B show the visual fields in a patient with fundus changes of compressive optic

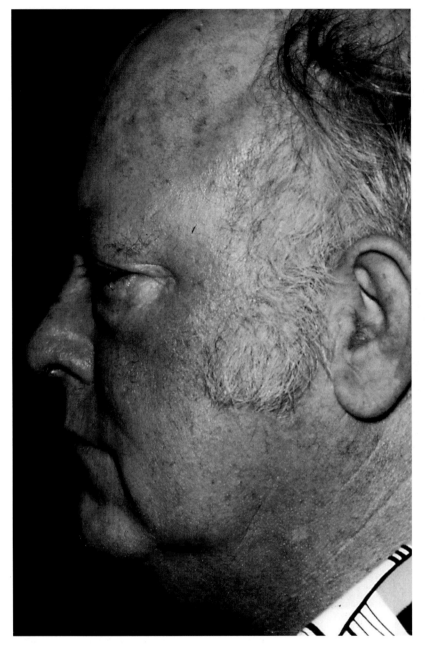

Figure 4-12. Minimal proptosis in a patient with severe thyroid optic neuropathy.

neuropathy (Figure 4-14C and D). The patient had a visual acuity of 20/25 OU. The technician had not taped the droopy upper eyelids nor placed a presbyopic correction in front of either eye. Performing the fields with just those changes produced a very different result (Figure 14-4E and F). Usually these patients have color defects, scotomas, pupillary abnormalities (an afferent pupil defect), and abnormalities on visual evoked potential (VEP) tests. Niegel and colleagues noted abnormal papillary responses in 34% of cases, with VEP changes in 94% and color vision alterations in 64%.[139]

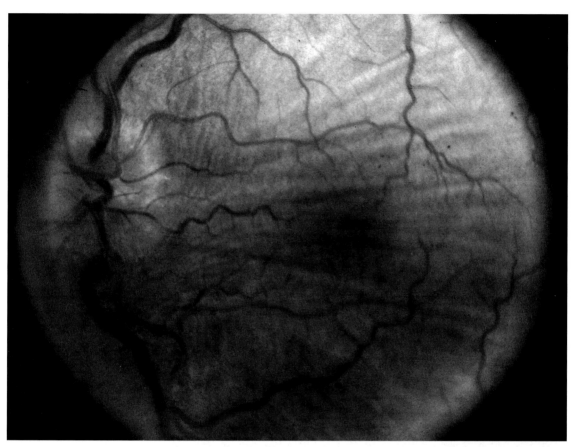

Figure 4-13. Fundus photograph showing choroidal folds and optic disc edema in a patient with thyroid optic neuropathy.

Setala and coworkers found all 20 eyes with compression optic neuropathy had VEP abnormalities.[140] Approximately 80% have associated extraocular muscle dysfunction. Feldon and colleagues noted saccadic velocities were diminished in almost all of these patients.[141] Common visual field defects in order of frequency are central scotomas, arcuate or altitudinal defects, paracentral scotomas, or generalized constriction.[142,143] Ancillary tests and studies useful in the evaluation of thyroid ophthalmopathy patients with decreased vision include VEP, pupillography, contrast sensitivity test, ultrasonography, CT, and MRI.[144,145] As discussed in Chapter 6, the pathophysiology of optic neuropathy appears to be an apical compression of the nerve by enlarged extraocular muscles.[138] In about 5% of cases there is just traction on a relatively short optic nerve that produces visual loss or inflammation in the optic nerve sheath accounting for diminished acuity.[146] Figure 4-15 shows a patient referred for orbital decompression because of presumed apical crowding of the optic nerve. There was only inflammation demonstrable with fluid in the optic nerve sheath. This inflammation responded completely to a short course of high-dose steroids. In approximately 30%, apical compression of the optic nerve is unilateral. Rarely, compression

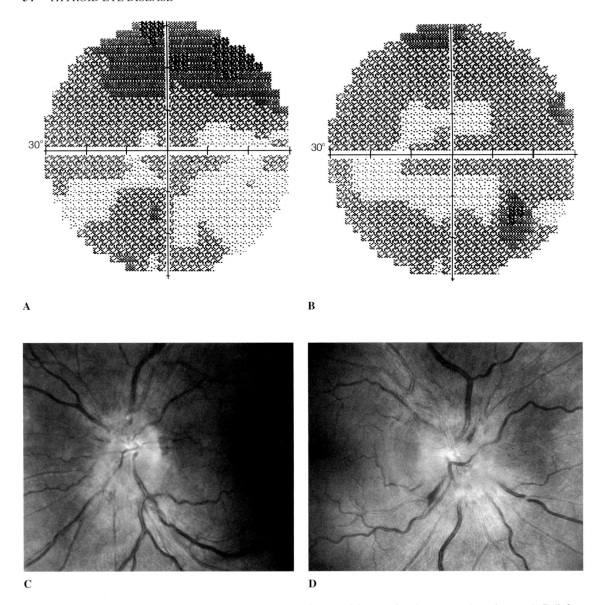

A   B

C   D

Figure 4-14. Visual field changes can be spurious, especially with technicians performing automatic perimetry. A, B (left eye, right eye). Marked visual field constriction. C, D. While the patient has compressive optic neuropathy changes (C = left eye, D = right eye) the visual acuity is 20/25 OU. E, F. Taping both upper lids and using presbyopic correction the fields improved markedly (E = right visual field, F = left visual field).

neuropathy can develop as long as 12 years after eye findings have stabilized.[147] In addition to typical MRI and CT findings (see below), ultrasonography often demonstrates evidence of nerve enlargement, with doubling of the optic nerve outline and other abnormalities.[43,48,105,138,148]

Other grading systems have been devised to assess thyroid eye disease severity and monitor its response to therapy. The evolution of this process is nicely summa-

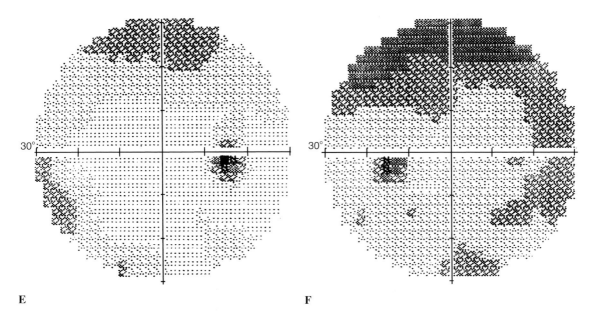

E   F

rized elsewhere.[149] Van Dyk, Donaldson, and others have tried to modify the NO SPECS system.[150,151] All of these grading systems suffer from two unavoidable flaws. First, patients do not have a uniform progression from one disease component to the next; as an example, not all patients with class 6 disease have proptosis. Second, a numerical score for components of thyroid orbitopathy does not take into account the relative importance of different disease components—i.e., soft-tissue swelling is not equivalent to visual loss yet some systems grade it as if it were. Donaldson et al. have attempted to make this classification more quantitative and assigned severity scores of 1 (minimal), 2 (moderate), or 3 (marked) to classes 2 through 6, with a maximum severity score of 15[150] (Table 4-6). Two patients with identical scores could have blindness in one case and only cosmetic deficits in the other. Other workers have tried to alter Donaldson's system or add scores for patients' subjective symptoms.[152,153]

Several groups of investigators have commented on the problems of current classification systems.[152–157] Mourits and colleagues noted that even endocrinologists or ophthalmologists in the same institution obtained variable results when evaluating a patient's status with the NO SPECS classification—the kappa value between two endocrinologists was only 0.48.[156] These investigators from Amsterdam proposed a quantitative means to measure motility disturbances.[156] The patient is asked to track a fixation light, and a calibrated arch is used to read the excursion of the eyes at the point the light reflex disappears from the center of the pupil.[156]

A consensus conference of endocrinologists and ophthalmologists from several continents proposed retaining the NO SPECS classification for description, but to use quantitative measures for eyelid, motility, proptosis, and visual function as a means of evaluating treatment response. As examples, optic nerve function can be quantified on the basis of acuity, visual fields, and color vision. In addition, an activity score based on pain, injection, erythema, and swelling is used.[157] Even with this newer consensus system, the ability to grade inflammation is untested and subjective.

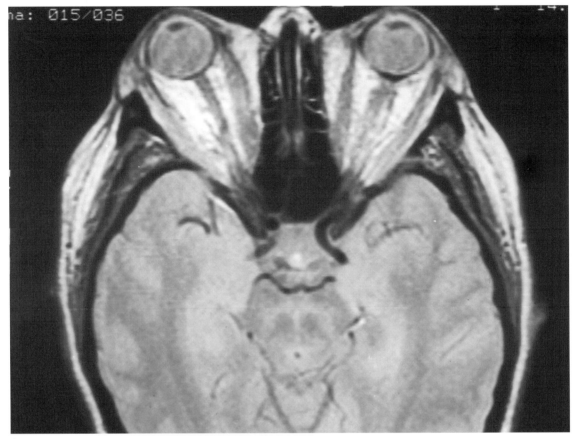

A

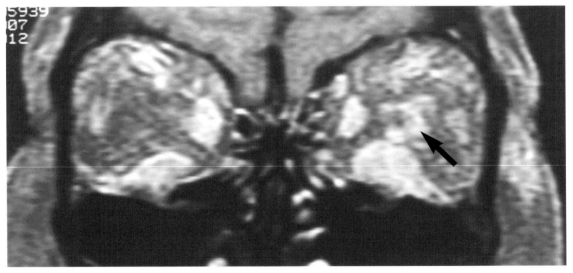

B

Figure 4-15. Axial (A) and coronal (B) magnetic resonance scans demonstrating perioptic nerve inflammation with fluid inside the sheath (arrow) as a cause of visual decrease. The patient was referred for orbital decompression but responded nicely to high-dose oral steroids.

Table 4-6. Ophthalmopathy Index*

Class	Definition	Score
Class 2	(S) soft tissue	1, 2, 3
Class 3	(P) proptosis	1, 2, 3
Class 4	(E) extraocular muscle	1, 2, 3
Class 5	(C) cornea	1, 2, 3
Class 6	(S) sight loss	1, 2, 3

*The scores in each category are summed to establish an ophthalmopathy index. Each class/component scored as 1 (minimal), 2 (moderate), or 3 (marked), except proptosis (class 3). Proptosis is scored as 1 (20.0–23.0 mm), 2 (> 23.0–27.0 mm) or 3 (> 27.0 mm).
Source: Modified from SS Donaldson, MA Bagshaw, JP Kriss. Supervoltage orbital radiotherapy for Graves' ophthalmopathy. J Clin Endocrinol Metab 1973;37:276.

REFERENCES

1. Cohn H. Messungen der prominenz der augen mittelst eines neuen instrumentes, des exophthalmometers. Klin Monatsbl Augneheilkd 1867;5:339.
2. Day RM. Ocular manifestations of thyroid disease: current concepts. Trans Am Ophthalmol Soc 1959;57:572.
3. Hertel E. Ein einfaches exophthalmometer. Arch Ophthalmol 1905;60:171.
4. Luedde WH. An improved transparent exophthalmometer. Am J Ophthalmol 1938;21:426.
5. Murphy ES. Improvised exophthalmometer. Arch Ophthalmol 1943;29:844.
6. Knudtzon K. On exophthalmometry. Acta Psychiatr Neurol 1949;24:523.
7. Drescher EP, Benedict WL. Asymmetric exophthalmos. Arch Ophthalmol 1950;44:109.
8. Ruedemann AD. Exophthalmos. Cleve Clin Q 1937;4:66.
9. Rundle FF. Some observations on exophthalmos. West J Surg 1947;55:578.
10. Streeten DHP, Anderson GH Jr, Reed GF, Woo P. Prevalence, natural history and surgical treatment of exophthalmos. Clin Endocrinol 1987;27:125.
11. Musch DC, Frueh BR, Landis JR. The reliability of Hertel exophthalmometry. Ophthalmology 1985;92:1177.
12. Frueh BR, Garber F, Grill R, Musch DC. Positional effects on exophthalmometer readings in Graves' eye disease. Arch Ophthalmol 1985;103:1355.
13. Pope RM. Unusual complication of use of Hertel exophthalmometer in a patient with Graves' ophthalmopathy. Br Med J 1989;298:365.
14. Segal RL, Rosenblatt S, Eliasoph I. Endocrine exophthalmos during lithium therapy of manic-depressive disease. N Engl J Med 1973;289:136.
15. Sumerskill WH, Molnar GD. Eye signs in hepatic cirrhosis. N Engl J Med 1962;266:1244.
16. Ivy HK. Medical approach to ophthalmopathy of Graves' disease. Mayo Clin Proc 1972;47:980.
17. Pochin EE. Mechanism of lid retraction in Graves' disease. Clin Sci 1939;4:91.
18. Resnick JS, Engel WK. Myotonic lid lag in hypokalemic periodic paralysis. J Neurol Neurosurg Psychiatry 1967;30:47.
19. Buffam FV, Rootman J. Lid retraction—its diagnosis and treatment. Int Ophthalmol Clin 1978;18:75.
20. Bartley GB. The differential diagnosis and classification of eyelid retraction. Ophthalmology 1996;103:168.
21. Grove AS Jr. Evaluation of exophthalmos. N Engl J Med 1975;292:1005.
22. Henderson JW, Campbell RJ, Farrow GM, Garrity JA. Orbital Tumors (3rd ed). New York: Raven, 1994.
23. Reese AB. Expanding lesions of the orbit. Trans Ophthalmol Soc UK 1971;91:85.
24. Parry CH. Enlargement of thyroid gland in connection with enlargement or palpitation of the heart. Collections from unpublished writings of the late Caleb Hillier Parry (Vol 2). London: Underwoods, 1825;111.

25. Von Graefe HA. Vortrag ueber die basedow'sche krankheit. Klin Monatsbl Augenheilkd 1864;2:183.

26. Moebius PJ. Ueber das V grafe'sche symptom und eine störung der convergenz. Schmidt's Jahrbucher Ges Med 1883;200:100.

27. Warner F. Ophthalmoplegia externa complicating a case of Graves' disease. Br Med J 1882;2:843.

28. Wilson LB. Cited by WA Plummer, RM Wilder. Etiology of exophthalmos; constitutional factors, with particular reference to exophthalmic goiter. Arch Ophthalmol 1935;13:833.

29. Cooper W. On protrusions of eyes in connection with anemia, palpitation and goitre. Lancet 1849;1:55.

30. Zondek H. In Kurzes Handbuch der Ophthalmologie (Vol 7). Berlin: Springer, 1932;375.

31. Willard LM. Two cases of exophthalmic goiter with ocular muscle complications. Ophthalmology 1915;11:338.

32. Lebensohn JE. The eye signs of Graves' disease. Am J Ophthalmol 1964;57:680.

33. Gifford H. A new eye-symptom in Graves' disease. Ophthalmic Res 1906;15:249.

34. Joffroy A. Nature et traitement du goitre exophtalmique. Prog Med Par 1893 (2S);18:477.

35. Von Stellwag C. Ueber gewisse innervationsstoerungen bie der basedow'schen krankheit. Wien Med Wchnschr 1869;737.

36. Rosenbach O. Ein häufig vorkommendes symptom der neurasthenie. Centralbl f Nervenh Leipz 1886;ix:513.

37. Loewi O. Ueber eine neue funktion des pankreas und ihre beziehung zum diabetes mellitus. Arch Exp Pathol Pharmakol Leipz 1888;59:83.

38. Neumann M. Herzleiden mit anschwellung der schilddruese und exophthalmos. Dtsch Klin 1853;5:269.

39. Rosin H, Jellinck S. Ueber farbekraft und eisengehalt des menschlichen blutes. Z Klin Med Berl 1900;39:109.

40. Kocher T. Die funktionelle diagnostik bei schilddrusenerkrankungen. Ergeb Chir Orthop 1911;3:1.

41. Givner I, Bruger M, Lowenstein O. Exophthalmos and associated ocular disturbances in hyperthyroidism. Arch Ophthalmol 1947;37:211.

42. Purnell EW. B-mode orbital ultrasonography. Int Ophthalmol Clin 1969;9:643.

43. Coleman DJ, Jack RL, Franzen LA, Werner SC. High resolution B-scan ultrasonography of the orbit. V. eye changes of Graves' disease. Arch Ophthalmol 1972;88:465.

44. Forrester JV, Sutherland GR, McDougall IR. Dysthyroid ophthalmopathy: orbital evaluation with B-scan ultrasonography. J Clin Endocrinol Metab 1977;45:221.

45. Purnell EW. Ultrasonic Interpretation of Orbital Disease. In KA Gitter, AH Keeney, LK Sarin, D Major (eds), Ophthalmic Ultrasound. St. Louis: Mosby, 1969;249.

46. Shammas HJ, Minckler DS, Ogden C. Ultrasound in early thyroid orbitopathy. Arch Ophthalmol 1980;98:277.

47. Werner SC, Coleman DJ, Franzen LA. Ultrasonographic evidence of a consistent orbital involvement in Graves' disease. N Engl J Med 1974;290:1447.

48. Skalka HW. The use of ultrasonography in the diagnosis of endocrine orbitopathy. Neurol Ophthalmol 1980;1:109.

49. Hodes BL, Stern G. Contact B-scan echographic diagnosis of ophthalmopathic Graves' disease. J Clin Ultrasound 1975;3:255.

50. Wessely K. Discussion. Ber Ophthalmol Ges 1918;41:80.

51. McNutt LC, Kaefring SL, Ossoinig KC. Echographic Measurement of Extraocular Muscles. In D White, R Brown (eds), Ultrasound in Medicine (Vol 3). New York: Plenum, 1977;927.

52. Pohjanpelto P. The thyroid gland and intraocular pressure: tonographic study of 187 patients with thyroid disease. Acta Ophthalmol 1968 (Suppl);97:11.

53. Braley AE. Malignant exophthalmos. Am J Ophthalmol 1953;36:1286.

54. Gamblin GT, Harper DG, Galentine P, et al. Prevalence of increased intraocular pressure in Graves' disease—evidence of frequent subclinical ophthalmopathy. N Engl J Med 1983;308:420.

55. Cheng H, Perkins ES. Thyroid disease and glaucoma. Br J Ophthalmol 1967;51:547.

56. Brailey WA, Eyre JWH. Some cases of exophthalmic goitre associated with increased intraocular tension. Guy's Hosp Rep 1897;54:65.

57. Moster ML, Bosley TM, Slavin ML, Rubin SE. Thyroid ophthalmopathy presenting as superior oblique paresis. J Clin Neuroophthalmol 1992;12:94.

58. Keyes JEL, Parisi PJ. Malignant exophthalmos with glaucoma. Trans Am Acad Ophthalmol 1953;57:177.

59. Lyons DE. Postural changes in IOP in dysthyroid exophthalmos. Trans Ophthalmol Soc UK 1971;91:799.

60. Friess HG, Klima G, Hesse W, et al. Die blickrichtungstonometrie als hilfsmittel zur fruhdiagnose der endokrinen ophthalmopathie. Klin Monatsbl Augenheilkd 1986;189:416.

61. Allen C, Stetz D, Roman SH, et al. Prevalence and clinical associations of intraocular pressure changes in Graves' disease. J Clin Endocrinol Metab 1985;61:183.

62. Gamblin GT, Galentine P, Chernow B, et al. Evidence of extraocular muscle restriction in autoimmune thyroid disease. J Clin Endocrinol Metab 1985;61:167.

63. Nordyke RA, Gilbert FI Jr, Harada ASM. Graves' disease. Influence of age on clinical findings. Arch Intern Med 1988;148:626.

64. Blomfield GW, Ecker H, Fisher M, et al. Treatment of thyrotoxicosis with [131]I: a review of 500 cases. Br Med J 1959;1:63.

65. Jacobson DH, Gorman CA. Endocrine ophthalmopathy: current ideas concerning etiology, pathogenesis and treatment. Endocr Rev 1984;5:200.

66. Jones IR. The pathogenesis and treatment of Graves' ophthalmopathy. Postgrad Med J 1987;63:731.

67. Bartley GB, Fatourechi V, Kadrmas EF, et al. The incidence of Graves' ophthalmopathy in Olmstead County, Minnesota. Am J Ophthalmol 1995;120:511.

68. Bartels EC. Thyroid Function in Patients with Progressive Exophthalmos: Study of 117 Cases Requiring Orbital Decompression. In R Pitt-Rivers (ed), Advances in Thyroid Research. New York: Pergamon, 1961;163.

69. Mulvany JH. The exophthalmos of hyperthyroidism (part I). Am J Ophthalmol 1944;27:589.

70. Marine D. Studies on pathological physiology of exophthalmos of Graves' disease. Ann Intern Med 1938;12:443.

71. Thomas HM Jr, Woods AC. Progressive exophthalmos following thyroidectomy. Bull Johns Hopkins Hosp 1936;59:99.

72. Means JH. Hyperophthalmopathic Graves' disease. Ann Intern Med 1945;23:779.

73. Dobyns BM. Present concepts of the pathologic physiology of exophthalmos. J Clin Endocrinol 1950;10:1202.

74. Moran RE. Decompression of the orbit for exophthalmos. Trans Am Goiter Assoc 1953;8:52.

75. Sugrue D, McEvoy M, Feely J, Drury M. Hyperthyroidism in the land of Graves': results of treatment by surgery, radioiodine and carbimazole in 837 cases. QJM 1980;49:51.

76. Perros P, Crombie AL, Matthews JNS, Kendall-Taylor P. Age and gender influence the severity of thyroid-associated ophthalmopathy: a study of 101 patients attending a combined thyroid-eye clinic. Clin Endocrinol 1993;38:367.

77. Metz HS, Woolf PD, Patton ML. Endocrine ophthalmopathy in adolescence. J Pediatr Ophthalmol Strabismus 1982;19:58.

78. Young LA. Dysthyroid ophthalmopathy in children. J Pediatr Ophthalmol Strabismus 1979;16:105.

79. Uretsky SH, Kennerdell JS, Guta JP. Graves' ophthalmopathy in childhood and adolescence. Arch Ophthalmol 1980;98:1963.

80. Bram I. Exophthalmic goiter in children: comments based upon 128 cases in patients of 12 and under. Arch Pediatr 1937;54:419.

81. Stout AU, Borchert M. Etiology of eyelid retraction in children: a retrospective study. J Pediatr Ophthalmol Strabismus 1993;30:96.

82. Shields CL, Nelson LB, Carpenter GC, Shields JA. Neonatal Graves' disease. Br J Ophthalmol 1988;72:424.

83. Wiersinga WM, Smit T, Van der Gaag R, Koornneeff L. Clinical presentation of Graves' ophthalmopathy. Ophthalmic Res 1989;21:73.

84. Sanders MD, Brown P. Acute presentation of thyroid ophthalmopathy. Trans Ophthalmol Soc UK 1986;105:720.

85. Gorman CA. The presentation and management of endocrine ophthalmopathy. J Clin Endocrinol Metab 1978;7:67.

86. Kriss JP, McDougall IR, Donaldson SS. Graves' Ophthalmopathy. In DT Krieger, CW Borden (eds), Theory in Endocrinology. Philadelphia: BC Decker, 1983.

87. Aranow H Jr, Day RM. Management of thyrotoxicosis in patients with ophthalmopathy: antithyroid regimen determined primarily by ocular manifestations. J Clin Endocrinol Metab 1965;25:1.

88. Werner SC, Day RM. Ocular Manifestations. In SH Ingbar, SC Werner (eds), The Thyroid. New York: Harper & Row, 1971;528.

89. Jones DI, Munro DS, Wilson GM. Observations on the course of exophthalmos after I-131 therapy. Proc R Soc Med 1969;62:15.

90. Werner SC, Coelho B, Quimby EH. Ten year results of I-131 therapy of hyperthyroidism. Bull N Y Acad Med 1957;33:783.

91. Hamilton RD, Mayberry WE, McConahey WM, Hanson KC. Ophthalmopathy of Graves' disease: a comparison between patients treated surgically and patients treated with radioiodide. Mayo Clin Proc 1967;42:812.

92. Hamilton HE, Schultz RO, De Gowinel EL. The endocrine eye lesion in hyperthyroidism. Arch Intern Med 1960;105:675.

93. Sloan LW. Systemic Correlations. In SC Werner (ed), The Thyroid. New York: Paul Hoeber, 1955;475.

94. Gorman CA. Temporal relationship between onset of Graves' ophthalmopathy and diagnosis of thyrotoxicosis. Mayo Clin Proc 1983;58:515.

95. Fatourechi V, Pajouhi M, Fransway AF. Dermopathy of Graves' disease (pretibial myxedema). Medicine 1994;73:1.

96. Dallow RL. Evaluation of unilateral exophthalmos with ultrasonography: analysis of 258 consecutive cases. Laryngoscope 1975;85:1905.

97. Lavergne G. Pitfalls in the diagnosis of endocrine exophthalmy. Mod Probl Ophthalmol 1975;14:421.

98. Pohjola S. Unilateral exophthalmos with special reference to endocrine exophthalmos with pseudotumor. Acta Ophthalmol 1964;42:456.

99. Wende S, Aulich A, Nover A, et al. Computed tomography of orbital lesions. Neuroradiology 1977;13:123.

100. Bowden AN, Ross FC. Investigation of endocrine exophthalmos. Proc R Soc Med 1969;62:13.

101. Reibaldi A, Avitabile R, Uva MG, Tritto M. Utility of ultrasound in unilateral endocrine exophthalmos. Orbit 1987;6:43.

102. Enzmann DR, Donaldson SS, Kriss JP. Appearance of Graves' disease on orbital computed tomography. J Comput Assist Tomogr 1979;3:815.

103. Sattler H. Basedow's Disease. New York: Grune & Stratton, 1952;27.

104. Rapoport B, Greenspan FS, Filetti S, Pepitone M. Clinical experience with a human thyroid cell assay for thyroid-stimulating immunoglobulin. J Clin Endocrinol Metab 1984;58:332.

105. Char DH, Norman D. The use of computed tomography and ultrasonography in the evaluation of orbital masses. Surv Ophthalmol 1982;27:49.

106. O'Brien CS, Leinfelder PJ. Unilateral exophthalmos: etiologic and diagnostic studies in 82 consecutive cases. Am J Ophthalmol 1935;18:123.

107. Rundle FF, Wilson CW. Asymmetry of exophthalmos in orbital tumor and Graves' disease. Lancet 1945;1:51.

108. Saltzman SL, Mellicker MC. Unilateral exophthalmos as a forerunner of thyrotoxicosis. Am J Ophthalmol 1951;34:372.

109. Moss HM. Expanding lesions of the orbit: a clinical study of 230 consecutive cases. Am J Ophthalmol 1962;54:761.

110. Sattler H. Die basedow'sche krankheit. Graefe-saemisch Handbuch Gesamten Augenheil Kunde Augenh 1909;9:1.

111. Pequegnat EP, Mayberry WE, McConahey WM, Wyse EP. Large doses of radioiodide in Graves' disease: effect on ophthalmopathy and long-acting thyroid stimulator. Mayo Clin Proc 1967;42:802.

112. Marcocci C, Bartalena L, Bogazzi F, et al. Studies on the occurrence of ophthalmopathy in Graves' disease. Acta Endocrinol (Copenh) 1989;120:473.

113. Eden KC, Trotter WR. Lid-retraction in toxic diffuse goitre. Lancet 1942;2:385.

114. Hamed LM, Lessner AM. Fixation duress in the pathogenesis of upper eyelid retraction in thyroid orbitopathy. Ophthalmology 1994;101:1608.

115. Small RG. Enlargement of levator palpebrae superioris muscle fibers in Graves' ophthalmopathy. Ophthalmology 1989;96:424.
116. Feldon SE, Levin L. Graves' ophthalmopathy: V. Aetiology of upper eyelid retraction in Graves' ophthalmopathy. Br J Ophthalmol 1990;74:484.
117. Yamamoto K, Itoh K, Yoshida S, et al. A quantitative analysis of orbital soft tissue in Graves' disease based on B-mode ultrasonography. Endocrinol Jpn 1979;26:255.
118. Yamamoto K, Saito K, Takai T, Yoshida S. Diagnosis of exophthalmos using orbital ultrasonography and treatment of malignant exophthalmos with steroid therapy, orbital radiation, and plasmapheresis. Prog Clin Biol Res 1983;116:189.
119. Amino N, Yuasa T, Yabu Y, et al. Exophthalmos in autoimmune thyroid disease. J Clin Endocrinol Metab 1980;51:1232.
120. Brownlie BEW, Newton OAG, Singh SP. Ophthalmopathy associated with primary hypothyroidism. Acta Endocrinol 1975;79:691.
121. Fox RA, Schwartz TB. Infiltrative ophthalmopathy and primary hypothyroidism. Ann Intern Med 1967;67:377.
122. Wyse EP, McConahey WM, Woolner LB, et al. Ophthalmopathy without hyperthyroidism in patients with histologic Hashimoto's thyroiditis. J Clin Endocrinol Metab 1968;28:1623.
123. Leiter L, Seidlin SM, Marinelli LD, Baumann EJ. Adenocarcinoma of the thyroid with hyperthyroidism and functional metastases. J Clin Endocrinol Metab 1946;6:247.
124. Hunt WB Jr, Crispell KR, McKee J. Functioning metastatic carcinoma of the thyroid producing clinical hyperthyroidism. Am J Med 1960;28:995.
125. Jacobson DR, Fleming BJ. Case report: Graves' disease with ophthalmopathy following radiotherapy for Hodgkin's disease. Am J Med Sci 1985;217.
126. Vana S, Nemec J. Endocrine ophthalmopathy. Diagnosis and longtime evaluation from the endocrine view. Radiobiol Radiother 1987;28:552.
127. Vargas ME, Warren FA, Kupersmith MJ. Exotropia as a sign of myasthenia gravis in dysthyroid ophthalmopathy. Br J Ophthalmol 1993;77:822.
127a. Sekhar GC, Lemke BN, Singh SK. Cystic lesions of the extraocular muscles. Ophthal Plast Reconstr Surg 1996;12:199.
128. Kadramas EF, Bartley GB. Superior limbic keratoconjunctivitis. Ophthalmology 1995;102:472.
129. Werner SC. Classification of eye changes of Graves' disease. J Clin Endocrinol 1969;29:982.
130. Werner SC. Modification of the classification of the eye changes of Graves' disease: recommendations of the Ad Hoc Committee of the American Thyroid Association. J Clin Endocrinol Metab 1977;44:203.
131. Miller NR (ed). Walsh and Hoyt's Clinical Neuro-Ophthalmology (4th ed, Vol 2). Baltimore: Williams & Wilkins, 1985;716.
132. Mein J. The orthoptic management of exophthalmic ophthalmoplegia. Am Orthopt J 1968;18:52.
133. Trobe JD, Glaser JS, Laflamme P. Dysthyroid optic neuropathy. Arch Ophthalmol 1978;96:1199.
134. Dannis P, Bastenie P. Les atteintes due nerf optique au cours des exophtalmies oedemateuses endocriniennes. Ophthalmologica 1953;126:65.
135. Wagner HP. Lesions of the optic nerve and exophthalmos of endocrine origin. Am J Med Sci 1956;232:226.
136. Winstanely J. Visual Field Defects in Dysthyroid Eye Disease and Their Management. In JS Cante (ed), Proceedings of the Second WM McKenzie Memorial Symposium, St. Louis: Mosby, 1972;230.
137. Panzo GJ, Tomsak RL. A retrospective of 26 cases of dysthyroid optic neuropathy. Am J Ophthalmol 1983;96:190.
138. Kennerdell JS, Rosenbaum AE, El Hoshy MH. Apical optic nerve compression of dysthyroid optic neuropathy on computed tomography. Arch Ophthalmol 1981;99:807.
139. Niegel JM, Rootman J, Belkin RI, et al. Dysthyroid optic neuropathy. Ophthalmology 1988;95:1515.
140. Setala K, Raitta C, Valimaki M, et al. The value of visual evoked potentials in optic neuropathy of Graves' disease. J Endocrinol Invest 1992;15:821.
141. Feldon SE, Levin L, Liu SK. Graves' ophthalmopathy. Correlation of saccadic eye movements with age, presence of optic neuropathy and extraocular muscle volume. Arch Ophthalmol 1990;108:1568.

142. Gasser P, Flammer J. Optic neuropathy of Graves' disease. Ophthalmologica 1986;192:22.

143. Rosen CE, Burde RM. Pathophysiology and Etiology of Graves' Ophthalmopathy. In SA Falk (ed), Thyroid Disease: Endocrinology, Surgery, Nuclear Medicine and Radiotherapy New York: Raven, 1990;255.

144. Char DH. The ophthalmopathy of Graves' disease. Med Clin North Am 1991;75:97.

145. Suttorp-Schulten MSA, Tijssen R, Mourits MPH, Apkarian P. Contrast sensitivity function in Graves' ophthalmopathy and dysthyroid optic neuropathy. Br J Ophthalmol 1993;77:709.

146. Anderson RL, Tweeten JP, Patrinely JR, et al. Dysthyroid optic neuropathy without extraocular muscle involvement. Ophthalmic Surg 1989;20:568.

147. Chou P-I, Feldon SE. Late onset dysthyroid optic neuropathy. Thyroid 1994;4:213.

148. Skalka HW. Perineural optic nerve changes in endocrine orbitopathy. Arch Ophthalmol 1978;96:468.

149. Bartley GB. Evolution of classification systems for Graves' ophthalmopathy. Ophthal Plast Reconstr Surg 1995;11:229.

150. Donaldson SS, Bagshaw MA, Kriss JP. Supervoltage orbital radiotherapy for Graves' ophthalmopathy. J Clin Endocrinol Metab 1973;37:276.

151. Van Dyk HJL. Orbital Graves' disease: a modification of the NO SPECS classification. Ophthalmology 1981;88:479.

152. Kahaly G, Schrezenmeir J, Krause U, et al. Cyclosporin and prednisone v. prednisone in treatment of Graves' ophthalmopathy: a controlled, randomized and prospective study. Eur J Clin Invest 1986;16:415.

153. Bartalena L, Marcocci G, Bogazzi R, et al. A new ophthalmopathy index for quantitation of eye changes of Graves' disease. Acta Endocrinol (Copenh) 1989;121:190.

154. Gorman C. Clever is not enough: NO SPECS is form in search of function. Thyroid 1991;1:353.

155. Frueh BR. Why the NO SPECS classification of Graves' eye disease should be abandoned, with suggestions for the characterization of this disease. Thyroid 1992;2:85.

156. Mourits M, Prummel MF, Wiersinga WM, Koornneef L. Measuring eye movements in Graves' ophthalmology. Ophthalmology 1994;101:1341.

157. Pinchera A, Wiersinga W, Glinoer D, et al. Classification of eye changes of Graves' disease. Thyroid 1992;2:235.

5

Differential Diagnosis and Imaging Studies

DIFFERENTIAL DIAGNOSIS

Orbital diseases that most closely simulate endocrine ophthalmopathy produce inflammation or infiltration of the extraocular muscles. Table 5-1 lists some conditions that can produce magnetic resonance imaging (MRI) or computed tomography (CT) evidence of enlarged extraocular muscles. These disorders include idiopathic orbital myositis, orbital inflammations (pseudotumor), sarcoid, Wegener's granulomatosis, metastases to the extraocular muscles, carotid-cavernous fistula, sphenoid ridge meningioma, amyloid, primary tumors, infection, lymphoma, leukemia, multiple myeloma, inflammatory bowel disease, Lyme disease, giant cell polymyositis, paraneoplastic processes, and orbital pathology associated with other collagen vascular diseases.[1–18]

Unlike thyroid eye diseases, inflammatory simulating lesions commonly begin with acute onset, often with deep, boring pain, diplopia, and ptosis.[11,19–40] Table 5-2 lists some of the clinical features that help differentiate thyroid eye disease from more frequent simulating lesions. Patients with carotid-cavernous fistulas or other arteriovenous malformations often note the abrupt onset of symptoms, such as a "buzzing sound," that suggest abnormal vascular communication.[41–44] Patients with lesions metastatic to the eye muscles frequently have a history of a primary malignancy; however, especially with renal and lung carcinoma, it is more common for the ophthalmologist to see ocular manifestations before the discovery of the primary neoplasm.[5,34–40,45–48]

Other causes of muscle enlargement, such as primary tumors, nonthyroid endocrine disorders, amyloidosis, contiguous infections, drugs, and systemic autoimmune processes, are rare.[49–57] Rhabdomyosarcoma, the most common primary orbital malignancy of childhood, usually occurs in a younger age group than does thyroid eye disease.

A sudden onset is atypical for Graves' ophthalmopathy, although I have rarely observed this presentation pattern with endocrine exophthalmos.[58] The history is useful in differentiating thyroid ophthalmopathy from other causes of lid or orbital pathology. More than 75% of patients with thyroid eye disease have signs or symptoms of hyperthyroidism at the time of diagnosis. As discussed in Chapter 2, these

Table 5-1. Imaging (Computed Tomography/Magnetic Resonance) Differential Diagnosis of Enlarged Extraocular Muscles

1. Thyroid orbitopathy
2. Myositis
   a. Idiopathic isolated disease
   b. Orbital pseudotumor with "spill-over"
   c. Myositis associated with systemic disease
      1. Collagen vascular disease: systemic lupus erythematosus
      2. Sarcoidosis
      3. Giant cell polymyositis (myocarditis and orbital myositis)
      4. Lyme disease
      5. Trichinosis
      6. Wegener's granulomatosis[136]
      7. As a sequel of viral infection
      8. Echinococcus cyst
      9. Histiocytosis syndromes
3. Enlarged muscles secondary to vascular abnormalities[133]
   a. Carotid-cavernous fistula
   b. Dural-sinus fistula
   c. Angioma
4. Primary tumors of the muscle
   a. Rhabdoma
   b. Rhabdomyosarcoma
   c. Hemangiopericytoma
   d. Intramuscular dermoid cyst
   e. Alveolar soft part sarcoma
   f. Malignant nonchromaffin paraganglioma
5. Lymphoid processes
   a. Acute leukemias
   b. Lymphomas
   c. Benign lymphoid deposits
   d. Multiple myeloma[140]
6. Metastases
   a. Breast carcinoma
   b. Cutaneous melanoma
   c. Contralateral uveal melanoma
   d. Lung carcinoma
   e. Neuroblastoma
   f. Pancreatic carcinoma
   g. Carcinoid
   h. Seminoma
   i. Bladder carcinoma
   j. Prostate carcinoma[137]
   k. Zollinger-Ellison[134]
   l. Colon carcinoma
   m. Gastric carcinoma[139]
   n. Rhabdomyosarcoma[135]
   o. Miscellaneous metastases
7. Miscellaneous processes
   a. Amyloidosis
   b. After local anesthesia for intraocular surgery
   c. Acromegaly
   d. Lithium
   e. Steroids (endogenous or exogenous)[138]
   f. Other drugs

Table 5-2. Clinical Parameters Useful to Differentiate Thyroid Orbitopathy from Other Simulating Lesions

Parameter	Thyroid Orbitopathy	Carotid-Cavernous Fistula	Metastases	Pseudotumor/ Myositis
History	Graves' disease	Hypertension; inflammatory symptoms	Primary tumor; head trauma	Rarely systemic
Bilateral	Common	Rare	Uncommon	Less common
Acute onset	Rare	Common	Less common	Common
Sharp pain	Rare	Uncommon	Uncommon	Common
Conjunctival vessel pattern	Over insertions	Arteriolar	None	Diffuse
Muscles involved	IR>MR>LR>SR	Nonspecific	Nonspecific	Nonspecific
Muscle function	Restrictive	Usually normal	Restrictive or paretic	Pain, early paresis with globe retraction

IR = inferior rectus; MR = medial rectus; LR = lateral rectus; SR = superior rectus.

include nervousness, heat intolerance, weight loss, emotional lability, cardiovascular instability, sweating, palpitations, and gastrointestinal disturbances. As discussed in Chapter 3, patients usually have one or more abnormalities on systemic tests.

Thyroid eye disease can also coexist with other systemic illnesses. I have observed thyroid ophthalmopathy patients with orbital metastases, demyelinating optic neuritis, and myasthenia gravis.[59–62] In a patient with thyroid eye disease with exotropia, especially if ptosis is also present, myasthenia must be ruled out (Figures 5-1 and 5-2).

Some eye signs are useful in differentiating simulating lesions from thyroid eye disease. Diffuse scleral inflammation (scleritis) is observed in many orbital pseudotumor patients but is not noted in patients with thyroid eye disease (Figure 5-3).[14,28–33] Optic nerve sheath meningiomas can mimic thyroid eye disease. These neoplasms usually occur in middle-aged women and begin with minimal to moderate proptosis and decreased vision.[1,14,63] Characteristic opticociliary shunt vessels are visible on the optic disc (Figure 5-4); this fundus finding does not occur in thyroid eye disease. In different forms of orbital inflammation (pseudotumor, myositis, or sarcoid) the proptosis and ptosis are often associated with erythema and heat over the lid and orbit. A patient with 3 mm of proptosis secondary to orbital myositis is shown in Figure 5-5. Note the ptosis and lid edema instead of the lid retraction characteristic of thyroid disease. As shown in Figure 11-2, thyroid patients have a tendency to develop relatively early onset levator disinsertion, and they may have ptosis, instead of eyelid retraction, in association with proptosis.

Carotid-cavernous fistulas are one of four types of arteriovenous fistulas that involve the cavernous sinus.[41–44,64] These rarely produce extraocular muscle enlargement, and those high-flow lesions that occur as a result of head trauma are not difficult to differentiate from thyroid eye disease. Patients with carotid-cavernous fistula have a characteristic external ocular appearance secondary to arterialization of the eye (Figure 5-6). In cases of high-flow lesions, the MRI or CT findings can usu-

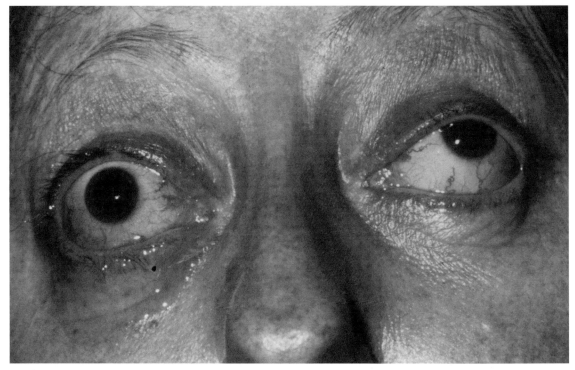

Figure 5-1. Exotropia in a patient with thyroid eye disease mandates an evaluation for myasthenia gravis.

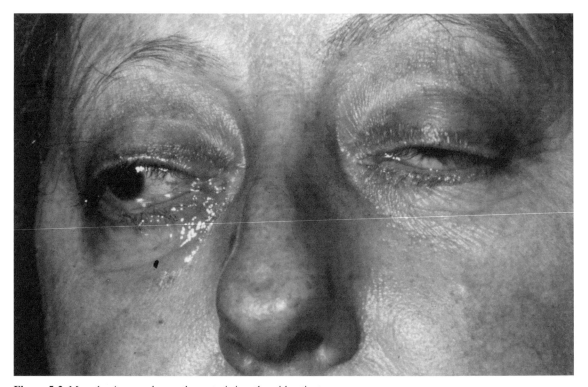

Figure 5-2. Myasthenia may also produce ptosis in a thyroid patient.

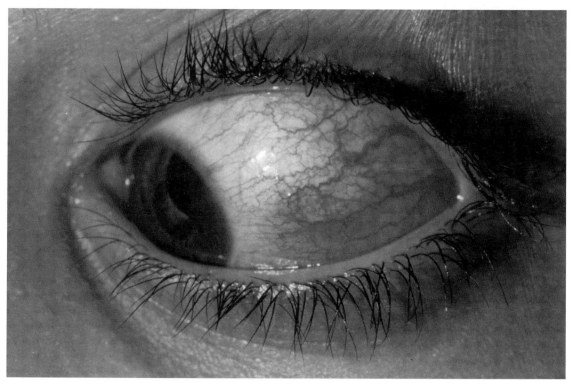

Figure 5-3. Diffuse scleritis in association with orbital pseudotumor.

Figure 5-4. Opticociliary shunt vessels in an optic nerve sheath meningioma (arrow).

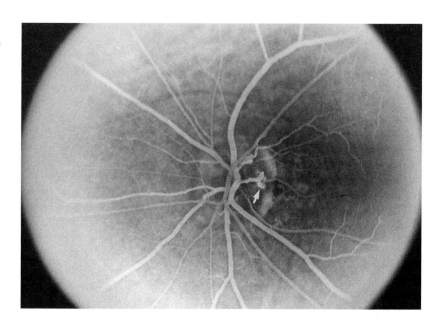

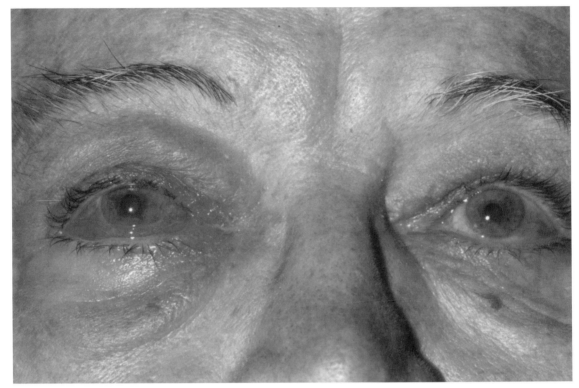

Figure 5-5. Lid inflammation and ptosis in association with proptosis in a patient with orbital pseudotumor.

ally differentiate arteriovenous malformations or carotid-cavernous fistulas from Graves' ophthalmopathy (Figure 5-7). Sometimes the findings in a spontaneous lesion are more subtle. The patient shown in Figure 5-8 is an older patient who was treated at another center for thyroid eye disease without effect. Figure 5-9 demonstrates enlargement of the extraocular muscles on axial CT. Figure 5-10 shows asymmetric enlargement of the superior ophthalmic vein. Clinically she had arterialization of the conjunctival vessels. She was treated with carotid massage, and one month later the vascular communication spontaneously closed (Figure 5-11).[41,42,44]

The imaging pattern is not always diagnostic. The CT shown in Figure 5-12 demonstrates a patient with thyroid eye disease with a very asymmetric superior ophthalmic vein simulating a vascular fistula. In contrast, Dr. William Hoyt and I shared a patient with neither clinical nor imaging evidence (CT and MRI) of a carotid-cavernous fistula who had thyroid compressive neuropathy. At surgery a vascular fistula was discovered and embolized. Currently if there is a question of a low-flow fistula, an MR angiogram is a reasonable screening test, although it has up to a 20% false-negative rate. If fistula diagnosis must be ruled out, then cerebral angiography is necessary.[65,66] We had another patient with a white eye, abnormal systemic thyroid tests, and a restrictive myopathy. An MR scan showed an enlarged unilateral superior ophthalmic vein and a fistula was diagnosed using angiography.

As previously mentioned, while some asymmetry in the degree of proptosis is not uncommon in thyroid eye disease, it is almost never greater than 7 mm, and usually is less than 3 mm. In contrast, depending on the stage of tumor develop-

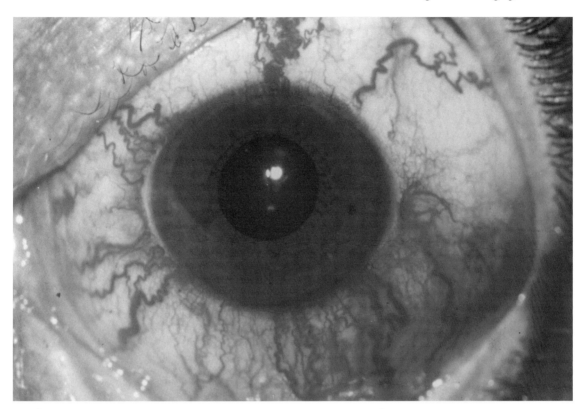

Figure 5-6. Anterior segment arterialization in a carotid-cavernous sinus fistula.

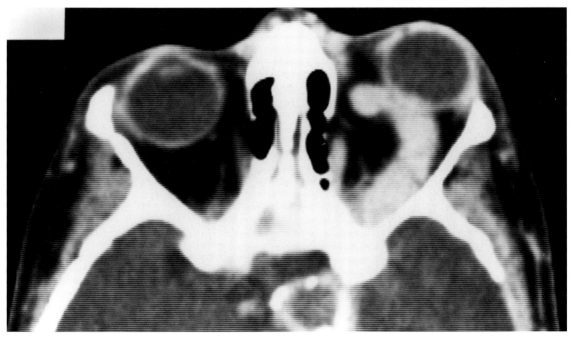

Figure 5-7. Computed tomography appearance of a high-flow carotid-cavernous fistula with enlarged superior ophthalmic vein.

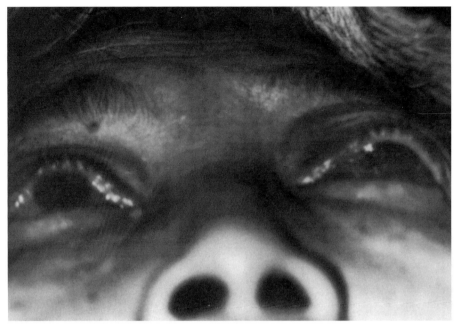

Figure 5-8. Patient with a spontaneous carotid-cavernous fistula treated elsewhere with high-dose steroids for presumed thyroid eye disease.

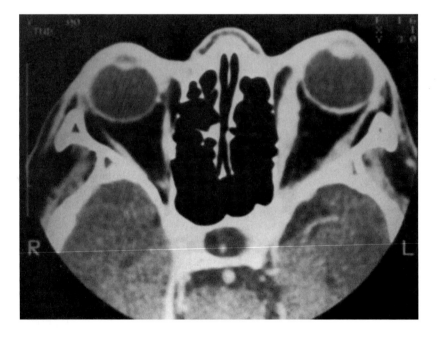

Figure 5-9. Axial computed tomography of patient shown in Figure 5-8 demonstrates enlargement of the recti muscles in a pattern consistent with thyroid eye disease.

ment, patients with orbital neoplasms may have greater degrees of orbital asymmetry (Figure 5-13). The proptosis direction is also a useful diagnostic observation. In thyroid ophthalmopathy the globe is usually displaced straight ahead. In lacrimal gland tumors the eye is pushed down and in, while with sinus disease or medial

Figure 5-10. More caudad axial computed tomography (CT) from Figure 5-9 shows asymmetric enlargement of the superior ophthalmic vein; CT and clinical picture diagnostic for a carotid-cavernous fistula.

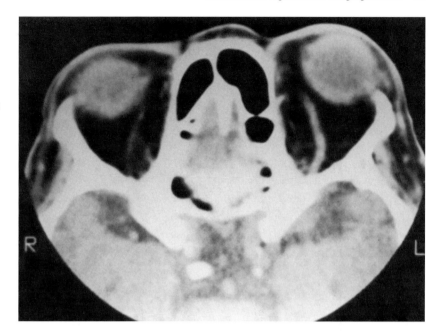

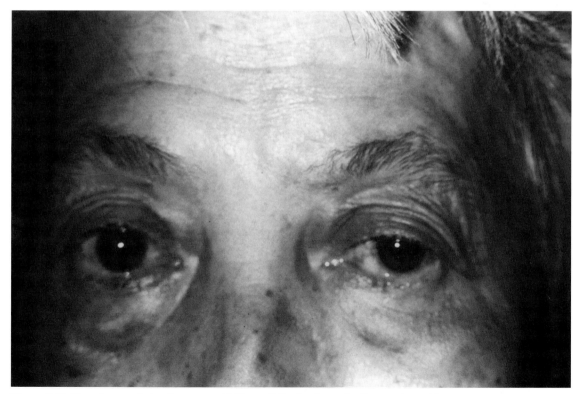

Figure 5-11. Complete resolution (compare with Figure 5-8) after 1 month of external carotid massage.

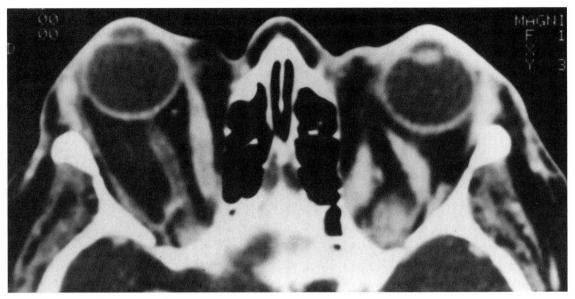

Figure 5-12. Asymmetric superior ophthalmic vein enlargement in a patient with thyroid orbitopathy can simulate the imaging pattern of a carotid cavernous fistula.

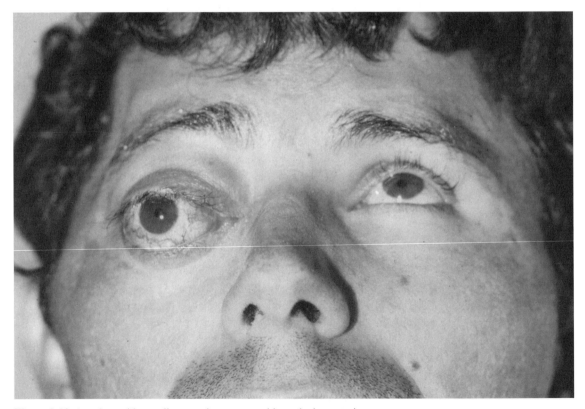

Figure 5-13. A patient with a malignant schwannoma with marked proptosis.

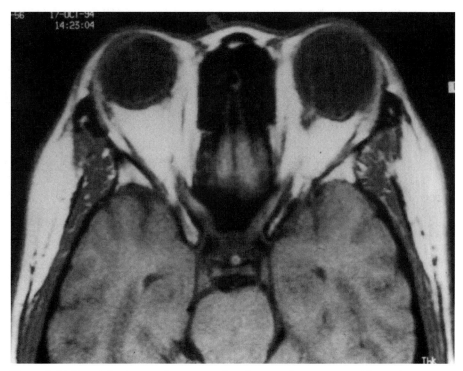

Figure 5-14. T_1-weighted magnetic resonance imaging scan demonstrates axial myopia as a cause of proptosis in a patient with abnormal thyroid function tests.

tumors the displacement may be down and out. The proptosis associated with vascular orbital tumors, unlike that of thyroid eye disease, varies with vascular pulsation or the Valsalva maneuver. Rarely, axial myopia can be confused for thyroid orbitopathy. Figure 5-14 shows a patient with abnormal thyroid function tests; the axial MR shows the correct diagnosis of axial myopia.

Orbital pseudotumors, which I arbitrarily define to encompass idiopathic inflammation myositis or benign lymphoid proliferations, can be difficult to differentiate from thyroid ophthalmopathy, especially when they present as an isolated myositis.[1,10,11,21,22,32,33] Orbital pseudotumors have four common presentation patterns: a lacrimal mass, a diffuse orbital inflammation, scleritis, and myositis.[1] Affected patients usually report an acute onset, often with a deep, boring pain, quite unlike the gritty foreign body sensation associated with thyroid eye disease (see Table 5-2). There is usually lid erythema and ptosis in association with proptosis. As discussed in reference 1, systemic laboratory evaluation of these patients is often useful. While these systemic studies by definition will be negative in a patient with isolated orbital myositis or an orbital pseudotumor, some patients with systemic etiologies will be diagnosed in this manner (see Table 5-1).

Patients with isolated myositis are often unable to perform ductions in the field of action of the involved muscle. Conversely, in thyroid myopathy the eye can move into the affected area but is restricted in ductions away from the muscle's field of action. In idiopathic orbital myositis, unlike thyroid eye disease, there is no propensity for inferior rectus muscle involvement; the patients who develop this entity are also usually younger than those with thyroid eye disease.

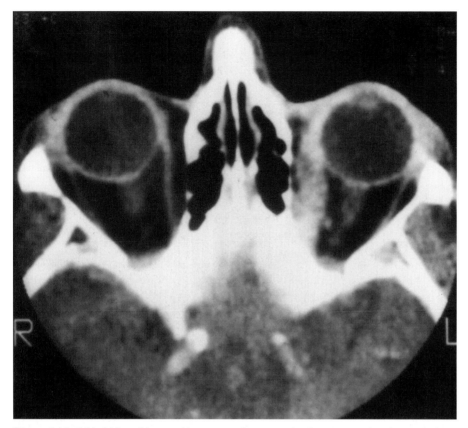

Figure 5-15. Orbital idiopathic myositis: computed tomography demonstrates involvement of entire medial rectus muscle including tendinous portion.

As discussed below, CT, MR and ultrasound patterns help distinguish orbital pseudotumors from thyroid eye disease. Table 5-1 lists causes of enlarged extraocular muscles observed on MR or CT. CT of idiopathic orbital myositis often demonstrates involvement of the entire muscle and tendon (Figure 5-15), although this is not always the case. Idiopathic myositis more commonly affects females; in one series there was a 2 to 1 ratio.[11] Siatkowski and colleagues reviewed 100 patients and noted that 68% had a single muscle involved; most frequently this was a horizontal rectus (62%). In that series they noted that only about one-half the patients had abnormal muscle function, and this was equally divided between restrictive and paretic dysfunction.[11] Moorman and Elston pointed out that eight of the nine patients they described had globe retraction on movement.[10] As discussed below, the CT or MR morphologic pattern of tendon involvement is typical for this entity, as is enhancement of the muscle with gadolinium on MRI (Figure 5-16). In my experience, virtually all the patients I have managed with this symptomatic problem have responded well to 100 mg of prednisone daily for 10 days.[1,10,67] Siatkowski and coworkers noted that 68% of their cases had a good response to systemic corticosteroids; however, 15% relapsed with that treatment.[11]

Myositis can develop in association with other systemic diseases. In some cases I have seen, the history and review of systems has made the diagnosis obvious,

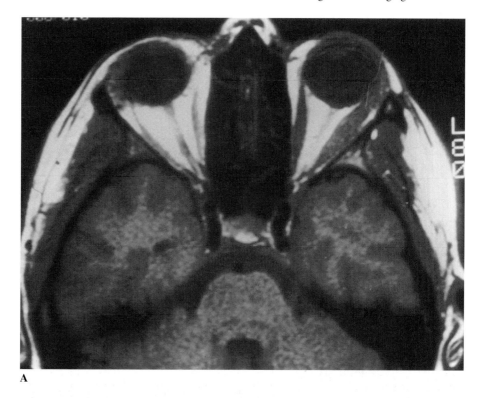

A

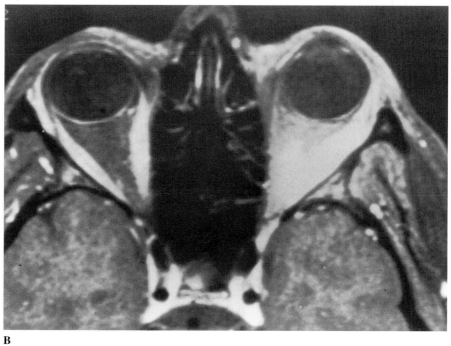

B

Figure 5-16. Axial magnetic resonance imaging without contrast (A) and with gadolinium (B) shows enhancement of the lateral rectus in a case of unilateral idiopathic myositis.

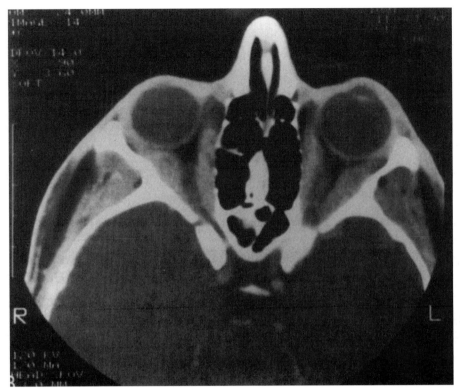

Figure 5-17. Axial computed tomography in a patient with sarcoid shows enlarged recti muscles in a pattern consistent with thyroid orbitopathy. (Reprinted with permission from WT Cornblath, V Elner, M Rolfe. Extraocular muscle involvement in sarcoidosis. Ophthalmology 1993;100:501.)

while in others the eye findings were the first manifestation of the systemic disease. Any patient who presents with myositis should have a complete history with emphasis on prior arthritis, skin rashes, fevers, sinus and respiratory problems, lymphadenopathy, weight changes, and exposure to ticks. I have seen two patients with symptomatic but undiagnosed systemic lupus erythematous who had myositis. Serop and colleagues reported a similar case of a 41-year-old woman with a 2-year history of unilateral enlargement of the lateral and inferior recti who was correctly diagnosed after seeking consultation because of her ocular symptoms.[12] Other reported causes of myositis in association with systemic inflammatory diseases include Wegener's granulomatosis, sarcoid (Figure 5-17), inflammatory bowel disease, Lyme disease, drugs, and giant cell polymyositis.[8,9,12–17,68] Friedland and coworkers reported on a patient who was receiving a calcium antagonist, diltiazem, and developed enlarged bilateral extraocular muscles; nearly identical side effects have also been reported with nifedipine.[68] Figure 5-18 shows a patient on long-term lithium with proptosis. The reason it is unilateral is that the patient was hit in the face by another person, causing a medial blow-out fracture. We have previously reported a necrotizing xanthogranuloma that involved the medial rectus muscle (Figure 5-19). These patients have a number of abnormal systemic findings.[69]

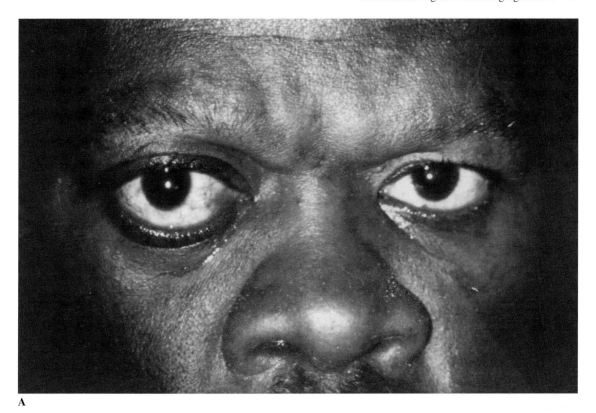

A

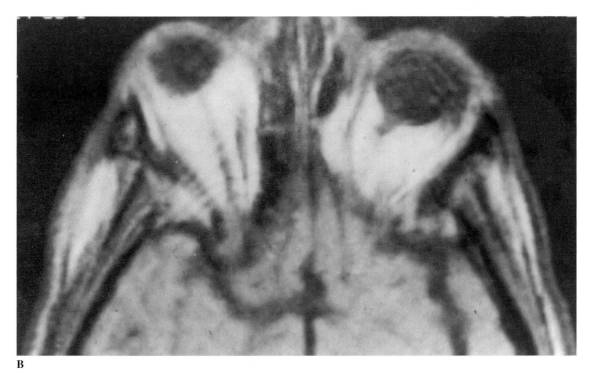

B

Figure 5-18. Lithium can produce exophthalmos, as shown in A. B is the patient's computed tomography scan. Note that he has had decompression of one orbit by a blow to the face.

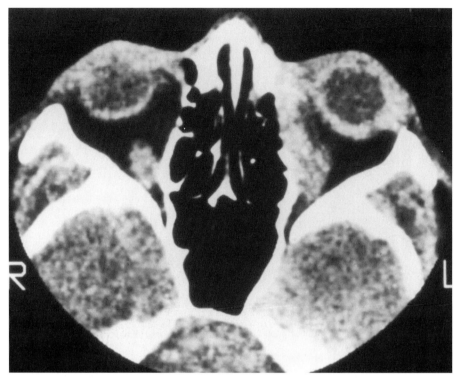

Figure 5-19. Axial computed tomography scan of medial rectus involvement with necrotizing xanthogranuloma.

Three cases of orbital myositis in association with giant cell myocarditis have been reported.[15,70,71] As shown in Figure 5-20, this patient presented with an orbital myositis that responded to corticosteroids, but later the patient developed cardiogenic shock.[15]

More typically, patients with a systemic inflammatory disease have stigmata of that process, then develop some eye findings. Figure 5-21 shows an axial CT of a child with classic Lyme disease who developed a medial rectus myositis.[17]

In patients with any systemic symptoms or a positive review of systems, as discussed above, we obtain a complete blood count, sedimentation rate, antineutrophil cytoplasmic antibodies (ANCA), LE prep, antinuclear antibodies, angiotensin-converting enzyme (ACE) assay and serum lysozyme.

Amyloid has rarely caused enlargement of extraocular muscles without systemic disease, and this diagnosis was only established on biopsy.[57] There have also been cases of systemic amyloidosis with involvement of the extraocular muscles in a similar pattern.[72] There also have been a number of cases reported in older patients, usually after periocular injection of local anesthesia for cataract surgery, who have developed a restrictive inferior rectus myopathy, occasionally with segmental thickening of the muscle.[73–75]

Table 5-3 shows some differentiating findings on MR or CT of thyroid eye disease and simulating conditions. On ultrasound examination, evidence of an associated scleritis is sometimes present with orbital pseudotumor (Figure 5-22), manifest as a "T-sign" indicating exudative fluid inside sub-Tenon's capsule.[19,32] Frequently in

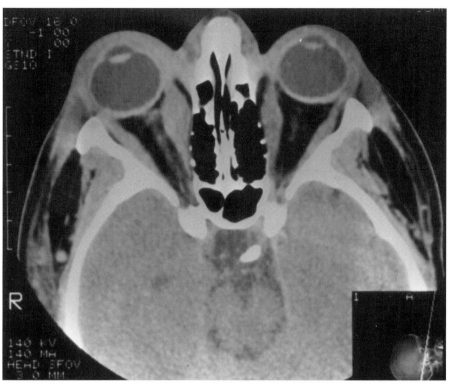

Figure 5-20. Axial computed tomography scan demonstrates an enlarged muscle with tendon involvement in a patient with giant cell polymyositis. (Courtesy of Martin Lieb, M.D. Reprinted with permission from ML Leib, JG Odel, MJ Cooney. Orbital polymyositis and giant cell myocarditis. Ophthalmology 1994;101:950.)

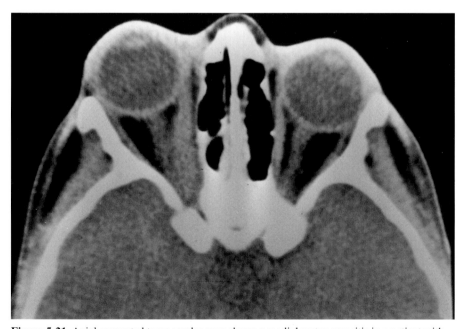

Figure 5-21. Axial computed tomography scan shows a medial rectus myositis in a patient with classic Lyme disease. (Courtesy of Martin Lieb, M.D. Reprinted with permission from KB Seidenberg, ML Leib. Orbital myositis with Lyme disease. Am J Ophthalmol 1990;109:13.)

Table 5-3. Imaging Characteristics of Thyroid Orbitopathy and Simulating Lesions

Parameter	Thyroid Orbitopathy	Pseudotumor/ Myositis	Carotid-Cavernous Fistula	Metastases
Muscle/tendon	Spares tendon	Involves both and enhances with contrast or GAD	Spares tendon	Involves both
Superior ophthalmic vein	Normal	Can be enlarged	Asymmetric	Normal
Orbital fat	Clear; increased volume	Often involved	Clear	Often involved
Lacrimal gland	Rarely enlarged	Often involved	Normal	Rarely involved
Orbital bones	Normal	Normal	Normal	Often invaded
Scleritis	Never	Common	Never	Rare

GAD = gadolinium.

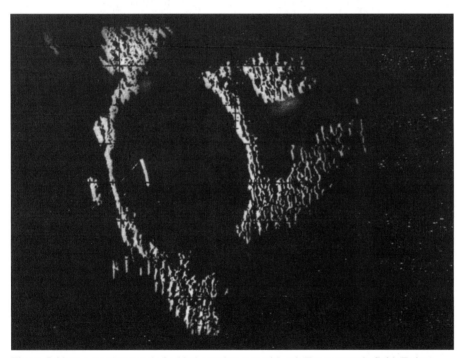

Figure 5-22. B-scan ultrasound of orbital pseudotumor with sub-Tenon capsule fluid (T-sign).

orbital pseudotumors, the orbital fat contiguous to the affected muscle is also involved (Figure 5-23).

Primary or metastatic neoplastic processes involving the extraocular muscles are uncommon. The most common primary extraocular muscle neoplasm is rhabdomyosarcoma, which usually affects children, an age group much less likely to develop thyroid eye disease.[11,51] Rare primary muscle neoplasms can involve the extraocular muscles; however, their CT findings are different from those of thyroid eye disease (Figure 5-24). Figure 5-25 shows an orbital hemangiopericytoma that

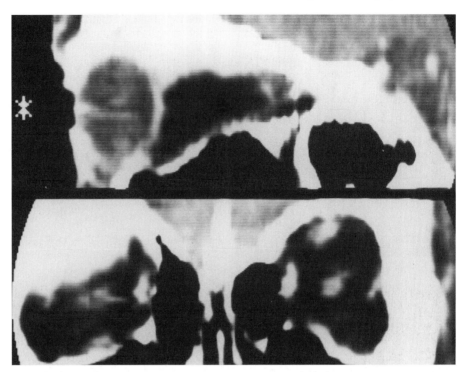

Figure 5-23. Parasagittal and coronal computed tomography reformations of orbital pseudotumor involving superior rectus fat and lacrimal gland.

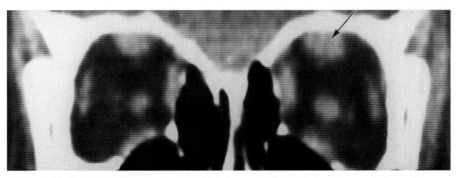

Figure 5-24. Orbital rhabdomyosarcoma of left levator and superior rectus muscle (arrow) on coronal reformation.

involved the medial rectus muscle. The clinical pattern, with only some alteration of muscle function on the basis of a mass effect, was sufficient to determine that this was not a myositis but rather a tumor.

In metastatic tumors, or lymphomas, the pattern of the tumefaction on CT is usually quite different from that of thyroid eye disease. Figures 5-26 through 5-32 show various systemic malignancies or hemorrhages that could simulate thyroid myopathy. Lymphomas can involve the extraocular muscles but almost always also infiltrate adjacent soft tissue (Figures 5-33 through 5-35). While lymphomas are difficult to

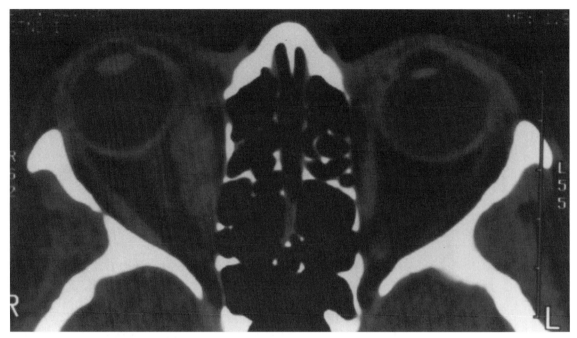

Figure 5-25. Axial computed tomography demonstrates an orbital hemangiopericytoma that involves the medial rectus.

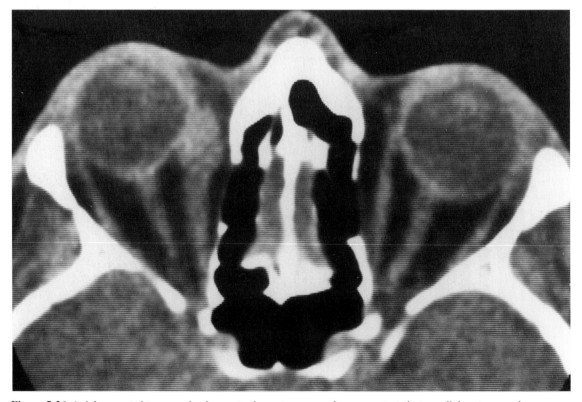

Figure 5-26. Axial computed tomography demonstrating cutaneous melanoma metastatic to medial rectus muscle.

Figure 5-27. Computed tomography demonstrating carcinoid metastatic to lateral rectus muscle on axial scan and coronal reformation.

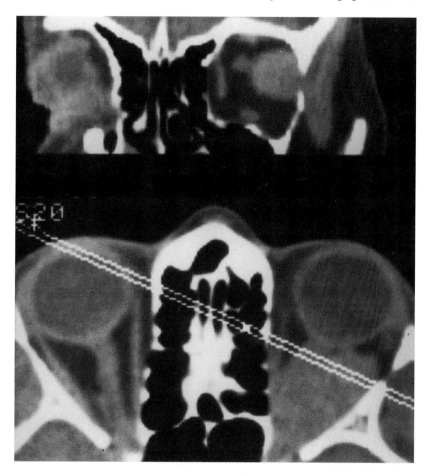

Figure 5-28. Computed tomography demonstrating hematoma in a cavernous hemangioma involving the medial rectus muscle on direct coronal scan.

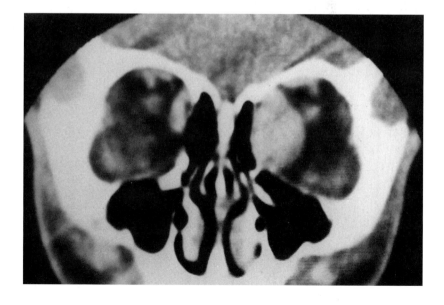

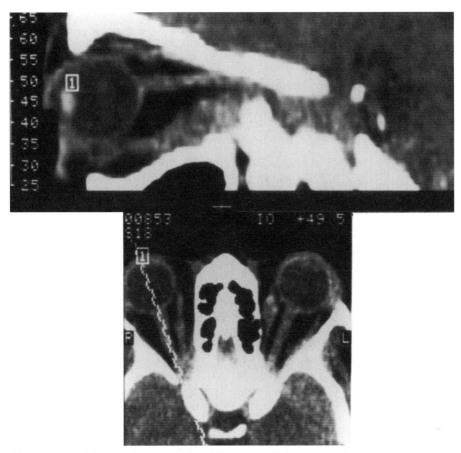

Figure 5-29. Axial computed tomography with parasagittal reformation showing adenocarcinoma of unknown site metastatic to multiple muscles.

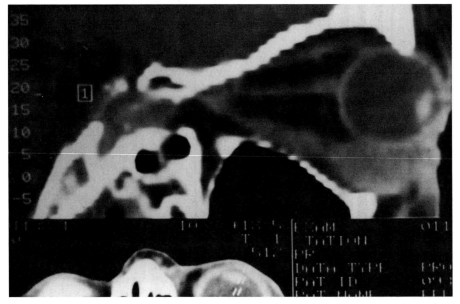

Figure 5-30. A cutaneous melanoma metastatic to the inferior rectus shown on parasagittal reformatted computed tomography.

Figure 5-31. Coronal magnetic resonance imaging of a breast carcinoma metastatic to the inferior rectus muscle.

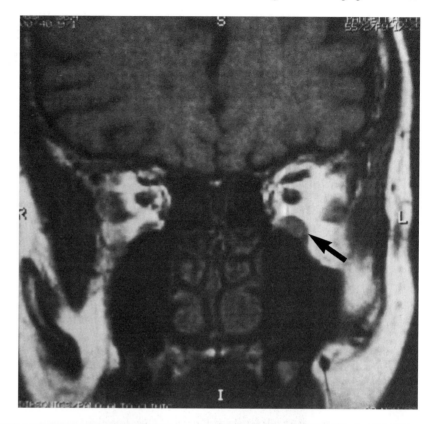

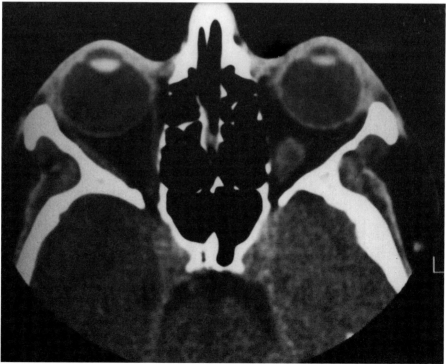

Figure 5-32. Axial computed tomography of case shown in Figure 5-31. Note "lumpy" muscle involvement.

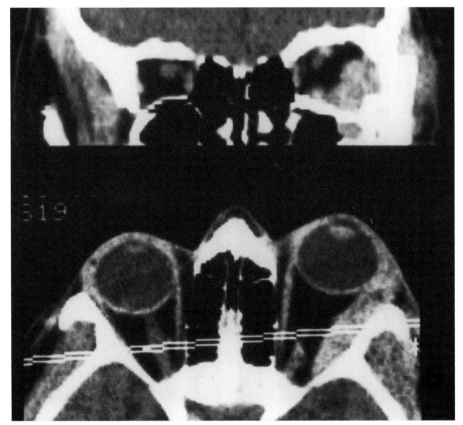

Figure 5-33. Lymphoma involving lateral rectus, orbital fat, and maxillary sinus on axial scan and coronal reformation.

distinguish from orbital pseudotumors, they generally are not a problem in the differential diagnosis of thyroid eye disease.[19] There is a random pattern of muscle involvement in the lymphoid processes as compared with thyroid orbitopathy. Leukemic infiltration of the extraocular muscles can present with a single muscle enlarged or, more commonly, involvement of all the muscles (Figures 5-35 and 5-36).

In acquired immunodeficiency syndrome (AIDS) patients, a number of unusual orbital presentations have developed. Figure 5-37 shows the CT scan of a young woman who presented with subacute esotropia with apparent enlargement of the medial rectus. On biopsy this was a low-grade bacterial infection of the muscle and contiguous area.

In addition to direct tumor involvement of the muscles, a paraneoplastic syndrome has been described. Harris and colleagues reported a patient with high-grade non-Hodgkin's disease who had enlargement and destruction of extraocular muscle fibers one year before the diagnosis of lymphoma (Figure 5-38).[14]

APPROACH TO DIAGNOSTIC EVALUATION

More than 75% of thyroid ophthalmopathy patients have a history of systemic thyroid disease or relatively characteristic eye findings, making the ocular diagnosis straightforward. In Chapter 2, the systemic evaluation of thyroid eye patients was discussed. I order,

Figure 5-34. T$_1$-weighted magnetic resonance imaging (MRI) (A) shows a systemic lymphoma that presented as a superior oblique myopathy. Parasagittal MRI (B) of the same case demonstrates superior oblique involvement.

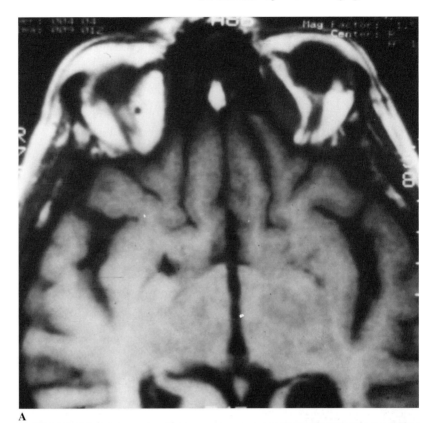

A

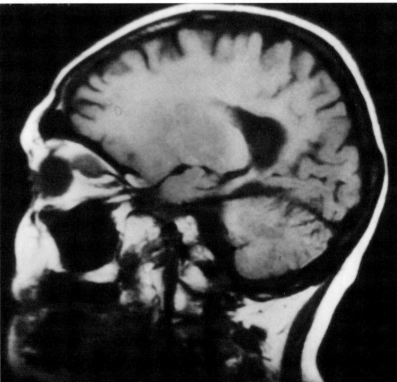

B

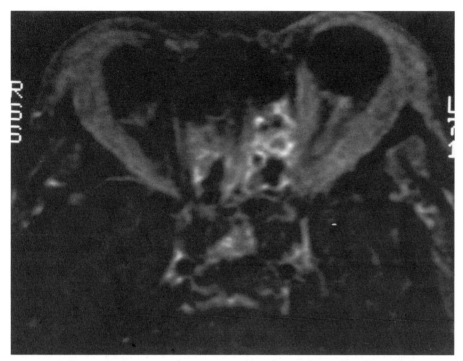

Figure 5-35. Axial magnetic resonance imaging shows several muscles involved in a patient with systemic lymphoma.

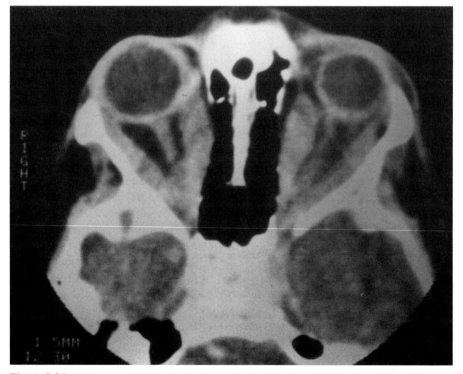

Figure 5-36. Axial computed tomography in a patient with leukemic infiltration of the extraocular muscles.

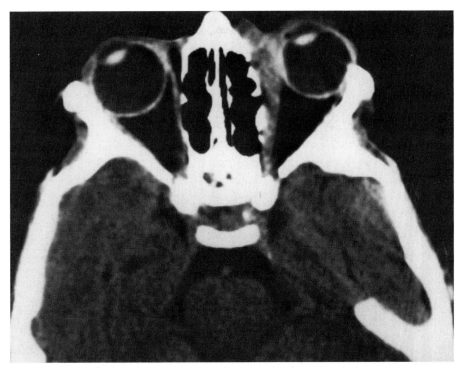

Figure 5-37. Axial computed tomography shows an area of infiltration in and around the medial rectus in a young woman with acquired immunodeficiency syndrome. The relatively sudden onset of diplopia with a negative brain scan 6 weeks before was consistent with a lymphoma; however, biopsy demonstrated an infectious etiology.

in the following sequence, until a positive result is obtained: serum thyroid-stimulating hormone (TSH) and antibody studies (anti-TSH receptor antibodies, antithyroglobulin, antithyroid peroxidase [anti-TPO] antibodies). Suspicious clinical findings and positive systemic tests are almost always sufficient to substantiate thyroid eye disease diagnosis.

In the minority of patients who present with eye signs before diagnosis of systemic thyroid disease or have euthyroid ophthalmopathy (see Chapter 3), establishing the correct diagnosis may be difficult. In addition to the history and physical findings discussed above, a number of ocular tests and orbital scans are useful. These studies may include the forced duction test (if an extraocular myopathy is present), ultrasonography, CT with computer reformation, and MR imaging and possibly indium-111 octreotide scans.

Technological advances in orbital scanning techniques have improved clinicians' ability to accurately diagnose and manage orbital tumefactions. I limit patient evaluation to routine ophthalmologic parameters unless there is more than 2 mm of proptosis (orbital asymmetry) or there is significant visual loss, diplopia, lid or conjunctival swelling, or ptosis in conjunction with lesser amounts of exophthalmos.

Especially in a cost-containment era, there are three indications for MR studies for patients with thyroid orbitopathy in the differential diagnosis. First, we use a CT or MR scan if the diagnosis (i.e., thyroid versus other cause of orbital disease) is uncertain. In a patient with classic thyroid orbitopathy with minimal eye symptoms we do not routinely obtain imaging tests. Second, in patients with thyroid disease and decreased vision, MR scans with fat saturation and gadolinium are indicated. In our ex-

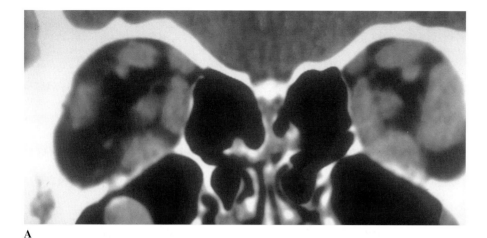

A

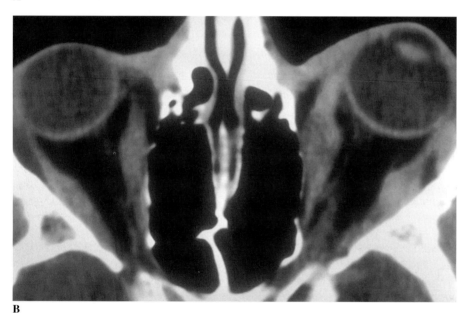

B

Figure 5-38. A. Coronal computed tomography shows enlargement of multiple extraocular muscles in a patient with a paraneoplastic syndrome. B. Axial view. Note on the same patient the relative sparing of most but not all muscle tendons. (Courtesy of Dr. G. Harris. Reprinted with permission from GJ Harris, ML Murphy, EW Schmidt, et al. Orbital myositis as a paraneoplastic syndrome. Arch Ophthalmol 1994;112:380.)

perience, the sensitivity of MR to detect and delineate the etiology of visual loss in these patients surpasses that possible with CT. As shown in Figure 5-39, MR can nicely detect compressive optic nerve changes and differentiate them from noncompressive neuropathy (see Figure 4-15). In addition we have also had one patient referred for optic nerve decompression where the MR demonstrated that the optic nerve was not compressed as well as showing on a spin-spin (T_2)-weighted image that the cause of visual decrease was one of several demyelinating plaques. Third, in cases of subacute thyroid orbitopathy in which it is uncertain whether medical, radiation, or surgical intervention is appropriate, spin-lattice (T_1)-weighted images and proton spectroscopic data may allow better delineation of inflammatory from fibrotic disease status than clinical evaluation. This latter usage is discussed in Chapters 8 and 9.

CT and ultrasonography are complementary diagnostic techniques that revolutionized the evaluation of orbital proptosis. Improvements in ultrasonography and axial CT supplemented by multiplanar computer-generated reformations make it possible to predict the location of most orbital pathology and occasionally to define the appropriate histology. Often the CT image or ultrasound pattern is sufficiently diagnostic to eliminate the need for orbital biopsy. Newer-generation, high-tesla, thin-section MR scans provide better anatomic detail than CT; however, the increased cost of these scans, especially since multiplanar techniques are needed, is a consideration in the 1990s. In most cases the added cost of MR scans is unnecessary. As discussed above, MR scans are indicated instead of CT where there is visual decrease or in patients where a therapeutic decision will be predicated on whether the patient is in the fibrotic versus inflammatory stage of thyroid orbitopathy, and that is uncertain from clinical evaluation.

COMPUTED TOMOGRAPHY

CT can distinguish normal and abnormal structures of different tissue density on the basis of differential x-ray absorptions (reviewed in reference 19). Retrobulbar fat absorbs x-rays to a lesser degree than water; it is imaged in CT as a black, low-density area that contrasts with the higher-density image of extraocular muscles and the optic nerve. CT's ability to differentiate these tissues is due to relative contrast differences greater than 14%; modern scanners can distinguish tissues with less than 1% contrast difference.

The presence of retrobulbar fat allows high spatial and density resolution of orbital structures. Inherent tissue differences in the orbit obviate the need for intravenous contrast unless a patient presents with visual loss. In this patient category, intravenous contrast may enhance such intracranial components as the optic nerve sheath or primary sphenoidal meningiomas.

In most institutions, orbital CT scans are routinely performed using 1- to 2-mm thick sections at 2-mm intervals in the axial plane. The individual volume elements (voxels) obtained from these axial slices can be reformatted in any plane to produce coronal, sagittal, paraxial, or parasagittal oblique images. These computer-reformatted images are generated after the patient has left the scanner and do not require additional exposure to ionizing radiation. In contrast to direct coronal scans, sagittal and coronal reformations avoid high spatial frequency artifacts from dental appliances and other metal implants. Multiplanar reformations enable the interested clinician to view a lesion in the optimum anatomic plane and assess its location relative to contiguous orbital, bone, sinus, and central nervous system structures.

Historically, the detection rate for orbital tumors with standard skull x-rays is approximately 35%. Plain skull films and complex motion geometric tomography provide bone images with only indirect information regarding soft-tissue disease. The soft tissues are directly imaged on CT. In my experience, and in other institutions, the false-negative and false-positive rates with CT scan are less than 3%.[1,76]

Images obtained on older CT equipment, especially first- and second-generation scanners, are suboptimal, with inferior spatial and density resolution. The value and accuracy of CT data depend on proper examination technique and the use of current-generation scanners.

In thyroid ophthalmopathy the imaging pattern is relatively characteristic (Tables 5-3 and 5-4). The orbital fat does not appear involved even though some pathologic

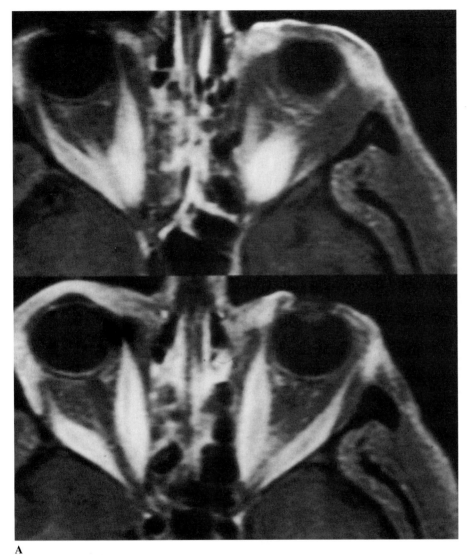

A

Figure 5-39. Magnetic resonance (MR) scans have better resolution that is useful in detection of compressive optic neuropathy. A shows an axial MR with fat saturation and gadolinium demonstrating compression. B demonstrates the same patient in a coronal scan.

studies have demonstrated lymphocytic infiltration.[23] The degree of orbital fat's involvement in thyroid ophthalmopathy, and to what extent its increase causes exophthalmos, are unresolved.

On imaging, the extraocular muscles appear to be the primary area of orbital involvement in thyroid eye disease (see Chapter 6). Some CT studies of thyroid ophthalmopathy patients have not noted orbital fat abnormalities, while others suggest that fat and muscle volume are increased.[19,77–81] The lacrimal gland can occasionally be enlarged. Extraocular muscle enlargement can be asymmetric in as many as 30% of the cases.[77] In a series of 116 patients with Graves' disease, Enzmann and coworkers noted definite enlargement of extraocular muscles in 85%.[77] The inferior rectus

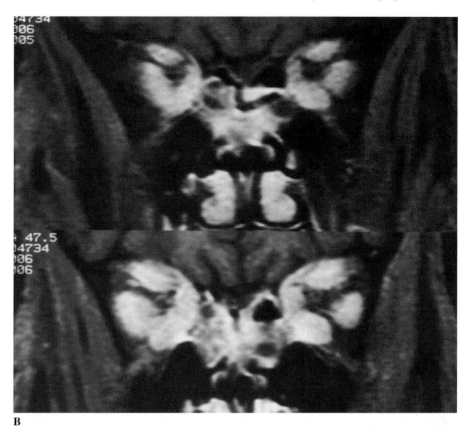

B

was enlarged in 77%, the superior rectus in 51%, and the lateral rectus in 80%. In another series of 80 CT examinations of thyroid eye patients, the inferior rectus was enlarged in 60%, the medial rectus in 50%, the superior rectus in 40%, and the lateral rectus in 22%.[82] Yoshikawa and coworkers performed CT scans on 349 thyroid patients. In their study the inferior rectus was enlarged in 43%, the medial rectus in 38%, the superior rectus in 29%, and the lateral rectus in 16%.[83] One muscle was enlarged in 31%, two muscles in 25%, three muscles in 24%, and all four recti in 21% of patients with ocular involvement.[83] These investigators also analyzed the pattern of

Table 5-4. Computed Tomography and Magnetic Resonance Findings
in Endocrine Exophthalmos

---

1. Enlarged extraocular muscles; tendinous insertion often spared
2. Normal orbital fat
3. Occasional slight bowing of medial orbital wall ("Coca-Cola" sign)
4. Occasional inferior rectus enlargement on axial scan; simulates an orbital tumor
5. Occasional compression of the optic nerve by enlarged extraocular muscles
6. Rare lacrimal gland enlargement
7. Intracranial fat prolapse with optic nerve compression
8. Absence of:
   a. Orbital masses
   b. Vascular engorgement
   c. Sinus involvement

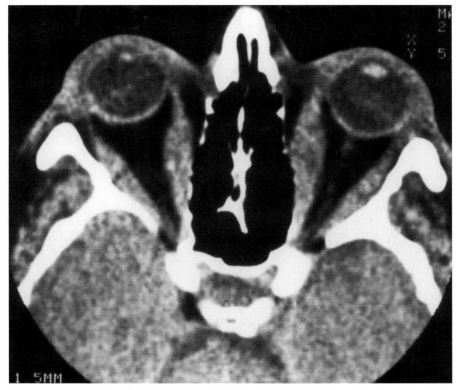

Figure 5-40. Axial computed tomography of endocrine exophthalmos; tendons of medial and lateral recti muscles are not enlarged.

muscle enlargement in 116 eyes with only one abnormal muscle and found it to be the inferior rectus in 57%, superior rectus in 22%, the medial rectus in 20%, and the lateral rectus in 1%.[83] In most studies, CT findings have correlated with clinical impressions of the severity of extraocular muscle enlargement.[23,80,84,85] Bilateral orbital involvement on CT scans is noted in approximately 50–75% of patients presenting with unilateral eye findings. Unlike patients with orbital myositis or orbital pseudotumor, evidence of muscle involvement on CT of thyroid orbitopathy is usually limited to the nontendinous portion of the muscle (see Figures 5-9 and 5-40).

Often several muscles are enlarged, especially at the orbital apex (Figure 5-41). The use of reformation improves delineation of the recti muscle involvement (Figure 5-42). In endocrine exophthalmos patients, there is no evidence of an orbital mass. In approximately 10% of thyroid ophthalmopathy patients referred for evaluation of a possible orbital tumor, the axial CT demonstrates an enlarged inferior rectus muscle that can simulate an apical neoplasm (Figure 5-43). Parasagittal computer reformation demonstrates the true nature of this lesion. For instance, Figure 5-44 with computer reformation of axial images reveals that the presumed apical mass is an enlarged inferior rectus muscle.[19,86–88] Some investigators believe that on axial CT the pattern of apical muscle enlargement often demonstrates a "paintbrush" margin, while most apical tumors have a sharp margin.[80] I have not found this sign to be a particularly useful finding.[19,89]

CT is also useful in thyroid eye disease patients to delineate the etiology of decreased vision. As discussed in Chapter 9, patients with thyroid optic neuropathy dis-

Figure 5-41. Axial computed tomography demonstrating apical enlargement of recti muscles in thyroid ophthalmopathy.

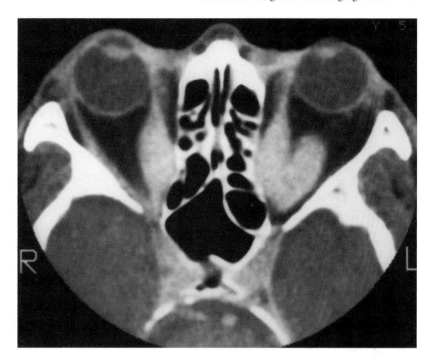

Figure 5-42. Axial computed tomography and coronal reformation. Coronal reformation demonstrates degree of recti muscle involvement at different levels of the orbit.

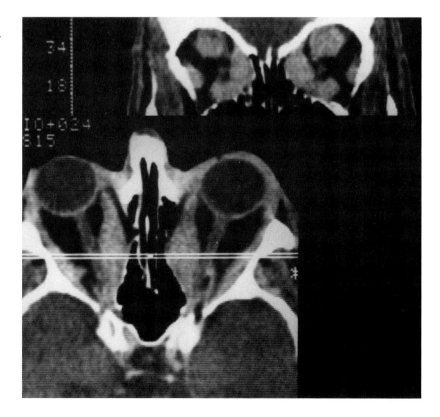

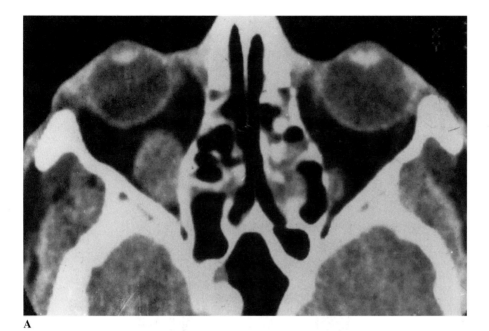

A

B

Figure 5-43. Axial computed tomography of enlarged inferior rectus muscle simulating apical tumor (A). Axial magnetic resonance imaging with enlarged inferior rectus muscles simulating apical mass lesions (B).

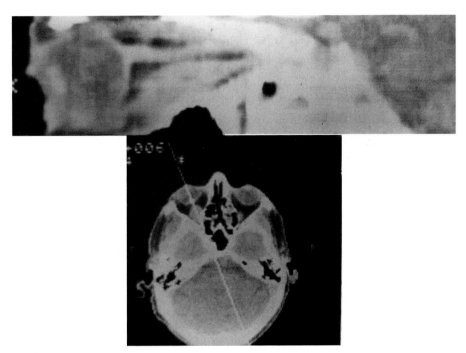

Figure 5-44. Parasagittal computer reformation of axial image in Figure 5-43 shows enlarged inferior rectus.

play enlarged extraocular muscles that cause a demonstrable compression of the nerve at the orbital apex (Figure 5-45).[19,90] Kennerdell and coworkers observed seven patients with optic neuropathy and noted enlarged apical extraocular muscles compressing the optic nerves in all cases.[90] Several investigators have noted that increased extraocular muscle volume or area on CT correlates with compressive optic neuropathy.[91–93] Feldon and coworkers have observed that increased muscle volume on CT was associated with optic nerve compression.[91] Hallin and Feldon also observed that

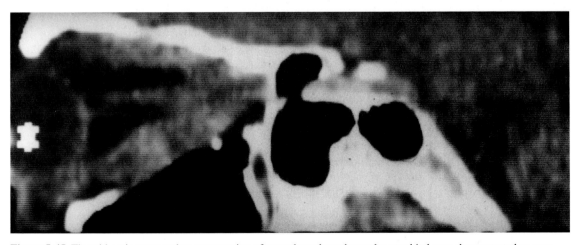

Figure 5-45. Thyroid optic neuropathy: compression of nerve by enlarged muscles at orbital apex demonstrated on computed tomography parasagittal reformation.

the area of the medial rectus muscle on a mid-axial scan correlated with total muscle volume (r = 0.88) and could be used to predict possible optic nerve compression. Barrett and coworkers studied 31 thyroid eye disease patients with high-resolution CT.[92] Coronal reconstruction of axial scans midway between the orbital apex and the posterior surface of the globe could be used to measure the area taken up by the extraocular muscles. This muscle index was helpful in differentiating patients with compressive optic neuropathy from those who did not have it. A muscle index greater than 67% was always associated with optic nerve disease, while an index of less than 50% was not.[92] Other findings that may be noted on CT are a dilated superior ophthalmic vein and abrupt angulation of the posterior muscle belly.[94] An additional sign of nerve compression is fat prolapse into the CNS.[94a] As discussed above (see Figure 5-39) MR scans show the optic nerve compression better than CT evaluation.

In patients with an orbital mass not involving the extraocular muscles, thyroid exophthalmos can be excluded as the primary cause of orbital pathology. An intraconal cavernous hemangioma, the most common benign neoplasm of adults, is shown in Figure 5-46.[95–97] In rare cases, patients can have a history of thyroid disease and diffuse orbital inflammation. Figure 5-47 demonstrates a patient with a history of treated hyperthyroidism who has a "unilateral orbital wipe-out" syndrome. I have seen five such cases in which the muscles are normal or slightly enlarged, but the major orbital pathology is a diffuse fibrosis of the orbital tissues. Orbital detail is obliterated on imaging studies.

In rare instances, muscle enlargement secondary to a metastatic tumor or lymphoma may simulate thyroid myopathy. In a number of centers, including my own, CT-directed fine-needle aspiration biopsy (FNAB) has been useful in such cases.[1,19,67,98,99] The patients in Figures 5-5, 5-30, 5-31, 5-33, and 5-34 had widespread malignancies that first became apparent after involvement of the extraocular muscle. Figure 5-48 demonstrates CT fine-needle placement for biopsy of a lymphoma involving the lateral rectus muscle. The major requirement for FNAB is an excellent cytologist. The morbidity associated with this procedure, in institutions with sufficient experience, is minimal.[1] A positive result is useful; however, a negative FNAB is not definitive since sampling errors or false-negative findings, especially with scirrhous metastases, are not uncommon.

ULTRASONOGRAPHY

Ultrasonography is a cost-effective screening test for the evaluation of thyroid exophthalmos patients. It is also an objective means to monitor anterior and midorbital therapeutic response, although I have not found that it adds sufficiently to clinical data as to be worthwhile. As Harrie has pointed out, there is sufficient variability in A-scan data to limit its patent use to determine whether fibrosis has developed.[100] My orbital surgery unit relies primarily on CT and MRI for the diagnosis of orbital tumors. Ultrasound is not as effective as CT in delineating the relationship of orbital pathology to contiguous structures, nor is it reliable in imaging lesions of the posterior orbit, nor those involving the bone walls.[19] As described in a number of publications, ultrasonography is usually performed with A-scan, B-scan, or both.[101,102] If a patient is suspected of having thyroid ophthalmopathy, ultrasonography may be used if an orbital scan is needed to confirm the diagnosis.[101–108] In one study, while enlargement of extraocular muscles was only noted clinically in 12% of patients, on ultrasonography this was detected in 95% of cases.[103]

Immersion B-scan ultrasound is the easiest image for the nonultrasonographer to visualize; enlarged extraocular muscles are quite clear (Figure 5-49 and Table 5-5).[104]

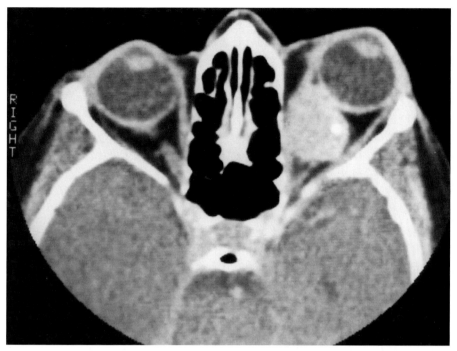

Figure 5-46. Axial computed tomography demonstrating intraconal cavernous hemangioma.

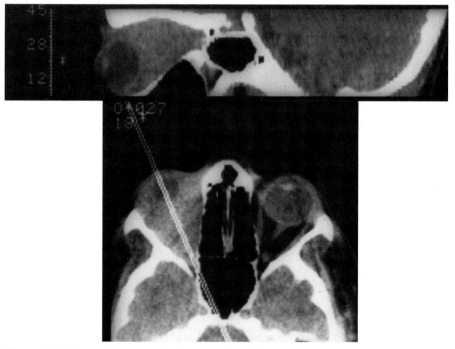

Figure 5-47. Computed tomography demonstrating obliteration of orbital detail in "unilateral orbital wipe-out" syndrome.

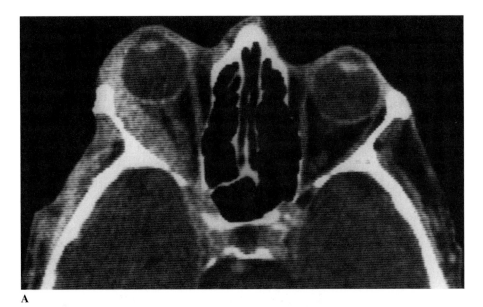

A

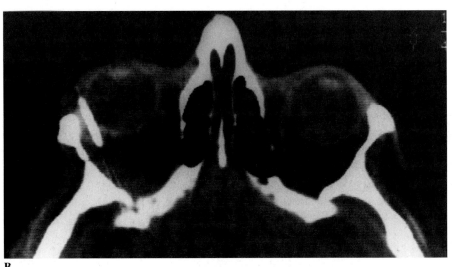

B

Figure 5-48. Axial computed tomography (CT) demonstrates lymphoma of lateral rectus muscle (A). Axial CT demonstrates accurate fine-needle biopsy placement in biopsy of enlarged muscle (B).

Quantitative A-scan echography, using a standardized Kretz unit, is most useful for determining if individual recti muscles are enlarged. Ultrasonographic characteristics of thyroid ophthalmopathy are shown in Table 5-5. McNutt et al. measured the A-scan maximum thicknesses of the different recti muscles in a group of patients with thyroid disease (see Table 5-5).[105] Most ultrasonographers believe that maximal muscle thickness above the ninety-fifth percentile, or a variance of more than 0.5 mm between the same muscles in the two orbits, is consistent with the diagnosis of thyroid eye disease.[106]

Figure 5-49. Diagram (A) and B-scan (B) demonstrate enlarged extraocular muscles.

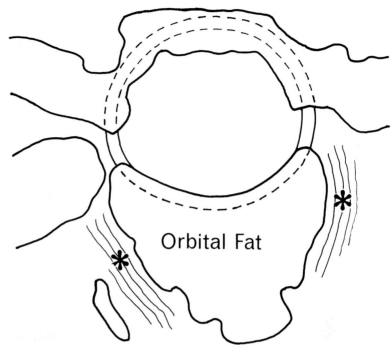

Orbital Fat

* enlarged recti

A

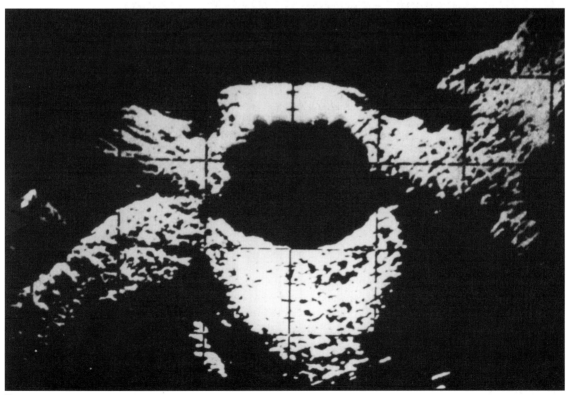

B

Table 5-5. Ultrasound Findings Suggestive of Endocrine Exophthalmopathy

B-scan:
1. Widening of echo-free area between orbital fat and bone
2. Increased delineation of extraocular muscle margin
3. Posterior scalloped/indented orbital fat secondary to muscle enlargement
4. "Doubling" of optic nerve sheath in thyroid optic neuropathy
5. No detectable neoplasm

A-scan:
1. Extraocular muscle enlargement (> 95th percentile)[105]
   a. Medial rectus > 5.20 mm
   b. Inferior rectus > 4.45 mm
   c. Lateral rectus > 5.12 mm
   d. Superior rectus > 4.80 mm

Shammas and coworkers observed that, even in patients referred for a diagnosis other than thyroid ophthalmopathy, thyroid eye disease could usually be correctly diagnosed with ultrasonography in patients with unilateral proptosis.[106] As mentioned earlier, the detection of extraocular muscle defects with ultrasonography is more sensitive than is clinical examination. In a study by Forrester et al., 20 of 32 patients (63%) without clinical eye disease had B-scan evidence of muscle enlargement.[107] Some ultrasound studies have routinely demonstrated enlarged optic nerves in thyroid eye disease; most studies have noted these findings rarely, usually in association with optic neuropathy.[105–113] An A-scan demonstrating an enlarged medial rectus muscle is shown in Figure 5-50. While a number of authors have suggested that A-scan ultrasound measurements of muscle thickness are highly accurate and reproducible, the nongeometric pattern of muscle enlargement can produce measurement errors on repeat ultrasound evaluations.[114] Color Doppler studies have also been performed in thyroid orbitopathy.

MAGNETIC RESONANCE IMAGES

MR scanning is a diagnostic imaging technique that does not use ionizing radiation. It is based on the principle that nuclei with an odd number of nucleons (protons and neutrons) behave as small magnets or dipoles. Hydrogen nuclei (protons) are ubiquitous, and their resonance is the basis of clinical MR imaging techniques. When the orbit is placed in a magnetic field there is a net alignment of protons. When exposed to radiofrequency (RF) excitation there is a reversal of polarity of some of these hydrogen nuclei, and they are raised to a higher energy level. When the RF is terminated, the protons return to the baseline polarity, and the emitted energy can be measured. This is called T_1 relaxation and is best measured immediately after RF termination. Differences in the rates of repolarization vary with the molecular environment and are partially the basis for tissue contrast in MRI. Exposure to RF excitation also initiates a uniform synchronous precession, or spin, among the protons. When the RF is terminated, this precession diminishes at differing rates for protons in different molecular environments. The energy emission measured from this event is called T_2 relaxation time. Since the RF-initiated events depend on the frequency and magnetic field strength, the location of these events in three-dimensional space

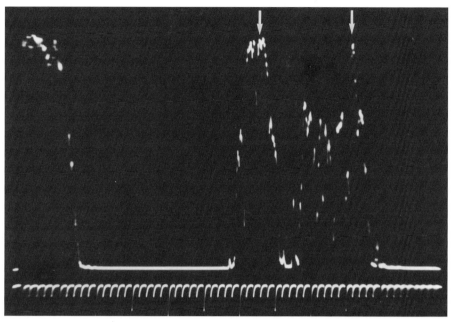

Figure 5-50. Enlarged rectus muscle (arrows) on A-scan.

can be determined by imposing a gradient (approximately 0.1 tesla [T] per centimeter) on the magnetic field and varying the RF.

Optimal current strength for clinical imaging is 1.5 T, although currently used scanners range from 0.15–4.5 T.[115–117] Optimal orbital anatomic detail is obtained with surface coils and thin section scans. Signal-to-noise ratio improves with increasing field strength. The components of the MR signal that form an image reflect proton density, T_1 relaxation, T_2 relaxation, and vascular flow, if present.

CT and MR image generation have a number of similarities. The relative intensity of the MR signal is displayed as a pixel matrix on a gray scale similar to CT. The major differences are the techniques and the tissue properties that are imaged. In CT, tissue density is related to the attenuation of x-rays. In MR, relative rates of remagnetization and loss of precessional frequency and proton density are responsible for signal intensity differences. These MR parameters are influenced by imaging techniques, field strength, and tissue magnetic susceptibility. MR intensity values are not related to a standard reference but rather to other tissues in the volume being imaged with a given set of imaging parameters.

In CT image generation, numbers are produced that are directly related to the x-ray attenuation in a finite volume of tissue represented by an individual number termed a *voxel*. The numerical representation of the MR image is the same as for CT; however, the physical property that results in the numerical value is the intensity of the RF signal of the perturbed hydrogen nuclei and that volume of tissue.

An MR signal is influenced by two major temporal factors. First, the alignment of protons in tissue varies at the time they are stimulated by the radiowaves and the magnetic field, and their initial status affects initial signal intensity and decay. Second, once the tissue protons are perturbed, they have a characteristic decay envelope.

Retrobulbar fat that has a short T_1 and medium T_2 relaxation will produce a relatively strong signal. Muscle is intermediate in signal intensity; cerebrospinal fluid and vitreous have long T_1 and T_2 relaxation times. Cortical bone is displayed as black (signal void) as there is no mobile hydrogen and therefore no MR signal.

Instrument parameters, repetition time (TR) and echo-time (TE), can be varied to emphasize T_1 or T_2 relaxation. TR indicates the time between excitations and usually ranges from 50 to 400 ms. The time after excitation at this resonant energy is TE and can range from 2.5 to 120.0 ms. Images with relative short TRs (<500 ms) and short TEs (<40 ms) are weighted. Images obtained with long TRs (approximately 2,000 ms) and long TEs (>60 ms) are T_2 weighted. T_1 and T_2 can also be measured as an absolute number.

The soft-tissue spatial resolution obtainable with proton MRI is greater than that obtained with high-resolution CT and shows greater tissue contrast. In some disease processes, MRI is more sensitive to alterations in water content or hydrogen concentration than is CT or other conventional imaging techniques. As an example, MRI demonstrates demyelinating plaques often not visible on CT images even after contrast material administration.[118]

There are some MRI data on thyroid ophthalmopathy.[116,119–128] The improved anatomic detail available on MRI scans of thyroid eye disease has yet to markedly alter our management of this disease, although the delineation of compressive optic neuropathy is easier with MRI than CT. Figures 5-39 and 5-51 show representative axial MR images in thyroid ophthalmopathy. MRI of optic nerves demonstrates compression better than CT (see Figure 5-45).

In comparative studies, Nianiaris and colleagues noted better identification of compressive optic neuropathy with MR as compared with CT.[122] Demer and Kerman noted that when ultrasound measurements of muscle thickness were compared with MR data, the accuracy of ultrasound was significantly less, and this problem was worse in muscles other than the inferior rectus.[124]

RADIONUCLEOTIDE SCANS

In a few centers, indium-111 nuclide scans have shown uptake of octreotide, a somatostatin analogue in both the orbit and thyroid.[129] Presently these orbital radionucleotide scan data seem to correlate with orbital inflammation, and the relative sensitivity versus other means to delineate inflammatory versus fibrotic changes remains to be determined.

FORCED DUCTION TESTS

The forced duction test was first described in ophthalmology almost 80 years ago.[130,131] It is useful in differentiating thyroid restrictive extraocular myopathies from other causes of ocular muscle dysfunction.[132] A schema of the forced duction test is shown in Figure 5-52. In adults the test is performed on an outpatient basis using topical anesthesia. Young children should be tested while under general anesthesia.

Forced duction testing of adults begins with a drop of topical tetracaine placed on the conjunctiva. The area of the muscle insertion is anesthetized by holding a cotton-tipped applicator soaked in either 4% cocaine or 4% lidocaine (Xylocaine) over it for approximately 1 minute. The muscle insertion is grasped with Bishop-Harmon forceps, and, with the patient's cooperation, the globe is rotated away from the muscle's field of action. The contralateral ocular muscle should also be tested as a baseline. Positive forced duction tests are observed in thyroid myopathy, idiopathic

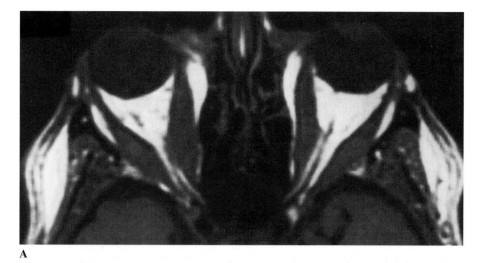

A

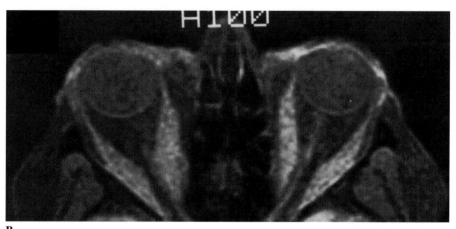

B

Figure 5-51. A T$_1$-weighted magnetic resonance imaging (A) shows enlarged extraocular muscles do not appear to compress the nerve. A fat saturation program demonstrates lack of compression along the nerve (B).

orbital myositis, muscle entrapment secondary to orbital blow-out fractures, and tumor infiltration of the muscles. A negative forced duction test in a muscle with strabismus argues against the diagnosis of a thyroid myopathy and suggests a non-restrictive myopathy such as that observed with cranial nerve palsies of various etiologies or ocular myasthenia gravis. In addition to the forced duction test findings, a restrictive myopathy is also evidenced by an increased intraocular pressure when the eye is rotated out of the muscle's field of action.

CONCLUSION

Diagnostic evaluation of patients presenting with thyroid eye disease is relatively straightforward. In the atypical patient who presents with proptosis or other eye signs without a history or the systemic laboratory findings of thyrotoxicosis, ophthalmo-

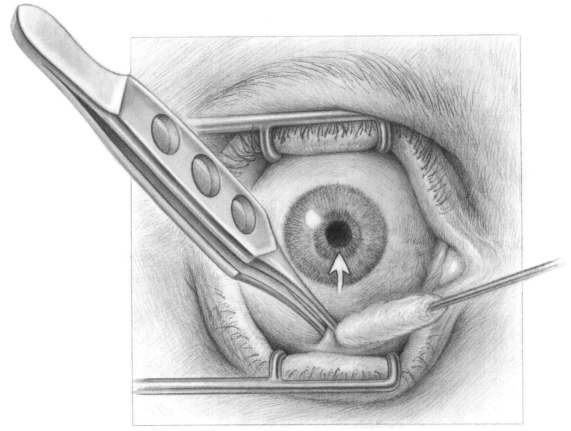

Figure 5-52. Schema of forced duction test of inferior rectus.

logic findings and orbital scans are extremely useful. In an atypical presentation, or to rule out an orbital tumor, CT or MR images are obtained. MR images should be obtained in patients with decreased vision or in cases requiring a better delineation of inflammatory versus fibrotic status of the disease process. In middle-aged and older patients, thyroid ophthalmopathy is a frequent cause of diplopia, and forced duction tests are useful to distinguish it from other causes of nonrestrictive ophthalmoplegia.

REFERENCES

1. Char DH. Clinical Ocular Oncology (2nd ed). Philadelphia: Lippincott-Raven, 1997.
2. Wilson JA, Von Haacke NP, Adams GGW, Dale BAB. Surgical decompression of the orbit. J R Coll Surg Edinb 1986;31:22.
3. Reifler DM, Holtzman JN, Ringel DM. Sphenoid ridge meningioma masquerading as Graves' orbitopathy. Arch Ophthalmol 1986;104:1591.
4. Capone A Jr, Slamovits TL. Discrete metastasis of solid tumors to extraocular muscles. Arch Ophthalmol 1990;108:237.
5. Slamovits TL, Burde RM. Bumpy muscles (clinical conference). Surv Ophthalmol 1988;33:189.

6. Westra WH, Gerald WL, Rosai J. Solitary fibrous tumor. Consistent CD34 immunoreactivity and occurrence in the orbit. Am J Surg Pathol 1994;18:992.

7. Howard GR, Nerad JA, Bonavolonta G, Tranfa F. Orbital dermoid cysts located within the lateral rectus muscle. Ophthalmology 1994;101:767.

8. Squires RH Jr, Zwiener RJ, Kennedy RH. Orbital myositis and Crohn's disease. J Pediatr Gastroenterol Nutr 1992;15:448.

9. Orssaud C, Poisson M, Gardeur D. Orbital myositis, recurrence of Whipple's disease. J Fr Ophtalmol 1992;15:205.

10. Moorman CM, Elston JS. Acute orbital myositis. Eye 1995;9:96.

11. Siatkowski RM, Capo H, Byrne SF, et al. Clinical and echographic findings in idiopathic orbital myositis. Am J Ophthalmol 1994;118:343.

12. Serop S, Vianna RN, Claeys M, De Laey JJ. Orbital myositis secondary to systemic lupus erythematosus. Acta Ophthalmologica 1994;72(4):520.

13. Cornblath WT, Elner V, Rolfe M. Extraocular muscle involvement in sarcoidosis. Ophthalmology 1993;100:501.

14. Harris GJ, Murphy ML, Schmidt EW, et al. Orbital myositis as a paraneoplastic syndrome. Arch Ophthalmol 1994;112:380.

15. Leib ML, Odel JG, Cooney MJ. Orbital polymyositis and giant cell myocarditis. Ophthalmology 1994;101:950.

16. Purcell JJ, Taulbee WA. Orbital myositis after upper respiratory tract infection. Arch Ophthalmol 1981;99:437.

17. Seidenberg KB, Leib ML. Orbital myositis with Lyme disease. Am J Ophthalmol 1990;109:13.

18. O'Neil RA, Ngu SL, Prosser IW. Orbital lymphoma simulating thyroid ophthalmopathy. Letter to the Editor. AJR Am J Roentgenol 1994;162:734.

19. Char DH, Unsold R. Ocular and Orbital Pathology: Clinical Aspects. In TH Newton, AN Hasso, WP Dillon (eds), Modern Neuroradiology. Vol 3: Computed Tomography of the Head and Neck. Kentfield, IA: Clavadel Press, 1988.

20. Cassan SM, Divertie MD, Hollenhorst RW, Harrison EG Jr. Pseudotumor of the orbit and limited Wegener's granulomatosis. Ann Intern Med 1970;72:687.

21. Weinstein JS, Dresner SC, Slamovits TL, Kennerdell JS. Acute and subacute orbital myositis. Am J Ophthalmol 1983;96:209.

22. Wolter JR, Hoy JE, Schmidt DM. Chronic orbital myositis. Its diagnostic difficulties and pathology. Am J Ophthalmol 1966;62:292.

23. Trokel SL, Jakobiec FA. Correlation of CT scanning and pathologic features of ophthalmic Graves' disease. Ophthalmology 1981;88:553.

24. Richards AB, Skalka HW, Roberts FJ, Flint A. Pseudotumor of the orbit and retroperitoneal fibrosis. A form of multifocal fibrosclerosis. Arch Ophthalmol 1980;98:617.

25. Spalton DJ, Graham EM, Page NGR, Sanders MD. Ocular changes in limited forms of Wegener's granulomatosis. Br J Ophthalmol 1981;65:553.

26. Haynes BF, Fishman ML, Fauci AS, Wolff S. The ocular manifestations of Wegener's granulomatosis. Am J Med 1977;63:131.

27. Goldberg L, Tao A, Romano P. Severe exophthalmos secondary to orbital myopathy not due to Graves' disease. Br J Ophthalmol 1982;66:392.

28. Blodi FC, Gass JD. Inflammatory pseudotumor of the orbit. Br J Ophthalmol 1968;52:79.

29. Chavis RM, Garner A, Wright JE. Inflammatory orbital pseudotumor. A clinicopathological study. Arch Ophthalmol 1978;96:1817.

30. Jellinek EH. The orbital pseudotumor syndrome and its differentiation from endocrine exophthalmos. Brain 1969;92:35.

31. Birch-Hirschfeld A. Zur diagnostik und pathologie der orbitaltumoren (Ber Versmml Ophthalmol Ges 1905, 1906;Wiesb:127). Dtsch Ophthalmol Ges 1905;32:127.

32. Harr DL, Quencer RM, Abrams GW. Computed tomography and ultrasound in the evaluation of orbital infection and pseudotumor. Radiology 1982;142:395.

33. Slavin ML, Glaser JS. Idiopathic orbital myositis: report of six cases. Arch Ophthalmol 1982;100:1261.

34. Ashton N, Morgan G. Discrete carcinomatous metastases in the extraocular muscles. Br J Ophthalmol 1974;58:112.

35. Cuttone JM, Litvin J, McDonald JE. Carcinoma metastastic to an extraocular muscle. Ann Ophthalmol 1981;13:213.

36. Harris AL, Montgomery A. Orbital carcinoid tumor. Am J Ophthalmol 1980;90:875.

37. Rush JA, Waller RR, Campbell RJ. Orbital carcinoid tumor metastatic from the colon. Am J Ophthalmol 1980;89:636.

38. Sniderman HR. Orbital metastasis from tumor of the pancreas. Am J Ophthalmol 1942;25:1215.

39. Buys R, Abramson DH, Kitchin FD, et al. Simultaneous ocular and orbital involvement from metastatic bronchogenic carcinoma. Ann Ophthalmol 1982;14:1165.

40. Bedford PD, Daniel PM. Discrete carcinomatous metastases in the extrinsic ocular muscles. Am J Ophthalmol 1960;49:723.

41. Palestine AG, Younge BR, Piepgras DG. Visual prognosis in carotid-cavernous fistula. Arch Ophthalmol 1981;99:1600.

42. Merlis AL, Schaiberger CL, Adler R. External carotid-cavernous sinus fistula simulating unilateral Graves' ophthalmopathy. J Comput Assist Tomogr 1982;6:1006.

43. Oestreicher JH, Frueh BR. Carotid-cavernous fistula mimicking Graves' eye disease. Ophthal Plast Reconstr Surg 1995;11:238.

44. Goldberg RA, Garcia GH, Duckwiler GR. Combined embolization and surgical treatment of arteriovenous malformation of the orbit. Am J Ophthalmol 1993;116:17.

45. Green S, Som PM, Lavagnini PG. Bilateral orbital metastases from prostate carcinoma: case presentation and CT findings. AJNR Am J Neuroradiol 1995;16:417.

46. Hugkulstone CE, Winder S, Sokal M. Bilateral orbital metastases from transitional cell carcinoma of the bladder. Eye 1994;8:580.

47. Van Gelderen WFC. Gastric carcinoma metastases to extraocular muscles. J Comput Assist Tomogr 1993;17:499.

48. Goldberg RA, Rootman J, Cline RA. Tumors metastatic to the orbit: a changing picture. Surv Ophthalmol 1990;35(1):1.

49. Nirankari MS, Greer CH, Chaddah MR. Malignant non-chromaffin paraganglioma in the orbit. Br J Ophthalmol 1963;47:357.

50. Dal Pozzo G, Boschi MC. Extraocular muscle enlargement in acromegaly. J Comput Assist Tomogr 1982;6:706.

51. Knowles DM 2d, Jakobiec FA, Potter GD, Jones IS. Ophthalmic striated muscle neoplasms. Surv Ophthalmol 1976;21:219.

52. Amemiya T. Eosinophilic granuloma of the soft tissue in the orbit. Ophthalmologica 1981;182:42.

53. Morgan DC, Mason AS. Exophthalmos in Cushing's syndrome. Br Med J 1958;2:481.

54. Weidler WB. Acromegaly with extreme degree of exophthalmos. Boston Med Surg J 1916;174:506.

55. Cushing H. Basophil adenomas of pituitary body and their clinical manifestations (pituitary basophilism). Bull Johns Hopkins Hosp 1932;50:137.

56. Holmstrom GE, Nyman KG. Primary orbital amyloidosis localized to an extraocular muscle. Br J Ophthalmol 1987;71:32.

57. Erie JC, Garrity JA, Norman ME. Orbital amyloidosis involving the extraocular muscles. Arch Ophthalmol 1989;107:1428.

58. Sanders MD, Brown P. Acute presentation of thyroid ophthalmopathy. Trans Ophthalmol Soc UK 1986;105:720.

59. Ford HC, Delahunt JW, Teague CA. Squamous cell carcinoma of the eyelid masquerading as "malignant" ophthalmopathy of Graves' disease. Br J Ophthalmol 1983;67:596.

60. Cohen JS. Optic neuropathy of Graves' disease, hyperthyroidism, and ocular myasthenia gravis. Arch Ophthalmol 1973;90:131.

61. Vento JA, Slavin JD Jr, Reardon GE, Spencer RP. Graves' disease. Initial presentation with exophthalmos and solitary hot nodule. Clin Nucl Med 1986;11:404.

62. Bixenman WW, Buchsbaum HW. Multiple sclerosis, euthyroid restrictive Graves' ophthalmopathy, and myasthenia gravis. A case report. Graefes Arch Clin Exp Ophthalmol 1988;226:168.

63. Zakka KA, Summerer RW, Yee RD, et al. Opticociliary veins in a primary optic nerve sheath meningioma. Am J Ophthalmol 1979;87:91.

64. Hanneken AM, Miller NR, Debrun GM, Nauta HJW. Treatment of carotid-cavernous sinus fistulas using a detachable balloon catheter through the superior ophthalmic vein. Arch Ophthalmol 1989;107:87.

65. Uchino A, Hasuo K, Matsumoto S, Masuda K. MRI of dural carotid-cavernous fistulas. Comparisons with postcontrast CT. Clin Imaging 1992;16:263.

66. Hirabuki N, Fujita N, Hashimoto T, et al. Follow-up MRI in dural arteriovenous malformations involving the cavernous sinus: emphasis on detection of venous thrombosis. Neuroradiology 1992;34:423.

67. Char DH, Miller T. Orbital pseudotumor. Fine-needle aspiration biopsy and response to therapy. Ophthalmology 1993;100:1702.

68. Friedland S, Kaplan S, Lahav M, Shapiro A. Proptosis and periorbital edema due to diltiazem treatment [letter]. Arch Ophthalmol 1993;111:1027.

69. Char DH, LeBoit PE, Yung LJ, et al. Radiation therapy for ocular necrobiotic xanthogranuloma. Arch Ophthalmol 1987;105:174.

70. Klein BR, Hedges TR III, Dayal Y, Adelman LS. Orbital myositis and giant cell myocarditis. Neurology 1989;39:988.

71. Kattah JC, Zimmerman LE, Kolsky MP, et al. Bilateral orbital involvement in fatal giant cell polymyositis. Ophthalmology 1990;97:520.

72. Katz B, Leja S, Melles RB, Press GA. Amyloid ophthalmoplegia. Ophthalmoparesis secondary to primary systemic amyloidosis. J Clin Neuroophthalmol 1989;9:39.

73. Hamilton SM, Elsas FJ, Dawson TL. A cluster of patients with inferior rectus restriction following local anesthesia for cataract surgery. J Pediatr Ophthalmol Strabismus 1993;30:288.

74. Hunter DG, Lam GC, Guyton DL. Inferior oblique muscle injury from local anesthesia for cataract surgery. Ophthalmology 1995;102:501.

75. Munoz M. Inferior rectus muscle overaction after cataract extraction. Am J Ophthalmol 1994;118:664.

76. Forbes GS, Sheedy PF 2d, Waller RR. Orbital tumors evaluated by computed tomography. Radiology 1980;136:101.

77. Enzmann DR, Donaldson SS, Kriss JP. Appearance of Graves' disease on orbital computed tomography. J Comput Assist Tomogr 1979;3:815.

78. Donaldson SS, Bagshaw MA, Kriss JP. Supervoltage orbital radiotherapy for Graves' ophthalmopathy. J Clin Endocrinol Metab 1973;37:276.

79. Trokel SL, Hilal SK. Recognition and differential diagnosis of enlarged extraocular muscles in computed tomography. Am J Ophthalmol 1979;87:503.

80. Enzmann D, Marshall WH Jr, Rosenthal AR, Kriss JP. Computed tomography in Graves' ophthalmopathy. Radiology 1976;118:615.

81. Forbes G, Gorman CA, Gehring D, Baker HL Jr. Computer analysis of orbital fat and muscle volumes in Graves' ophthalmopathy. AJNR Am J Neuroradiol 1983;4:737.

82. Wiersinga WM, Smit T, Van der Gaag R, Koornneeff L. Clinical presentation of Graves' ophthalmopathy. Ophthalmic Res 1989;21:73.

83. Yoshikawa K, Higashide T, Nakase Y, et al. Role of rectus muscle enlargement in clinical profile of dysthyroid ophthalmopathy. Jpn J Ophthalmol 1991;35:175.

84. Inoue Y, Inoue T, Ichikizaki K, et al. The role of extraocular muscle in the development of dysthyroid ophthalmopathy. Jpn J Clin Ophthalmol 1978;32:901.

85. Feldon SE, Weiner JM. Clinical significance of extraocular muscle volumes in Graves' ophthalmopathy: a quantitative computed tomography study. Arch Ophthalmol 1982;100:1266.

86. Fledelius HC, Glydensted C. Ultrasonography and computed tomography in orbital diagnosis. Acta Ophthalmol 1978;56:751.

87. Susac JO, Martins AN, Robinson B, Corrigan DF. False diagnosis of orbital apex tumor by CAT scan in thyroid eye disease. Ann Neurol 1977;1:397.

88. Trokel SL, Hilal SK. Computerized axial tomography in patients with exophthalmos. Arch Ophthalmol 1976;94:867.

89. Brismar J, Davis KR, Dallow RL, Brismar G. Unilateral endocrine exophthalmos. Diagnostic problems in association with computed tomography. Neuroradiology 1976;12:21.

90. Kennerdell JS, Rosenbaum AE, El Hoshy MH. Apical optic nerve compression of dysthyroid optic neuropathy on computed tomography. Arch Ophthalmol 1981;99:807.

91. Feldon SE, Muramatsu S, Weiner JM. Clinical classification of Graves' ophthalmopathy. Identification of risk factors for optic neuropathy. Arch Ophthalmol 1984;102:1469.

92. Barrett L, Glatt HJ, Burde RM, Gado MH. Optic nerve dysfunction in thyroid eye disease: CT. Radiology 1988;167:503.

93. Spector G, Thawley SE. Management of Graves' Ophthalmopathy. In SA Falk (ed), Thyroid Disease: Endocrinology, Surgery, Nuclear Medicine and Radiotherapy. New York: Raven, 1990;265.

94. Niegel JM, Rootman J, Belkin RI, et al. Dysthyroid optic neuropathy. Ophthalmology 1988;95:1515.

94a. Birchall D, Goodall KL, Noble JL, et al. Ophthalmopathy: intracranial fat prolapse on CT images as an indicator of optic nerve compression. Radiology 1996;200:123.

95. Henderson JW. Orbital Tumors (2nd ed). New York: Brian Decker, 1980.

96. Reese AB. Expanding lesions of the orbit. Trans Ophthalmol Soc UK 1971;91:85.

97. Harris GJ, Jakobiec FA. Cavernous hemangioma of the orbit. J Neurosurg 1979;51:219.

98. Arora R, Rewari R, Betharia SM. Fine-needle aspiration cytology of orbital and adnexal masses. Acta Cytol 1992;36:483.

99. Zajdela A, Vielh P, Schlienger P, Haye C. Fine-needle cytology of 292 palpable orbital and eyelid tumors. Am J Clin Pathol 1990;93:100.

100. Harrie RP. A-scanning Graves' ophthalmopathy. Arch Ophthalmol 1993;100:1430.

101. Ossoinig K. Echography of the eye, orbit and periorbital region. In PH Arger (ed), Orbit Roentgenology. New York: Wiley, 1977;223.

102. Coleman DJ, Lizzi FL, Jack RL. Ultrasonography of the Eye and Orbit. Philadelphia: Lea & Febiger, 1977.

103. Atta HR, McCreath G, McKillop JH, et al. Ophthalmopathy in early thyrotoxicosis—relationship to thyroid receptor antibodies and effects of treatment. Scott Med J 1990;35:41.

104. Willinsky RA, Arenson AM, Hurwitz JJ, Szalai J. Ultrasonic B-scan measurement of the extraocular muscles in Graves' orbitopathy. J Can Assoc Radiol 1984;35:171.

105. McNutt LC, Kaefring SL, Ossoinig KC. Echographic Measurement of Extraocular Muscles. In D White, R Brown (eds), Ultrasound in Medicine (Vol 3). New York: Plenum, 1977;927.

106. Shammas HJ, Minckler DS, Ogden C. Ultrasound in early thyroid orbitopathy. Arch Ophthalmol 1980;98:277.

107. Forrester JV, Sutherland GR, McDougall IR. Dysthyroid ophthalmopathy: orbital evaluation with B-scan ultrasonography. J Clin Endocrinol Metab 1977;45:221.

108. Purnell EW. B-mode orbital ultrasonography. Int Ophthalmol Clin 1969;9:643.

109. Coleman DJ, Jack RL, Franzen LA, Erner SC. High resolution B-scan ultrasonography of the orbit. V. Eye changes of Graves' disease. Arch Ophthalmol 1972;88:465.

110. Purnell EQ. Ultrasonic Interpretation of Orbital Disease. In KA Gitter, AH Keeney, LK Sarin, D Major (eds), Ophthalmic Ultrasound. St. Louis: Mosby, 1969;249.

111. Werner SC, Coleman DJ, Franzen LA. Ultrasonographic evidence of a consistent orbital involvement in Graves' disease. N Engl J Med 1974;290:1447.

112. Skalka HW. The use of ultrasonography in the diagnosis of endocrine orbitopathy. Eur Ophthalmol 1980;1:109.

113. Hodes BL, Stern G. Contact B-scan echographic diagnosis of ophthalmopathic Graves' disease. J Clin Ultrasound 1975;3:255.

114. Holt JE, O'Connor PS, Douglas JP, Byrne B. Extraocular muscle size comparison using standardized A-scan echography and computerized tomography scan measurements. Ophthalmology 1985;92:1351.

115. Crooks LE, Hoenninger J, Arakawa M, et al. High-resolution of magnetic resonance imaging. Radiology 1984;150:163.

116. Moseley I, Brant-Zawdski M, Mills C. Nuclear magnetic resonance imaging of the orbit. Br J Ophthalmol 1983;67:333.

117. Hans JS, Benson JE, Bonstelle CT, et al. Magnetic resonance imaging of the orbit: preliminary experience. Radiology 1984;150:755.

118. Crooks LE, Ortendahl DA, Kaufman L, et al. Clinical efficiency of nuclear magnetic resonance imaging. Radiology 1983;146:123.

119. Morrice GD, Smith FW. Early experience with nuclear magnetic resonance (NMR) imaging in the investigation of ocular proptosis. Trans Ophthalmol Soc UK 1983;103:143.

120. Wiegand W. Darstellungs-und differenzierungsmöglichkeit von augenmuskelveranderungen bei endokriner orbitopathie und okularer myositis mit hilfe der kernspin-tomographie. Klin Monatsbl Augenheilkd 1986;189:214.

121. Troelstra A, Rijneveld WJ, Kooijman AC, Houtman WA. Correlation between NMR scans of extraocular muscles and clinical symptoms in Graves' ophthalmopathy. Doc Ophthalmol 1988;70:243.

122. Nianiaris N, Hurwitz JJ, Chen JC, Wortzman G. Correlation between computed tomography and magnetic resonance imaging in Graves' orbitopathy. Can J Ophthalmol 1994;29:9.

123. Inoue Y, Hagashide T, Yoshikawa K, Inoue T. Sagittal magnetic resonance imaging of dysthyroid ophthalmopathy. Eur J Ophthalmol 1993;3:31.

124. Demer JL, Kerman BM. Comparison of standardized echography with magnetic resonance imaging to measure extraocular muscle size. Am J Ophthalmol 1994;118:351.

125. Hosten VN, Schorner W, Lietz A, Wenzel KW. Der krankheitsverlauf bei der endokrinen orbitopathie. Fortschr Rontgenstr 1992;157:210.

126. Hosten N, Sander B, Cordes M, et al. Graves' ophthalmopathy: MR imaging of the orbits. Radiology 1989;172:759.

127. Ohnishi T, Noguchi S, Murakami N, et al. Extraocular muscles in Graves' ophthalmopathy: usefulness of T2 relaxation time measurements. Radiology 1994;190:857.

128. Utech CI, Khatibia U, Winter PF, Wulle KG. MR T2 relaxation time for the assessment of retrobulbar inflammation in Graves' ophthalmopathy. Thyroid 1995;5:185.

129. Mansi L, Rambaldi PR, Bizzarro A, et al. Indium-111 octreotide in Graves' disease and in the evaluation of active exophthalmos. Q J Nucl Med 1995;39:105.

130. Wolff J. The occurrence of retraction movements of the eyeball together with congenital defects in the external ocular muscles. Arch Ophthalmol 1900;29:297.

131. Dunnington JH, Berke RN. Exophthalmos due to chronic orbital myositis. Arch Ophthalmol 1943;30:446.

132. Oei TH, Verhagen WIM, Horsten GPM. Forced duction test in clinical practice. Ophthalmologica 1983;186:87.

133. Patrinely CR, Osborn AG, Anderson RL, Whiting AS. Computed tomographic features of nonthyroid extraocular muscle enlargement. Ophthalmology 1989;96:1038.

134. Liu GT, Schatz NJ, Curtin VT, Tse DT. Bilateral extraocular muscle metastases in Zollinger-Ellison syndrome. Arch Ophthalmol 1994;112:451.

135. Fekrat S, Miller NR, Loury MC. Alveolar rhabdomyosarcoma that metastasized to the orbit. Arch Ophthalmol 1993;111:1662.

136. Provenzale JM, Mukherji S, Allen NB, et al. Orbital involvement by Wegener's granulomatosis: imaging findings. AJR Am J Roentgenol 1996;166:929.

137. Green S, Som PM, Lavagnini PG. Bilateral orbital metastases from prostate carcinoma: case presentation and CT findings. AJNR Am J Neuroradiol 1995;16:417.

138. Fan CJ, Goh KL, Wang F. Steroid induced exophthalmos: a case report. Australas Radiol 1989;33:182.

139. Van Gelderen WFC. Gastric carcinoma metastases to extraocular muscles. J Comput Assist Tomogr 1993;17:499.

140. Akamizu T, Kohn LD, Mori T. Molecular studies on thyrotropin (TSH) receptor and anti-TSH receptor antibodies. Endocr J 1995;42:617.

6

Pathogenesis and Pathophysiology of Thyroid Ophthalmopathy

There are several theories explaining the development of thyroid ophthalmopathy; however, the nature of the shared thyroid-orbital antigen, the primary orbital cell important in the pathogenesis of this immune process, and the pathophysiology of thyroid eye disease remain to be elucidated. Almost all investigators consider ophthalmopathy to be a component of Graves' disease.[1]

No relationship has been proved between systemic hyperthyroidism and thyroid ophthalmopathy, but a large body of clinical data suggests not only a strong association but also that thyroid and orbital inflammation are two facets of the same disease. As discussed in Chapters 3 and 4, the majority of Graves' ophthalmopathy patients present with systemic thyroid disease before development of eye disease.[2–5] Orbital imaging studies of Graves' disease patients having little or no clinical evidence of eye disease reveal enlargement of extraocular muscles in most hyperthyroid patients.[6–10] While eye findings can occur before discovery of hyperthyroidism, there is usually a close temporal association. Gorman demonstrated that more than 80% of severe ophthalmopathy patients develop eye findings within 18 months before or after the discovery of systemic thyroid disease.[11] Amino and colleagues have shown in Japanese patients that there is a normal Gaussian distribution of exophthalmos in Graves' disease suggesting concordance with systemic hyperthyroidism.[12] Similar data have been demonstrated in a Dutch study of 90 untreated patients with Graves' ophthalmopathy. They noted that the age and sex distribution of thyroid eye and systemic hyperthyroid patients at their institution were nearly identical.[13]

Numerous observations refute a complete association between ophthalmopathy and thyroid disease. As mentioned above, eye findings can occur before or at any time after the discovery of thyroid disease.[14,15] The clinical manifestations of ophthalmopathy do not correlate with thyroid disease course or severity. As shown in Figure 4-9, eye findings can occur in patients who have neither Graves' disease nor evidence of thyroid gland inflammation. Similarly, thyroid-stimulating antibody levels, which often correlate with thyroid disease status and prognosis, do not correlate with eye findings.[16] While some patients with euthyroid ophthalmopathy develop hyperthyroidism, a significant percentage do not. However, almost all of these patients have some demonstrable immunologic reactivity toward thyroid antigens.[17] Finally, if ophthalmopathy is a feature of thyroid disease, it is puzzling that eye disease is often asymmetric and has a predilection for some recti muscles and not others.[18] While clinical examination more often reveals inferior and medial recti muscle involvement, careful computed tomography (CT), magnetic resonance imaging (MRI), or ultrasonographic study demonstrates that most, if not all, extraocular muscles are often involved in thyroid eye disease.[6–10]

HISTORY

There are many theories to explain thyroid ophthalmopathy development; most have proved to be incorrect. Some erroneous ideas still influence patient management, and the pathogenesis of this disorder remains unclear. While Parry first described an association between diffuse goiter and eye findings, von Basedow is credited with the concept that such eye findings occur as a consequence of thyroid disease. He hypothesized that thyroid ophthalmopathy is due to strumous hypertrophy of the orbital contents.[19] In 1849, Cooper postulated that exophthalmos results from orbital muscle laxity and venous congestion.[20] Jones et al. theorized that orbital edema was the cause of thyroid exophthalmos.[21–23]

Cervical autonomic sympathetic stimulation was a popular mid-nineteenth century theory accounting for thyroid ophthalmopathy. Bernard demonstrated that electrostimulation of the cervical sympathetics in animals caused widened palpebral fissures and as much as 4–5 mm of exophthalmos in dogs.[24] Krauss and Frund postulated that this autonomic nerve stimulation resulted in contraction of smooth muscle with resultant lid retraction, orbital venous dilation, and proptosis.[25] The inaccuracy of this concept for human thyroid eye disease was demonstrated by McLean and Norton.[26] They performed stellate ganglion blocks in three thyroid eye disease patients and noted no reversal of lid retraction; similarly, no change was observed after treatment with reserpine.[26] These findings demonstrate that factors in addition to sympathetic stimulation are important to eyelid changes in thyroid ophthalmopathy. Other theories explaining thyroid eye disease that have proved inaccurate include dilation of orbital blood vessels, relaxation of striated orbital muscles, simple orbital edema, and infectious factors.[27,28]

Many investigators have demonstrated that pituitary factors can cause exophthalmos in laboratory animals.[29] Review of that data by Smelser and Wybar revealed that the exophthalmic effect of these factors in the most commonly used animal, the guinea pig, was on the retrobulbar harderian gland, which does not exist in humans.[29–36]

When the concept of negative feedback suppression of the pituitary axis developed, it was postulated that hypothyroidism after Graves' disease would increase the release of pituitary factors and thus the chance of ophthalmopathy. Some investigators also theorized that there were increased thyrotropin (thyroid-stimulating hormone [TSH]) levels in malignant exophthalmos.[37–44] As discussed in Chapter 7, some data support the concept that hypothyroidism after treatment may increase the risk of thyroid eye disease.

A case report by Furth and colleagues demonstrated that eye findings could occur and progress in the absence of pituitary factors.[45] They reported a patient whose severe right-sided ophthalmopathy, unresponsive to orbital decompression, went into remission after total surgical hypophysectomy. The patient did well for 2½ years, during which time pituitary function was absent. Severe ophthalmopathy then developed in the previously uninvolved left orbit. Other investigators have demonstrated that TSH levels are not routinely elevated in patients with thyroid ophthalmopathy.[46]

Some investigators believed that ophthalmopathy was an organ-specific autoimmune disorder not caused by thyroid disease but by an abnormality in the immunologic homeostatic mechanism resulting in aberrant T cell reactivity toward the thyroid and extraocular muscles.[47–51] Winand and coworkers postulated that humoral immunity toward a TSH subunit resulted in extraocular muscle damage and disease development.[52,53] Kriss and colleagues hypothesized that reactivity toward a shared ocular-thyroid antigen such as TSH resulted in the development of thyroid ophthalmopathy.[54]

HISTOLOGIC STUDIES

The factors responsible for proptosis in thyroid eye disease have been debated for years. Investigators have performed numerous histologic studies on orbital tissues from Graves' ophthalmopathy patients.[2,55–66] Rundle and Pochin, for instance, demonstrated that proptosis developed as a result of an increase in the orbital contents; they showed that a 4-ml increase in orbital volume increased proptosis by 6 mm.[67]

Accumulated clinical, histologic, and radiographic data demonstrate that enlarged extraocular muscles are predominantly responsible for exophthalmos in thyroid eye disease (Figures 6-1 and 6-2). As discussed in Chapter 5, ultrasound, MRI, and CT have demonstrated the correlation of extraocular muscle enlargement with severity of ophthalmopathy.[68–70] Extraocular muscles differ in a number of ways from other skeletal muscles. Ringel and coworkers noted that the extraocular muscles had a higher innervation ratio and more variation in size and fiber type than skeletal muscles.[71] Carry and coinvestigators observed that extraocular muscles have significantly larger mitochondrial areas, and the volume of mitochondria varied between the coarse granular and fine extraocular muscle fibers; that parameter alone was not sufficient to delineate subgroups of extraocular muscles.[72]

In l886, Silcock first noted extraocular muscle changes in an autopsy study of a patient with thyroid ophthalmopathy.[73] He noted yellowish discoloration of the muscles with interfascicular fatty infiltration. Subsequently a number of other authors have observed extraocular muscle changes in thyroid eye disease—extraocular muscles were two to eight times enlarged, rubbery, dark red, edematous, and fibrotic. There is histologic evidence of numerous inflammatory cells (lymphocytes, neutrophils, and plasma cells) and mucopolysaccharide infiltration.[74–80] The typical inflammatory infiltration of an extraocular muscle is shown in Figure 6-3. Kroll and Kuwabara studied 19 muscles, all obtained at the time of lateral decompression, from 17 eyes of 10 patients.[81] On gross examination, these muscles were two to five times normal size. Orbital fat appeared normal. Most muscles had lymphocytic infiltration, macrophages, mast cells, and edema. In a few cases degenerative changes were observed on light and electron microscopic examination. Daicker studied a series of extraocular muscles in thyroid ophthalmopathy patients and noted that fatty infiltration of the muscle appeared to be the major constituent responsible for enlargement.[82] Mucopolysaccharide deposits, inflammatory infiltrates, proliferation of the endomysium, and fibrosis appeared less important in the development of enlarged muscles.[82]

Tallstedt and Norberg performed immunohistologic studies on five Graves' patients' extraocular muscles. They noted that the muscles themselves were not markedly affected by the disease process.[83] As other studies have shown, most of

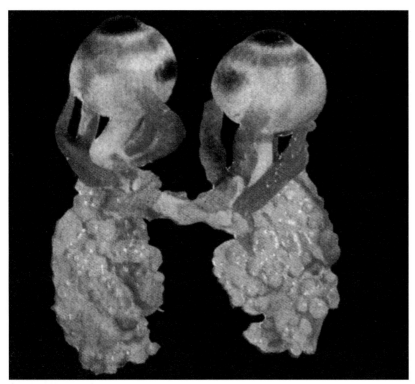

A

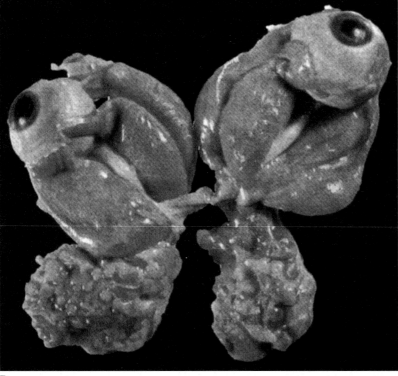

B

Figure 6-l. Normal (A) and enlarged extraocular muscles (B) in thyroid eye disease. (Reprinted with permission from T Levitt. The Thyroid. Edinburgh: Churchill Livingstone, 1954).

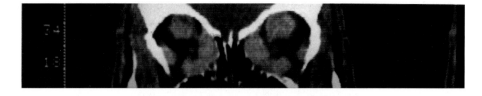

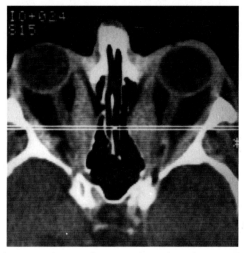

Figure 6-2. Computed tomography scan demonstrating enlarged extraocular muscles.

the increased volume was due to inflammatory cells and interstitial edema, with little intrinsic muscle cell damage.[83] In contrast, some other investigators have noted ultrastructural evidence of intrinsic muscle cell damage, including increased mitochondrial size and necrosis.[84]

An inherent problem with most histologic studies of extraocular muscle has been that the recti muscles are variably affected at different times in the disease process. Late in the course of thyroid eye disease, for instance, muscles can be fibrotic and relatively shrunken.[74–80] A fibrotic muscle is shown in Figure 6-4.

The importance of abnormal orbital fat in the development of severe ophthalmopathy has been extensively debated. Smelser and Ozanics demonstrated that orbital fat responded differently to pituitary extracts than adipose tissue from other areas of the body.[85] Riley reviewed the histologic data available from the Mayo Clinic and noted that inflammatory cells (lymphocytes, mast cells, and polymorphonuclear cells) and mucopolysaccharides were increased in the orbit.[86] Some investigators theorized that the presence of mucopolysaccharides secondary to this pathologic process resulted in an elevated water content with resultant orbital edema.[86–88] Riley's studies of orbital fat from decompression specimens revealed that connective tissue replaced fat, resulting in fibrosis and lipid deposition.[86] He postulated that the major change in the orbit of thyroid eye disease patients was due to increased secretory activity of fibroblasts. I have occasionally observed similar changes of only increased orbital connective tissue in a minority of patients requiring orbital decompression (Figure 6-5). Forbes and coworkers used CT imaging studies

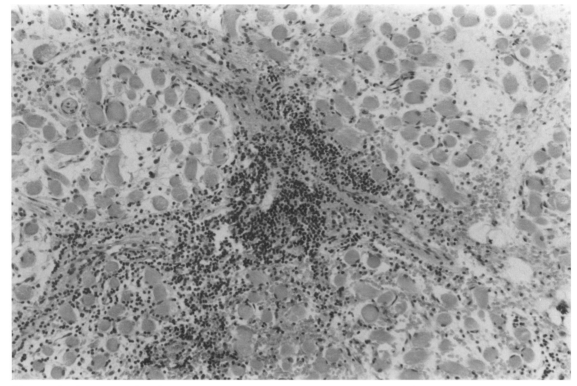

Figure 6-3. Histologic section of a rectus muscle in thyroid eye disease; note round cell infiltration.

to demonstrate only increased orbital connective tissue without muscle enlargement in about 9% of thyroid orbitopathy.[89]

In the majority of patients with orbital decompression I have operated on, the retrobulbar fat appears normal; in fact, the relatively normal condition of the orbital fat is important for a good response to a standard orbital decompression procedure. The orbital fat in thyroid ophthalmopathy patients also appears normal on MRI and CT examination (see Chapter 5).[69,90,91] Trokel and Jakobiec reported no inflammatory changes in orbital fat at the time of decompression,[69] nor could they find evidence of abnormal glycosaminoglycans. The importance of increased orbital fat volume in the production of proptosis associated with thyroid ophthalmopathy is unclear. Normal and increased fat volumes have been observed in patients with proptosis.[18,68,69,92–95]

IMMUNOLOGIC STUDIES

As discussed in Chapter 2, the role of immunogenetic factors in the development of both autoimmune thyroid disease and endocrine exophthalmos is uncertain. Human leukocyte antigen (HLA)-B8 and HLA-DR3 have been noted to be more frequent in patients with Graves' ophthalmopathy. In Hungarian patients HLA-B8 was noted in 68% and HLA-DR3 in 74% of those with eye disease.[96] In that study and one by

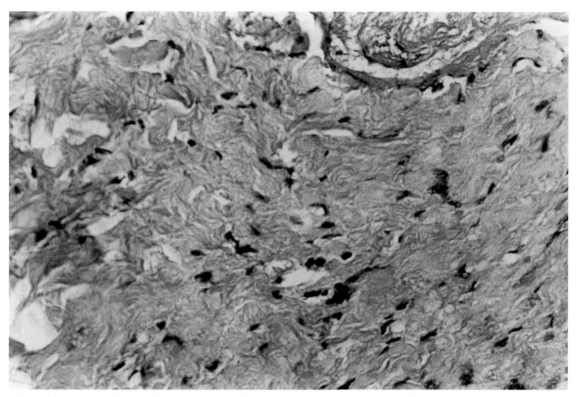

Figure 6-4. End-stage change of a rectus muscle in long-standing Graves' ophthalmopathy.

Farid, a stronger association between ophthalmopathy and HLA-B8 rather than HLA-DR3 was observed.[97] Sergott and coworkers noted that HLA-Bw35 was noted more frequently in thyroid eye disease patients displaying orbital inflammation, especially accompanied by severe extraocular involvement.[98] In Japanese patients a different set of HLA haplotypes is associated with Graves' disease.[99,100] In some European studies conflicting HLA data have been described with minimal correlation to thyroid eye disease.[101–103] As discussed in Chapter 2, there are a number of possible explanations for human HLA disease associations. Amino acid sequencing has demonstrated close homology between common bacterial antigens and HLA haplotypes, and this homology could result in loss of immunologic tolerance.[104] More recent studies have demonstrated that similarities in the antigenic structure are not always associated with amino acid homology.[105] In one study, molecular mimicry was shown in the absence of sequence homology.[105]

While it is clear that thyroid orbitopathy is an autoimmune disease, the nature of the pathogenetic antigen shared between the thyroid and the orbit, the relative importance of the cellular versus humoral immune response, and the primary orbital cell responsible for initiating a local ophthalmic autoimmune process remain to be elucidated.

As has been true with all laboratory techniques, there are inherent limitations with newer molecular biologic approaches. Three caveats illustrate these problems. First, in studies of thyroid antibodies, Quaratino and associates observed that amino acid

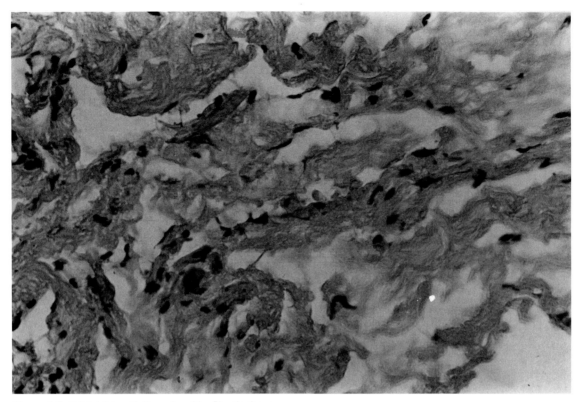

Figure 6-5. Orbital fat partially replaced by fibrotic tissue.

sequence homology may not predict the occurrence (or lack thereof) of a near identical immune response to two similar moieties, which is the basis of molecular mimicry.[105] Thus, while the ability to rapidly sequence a protein provides some useful
information, amino acid homology does not always indicate that there will be immune responses of a molecular mimicry type to nearly identical proteins. Second, the
ability to use material obtained from complementary deoxyribonucleic acid (cDNA)
libraries to determine the importance of a potential autoantigen is limited by the
markedly lesser antigenic stimulus of linear epitopes that do not have a normal surface configuration.[106] Third, the demonstration of messenger ribonucleic acid
(mRNA) for a given protein, using polymerase chain reaction (PCR) techniques,
while showing that a cell has the potential to produce that protein, does not show
that the actual protein is produced, that it is produced in the normal quantity, or that
it is not altered during production.[107]

Some of these molecular biology quandaries have affected the investigation
for the elusive thyroid-orbital antigen. Kriss and colleagues hypothesized that reactivity toward a shared orbital-thyroid antigen resulted in the development of
thyroid orbitopathy.[54] TSH is a G-protein with an antigenic large extracellular
portion and therefore has been suggested as a good shared antigen candidate.[108]
Earlier studies demonstrated TSH receptors (TSHrs) on orbital connective tissue
and muscle.[109–111] These older studies do not demonstrate the presence of TSHrs.
TSH will adhere to many substances, and its presence in the orbit does not prove

that the TSHr is expressed. Winand and coworkers postulated that a TSH subunit was exophthalmogenic, and interaction with an abnormal immunoglobulin bound to extraocular muscles was responsible for the development of thyroid orbitopathy.[52,53] Kohn and Winand noted that the presumed exophthalmogenic activity was in the beta fragment of approximately 50 amino acids. These later polypeptide fragments stimulated adenyl cyclase activity in orbital tissues.[52,53,112–116] Mullins and colleagues demonstrated thyroglobulin on orbital tissues and showed cellular immune response to it.[52,117] Several other candidate proteins that were considered included acetylcholinesterase and somatomedin C.[118–120] In a recent study, a small minority of thyroid orbitopathy patients (4 of 50) had antiacetylcholine receptor antibodies.[121]

Several workers have demonstrated mRNA for TSHr in orbital tissues.[122–127] At least three pieces of data are inconsistent with TSHr as the shared antigen. First, while some thyroid orbitopathy patients have antibodies against this antigen, they are neither of greater prevalence nor titer in Graves' disease patients with eye disease as compared with those who do not have eye findings.[123–125,128,129] However, in severe eye disease some studies have noted more antibodies that stimulate TSHr.[130] Second, if TSHr is the antigen, it is more difficult to explain the occurrence of eye findings in euthyroid orbitopathy patients. Third, these TSHr antibodies have not been demonstrated to increase fibroblast proliferation of extracellular matrix or damaged eye muscle.[131,132]

Further research has questioned if TSHrs are expressed in orbital connective tissue. While several laboratories have provided compelling PCR-based data for the mRNA of TSHr, there is a paucity of direct data demonstrating its presence.[107,124,125,133–136]

Bahn and colleagues noted a threonine for proline shift at codon 52 in the extracellular domain of TSH in some female thyroid eye patients, but its importance is uncertain.[137]

Elisei and colleagues did not find a known candidate, common antigen when they probed with Western blots orbital tissue using four thyroid orbitopathy patients' sera with reactivity to some known orbital antigens, using a lambda gt11 human eye muscle expression library.[106]

The orbital cell that is the primary site of thyroid-related autoimmunity is uncertain. There is a growing literature in which different groups argue in favor of the orbital fibroblast or the extraocular muscle cell.[84,107,138] In some sense this question is not, at present, terribly important. Clinically, the majority of symptoms and signs are due to alteration of the extraocular muscles. Whether the attack is directly on that tissue or is due to contiguous inflammation or a second messenger effect from neighboring fibroblasts does not alter the nature of the damage. Where the issue becomes important is that if only one of these two cell types is the primary site of autoimmunity, genetic therapy could be used to abort the onset of autoimmunity at that point. At present, this is not possible.

Historically, most studies of T cells, B cells, or soluble factors (immunoglobulins, immune complexes, and cytokines) in thyroid orbitopathy patients were performed on blood or its fractionated products.

The importance of these systemically circulating, antiorbital antibodies demonstrated in older studies in the pathophysiology of thyroid eye disease is unclear. Atkinson and colleagues have studied reactivity toward a crude homogenate of porcine orbital muscle that was cross-reactive with human orbital antigens.[139] They observed that 21 (64%) of 33 untreated Graves' ophthalmopathy patients had significant titers of antibodies toward this antigen, compared with 25% of treated, active ophthalmopathy patients (3 of 12), 17% of patients with inactive eye disease (3 of 18), and 3% of control subjects (1 of 40). The researchers failed to detect a correlation between antiorbital antibody titers and levels of TSH-binding inhibitory immunoglobulin (TBII), thyroglobulin, or microsomal antibodies.

Several investigators have shown that some ophthalmopathy patients have antibodies against a variety of orbital antigens.[140–142] Faryna and colleagues noted that 14 of 20 Graves' ophthalmopathy patients had an antihuman eye muscle membrane antibody.[140.] Follow-up studies by this group showed a good correlation between antibody titers and ophthalmopathy index.[143] Similarly, 30 of 40 ophthalmopathy patients had an antibody that bound to pig eye muscle and was not cross-reactive with TSH.[141,144] Other groups have noted some problems with these types of assays and those studies in particular. In a few studies, 30% of normal controls and 70% of ocular myasthenia gravis patients were also positive.[145,146] Other studies using similar methods have observed that most thyroid patients, irrespective of eye status, have antibodies toward shared thyroid and orbital antigens.[147] Some studies using the same methods as Kendall-Taylor or Faryna were unable to replicate their findings.[148–150]

Mengistu and others studied slightly different antibodies directed toward human eye muscle membranes and noted that 40 of 55 patients with ophthalmopathy had these immunoglobulins, and the titer correlated with clinical activity and length of disease.[151] This antigen appears to be a 64-kDa protein.[152]

Kodama and coworkers have used monoclonal antibody technology to study humoral immunologic alterations in thyroid eye disease. They produced murine monoclonal antibodies using eye muscle antigens as immunogens.[153] Most of the antibodies produced were specific for the cytosol (versus the membrane) component of eye muscle; one of them was cross-reactive with thyroid microsomes. Similar data have been produced by other groups.[154] These monoclonal antibodies were used to isolate and characterize an eye muscle antigen. Circulating autoantibodies against this particular antigen were detected in 17 of 23 (74%) patients with Graves' ophthalmopathy, 1 of 14 patients with Hashimoto's disease, and no patients with hyperthyroidism without eye findings. Kuroki and coworkers made mouse monoclonal antibodies to orbital antigens and observed that reactivity toward orbital antigens could be absorbed with thyroid membranes or thyroglobulin.[155] Waring and colleagues found that murine monoclonal antibodies directed against extraocular muscles were neither reactive with nor blocked by TSH.[156] Most data demonstrated little if any correlation between immune complexes and thyroid orbitopathy.[157,158]

Various aspects of systemic cellular immunity toward orbital antigens have been studied. A few investigators have noted nonspecific alteration in T cell subsets or natural killer cells.[159–162] The relevance of these T cell alterations to immunologic perturbations toward the thyroid and orbit is uncertain. Some groups have also noted antibody-dependent cellular cytotoxicity toward eye muscle antigens.[159–163] In one set of experiments there was cross-reactivity between the eye muscle and thyroid cell antigens.[163] Probable immune mechanisms for thyroid orbitopathy are shown in Figure 6-6 and Table 6-1.

Wall, Wenzel, and their respective colleagues, as well as other researchers, have noted that thyroid patients have in vitro cellular reactivity toward thyroid antigens, without apparent correlation or association with the level of eye disease.[164,165] Munro and coworkers studied migration-inhibiting factors (MIFs) with a crude human extraocular muscle antigen in patients with Graves' disease-related ophthalmopathy, patients with systemic hyperthyroidism but no ocular findings, and euthyroid ophthalmopathy patients.[166] All patients with ophthalmopathy had positive reactivity;

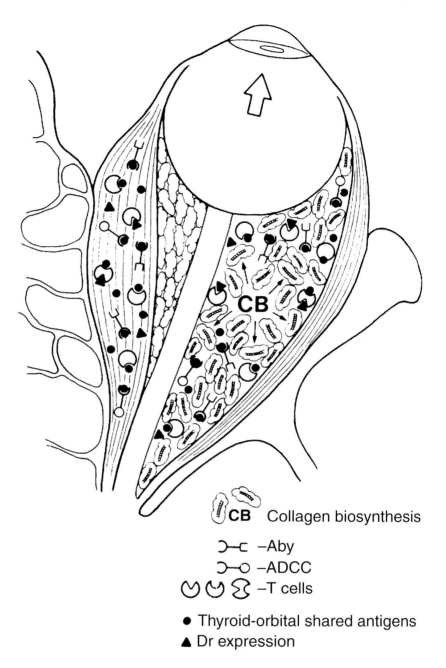

CB Collagen biosynthesis

)—c –Aby

)—o –ADCC

∪ ∪ ∽ –T cells

● Thyroid-orbital shared antigens

▲ Dr expression

Figure 6-6. Schematic mechanisms of immunologic mediated orbital change in thyroid eye disease.

however, one-third of patients with hyperthyroidism and no eye findings, and three of nine patients with euthyroid ophthalmopathy, also had positive MIF when tested with orbital antigens.[166] In a similar study, Mahieu and Winand noted positive MIF to thyroid and orbital antigens in six of 10 hyperthyroid patients who had no evidence of ophthalmopathy.[167,168]

Table 6-1. Immune Alterations in Graves' Ophthalmopathy

1. Immunogenetic: human leukocyte (HLA)-B, -DR and -DQ antigens
2. Cellular
   a. NK cells
   b. T cells (CD8 and CD4 subset perturbations)
   c. K cells (ADCC)
   d. CMI (migration-inhibiting factor, LS, cytotoxicity)
3. Humoral
   a. Reactivity to shared orbital-thyroid antigens
   b. Reactivity toward thyroid antigens
   c. Immunoglobulins that promote collagen biosynthesis
   d. Cytotoxic antibodies

Blau and coworkers studied cell-mediated cytotoxicity toward human autopsy extraocular muscle and control tissue. The reactivity of peripheral blood lymphocytes from an elderly, treated hyperthyroid patient with eye disease and high levels of antithyroglobulin was compared to that of a normal control. The patient had significantly more cytotoxicity against eye muscle than did the control—a reactivity undiminished by the addition of thyroglobulin.[169]

Two recent studies have demonstrated systemic signs of immunologic activation in thyroid eye disease patients. Interleukin (IL)-2 receptor activation has been noted in approximately 50% of thyroid eye disease patients. Several adhesion molecules important in lymphocyte transportation to reach an inflamed orbit have also been demonstrated in some of these patients.[170, 171]

Several groups have used cloning techniques on orbital decompression specimens from thyroid eye disease patients to analyze antigen arrays and T cell and B cell repertoires and their products. Some of these factors are shown with plausible pathways for thyroid orbitopathy in Figure 6-7. T cells are normally present in the orbit with equal numbers of CD8 cells and CD4 cells.[83,172,173] Many of the infiltrating T cells present in thyroid orbitopathy are activated memory cells.[173]

DeCarli and colleagues used IL-2 to propagate T cells from four orbital decompressions and compared these clones to those in the peripheral blood.[174] There was a reversal in the normal T cell CD4 to CD8 cell ratio. The profile of cytokines from orbital T cells predominantly includes IL-2, interferon (IFN)-gamma, and tumor necrosis factor (TNF)-alpha.[174] In another study, six T cell lines were grown from the orbital biopsies of two thyroid patients; these cell cultures were driven by IL-2, and the array of cytokines produced in vitro was analyzed.[175] These authors observed, as others before them, that these T cells are predominantly CD8+ and are mainly memory cells, probably with the IL-10 production-suppressing cytotoxicity.[176]

The nature of orbital B cells and their products has been studied by several investigators. Jaume and colleagues analyzed the array of immunoglobulin genes from the orbit of a thyroid orbitopathy patient with active disease.[177] They noted a very restricted repertoire of the genes that control immunoglobulin construction. These findings are similar to the restriction of heavy and light chains seen in the synovium of active rheumatoid arthritis.[177] In that study, 14 of 15 kappa clones were virtually identical. In a subsequent study, more diversity of lambda genes was noted; however, 12 of 15 clones were related to two family III germline genes.[178]

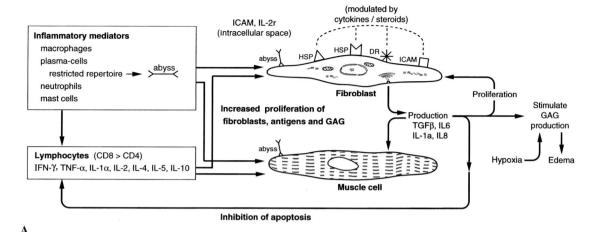

A

Figure 6-7. A. Plausible pathways for cytokines and other soluble factors in thyroid orbitopathy. B. The effect of the cytokines on both the muscles (enlargement) and on fibroblasts (augmented inflammation, increased GAG production and increased fibroblasts) results in proptosis, muscle enlargement and apical compression. Arrows demonstrate apical enlargement of muscles producing compression of the optic nerve.

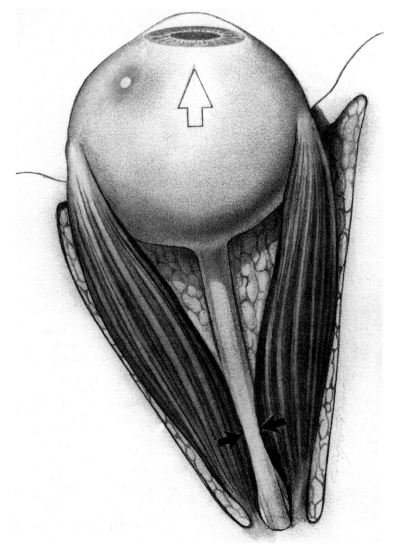

B

One of the V lambda genes had a high degree of homology with a monoclonal antibody to thyroglobulin.[179] As the authors point out, these B cell findings do not elucidate a primary versus secondary role of antibodies in the pathophysiology of thyroid orbitopathy.[178]

Intuitively, the muscle cell would appear to be a more likely target, since clinically and on imaging, the muscles are almost always involved in thyroid orbitopathy, while orbital fat less frequently shows signs of either lymphocytic infiltration or isolated volume expansion. In contrast, most histologic studies show little or no damage to the intrinsic muscle cells during the acute phase of thyroid orbitopathy when most inflammation is noted in the perimysial compartment between the muscle cells.

Some workers have studied a 64-kDa antigen shared between the eye muscle and the thyroid gland.[180] This antigen has 63% nucleotide homology with tropomodulin that binds tropomyosin.[181] In-depth analyses of that 64-kDa antigen with cloned eye muscle cDNA library demonstrated wider tissue distribution than just the thyroid and orbital tissues.[182,183] In several studies, minimal correlation between patients' serologic reactivity toward this 64-kDa antigen and thyroid eye disease status has been demonstrated, although Fall and colleagues have shown a better correlation when gentler separation techniques were used.[184–187] Antibody reactivity toward this 64-kDa antigen is probably a secondary phenomenon. More frequent reactivity in patients with only thyroid disease suggests it is a marker of thyroid autoimmunity, even though there is some cross-reactivity with orbital antigens.[188–190] Other investigators have not found that this antigen elicits a demonstrable T cell response.[191]

An intriguing negative study was performed with the middle ear musculature of five thyroid eye disease patients since these ear muscles are very similar in structure to the recti muscles. No evidence of middle ear muscle abnormalities was noted.[192]

There are more laboratory data consistent with the hypothesis that orbital fibroblasts are the primary focus for the inflammatory changes that occur in thyroid-related orbital disease. Most data suggest that HLA-DR antigens and intracellular adhesion molecule (ICAM) are present on orbital connective tissue in contrast to muscle cells.[108,171,193,194,194a] Several groups have shown that orbital fibroblasts are perturbed by and can alter intraorbital immune responses.[138] Most of the perturbing lymphocytes are CD4 and CD8 T cells that can produce several cytokines, including IL-2, IL-4, IL-5, IL-10, IFN-γ, TNF-α, and IL-1α. All of these cytokines have been demonstrated in the orbital connective tissues obtained from orbital decompression specimens.[195,196] The cytokines profile is more typical of a CD8 T cell—the reason these cells probably are not cytotoxic is because they also express IL-10.[174] Orbital connective tissue can produce autonomously or as a result of inflammation IL-1α, IL-6, and IL-8.[107]

Cytokines and corticosteroids can modulate fibroblast cell surface antigens, including heat shock protein, intercellular adhesion molecules, and HLA-D (class II) antigens.[138,197,198] The increased expression of these cell surface molecules can up-regulate a local immune or inflammatory response and allow the fibroblast to serve as an antigen presentation site. If the orbital fibroblast is the primary site of the autoimmune response, the immunologic perturbations in and around it could affect inflammation and fibrosis of the contiguous extraocular muscles. Fluid in the area would result in edema. Fibrosis of the extraocular muscles could be due to chronic compression and contiguous inflammation.[107] In addition to enlarged muscles, there is usually some increase in background orbital connective tissue. This process, once initiated, may be self-sustaining since fibroblast proliferation is stimulated by several cytokines, including IL-1α, IL-4, insulin-like growth factor, tumor growth factor-beta, and platelet-derived growth factors.[199]

In addition, the above cytokines, antibodies, and other inflammatory factors can increase glycosaminoglycan (GAG) production by the orbital fibroblasts.[138,200–204] GAG is a linear heteroglycan chain previously termed mucopolysaccharides that, after its release by the fibroblast, links with other proteins to form proteoglycans.[205] There are increased levels of GAG in the serum and urine in untreated patients.[202] GAG is a hydrophilic molecule whose production directly increases orbital volume and imbibes extracellular fluid with resultant edematous changes in the orbital connective tissue.[205,206]

Hypoxia also increases GAG production, and this could be a potential explanation for the epidemiologic data that has demonstrated an association between the eye disease and smoking.[207] Several studies demonstrated that smoking is associated with thyroid orbitopathy and that heavy smokers are likely to have severe disease.[208–214,214a] While there are several speculative mechanisms, including altered immunity, hypoxia, and effects on the thyroid gland function as the reasons for an association between smoking and thyroid eye disease, the nature of that association remains unclear.

Three cardinal questions remain about the initiation of thyroid orbitopathy. First, what is the pathogenic shared antigen? Second, why are there a number of incongruities in the clinical pattern given the shared thyroid gland-orbital antigen? These incongruities include the more frequent involvement of the inferior recti, compared to other muscles, orbital asymmetry, and the rarity of this disease in non-Graves' thyroid disease. Third, what is the role of primary and secondary orbital vascular engorgement? Feldon and others documented increased size of the superior ophthalmic vein on imaging studies and proposed that a decrease in orbital venous outflow might be important in the etiology and maintenance of orbital swelling.[215,216] Others believe orbital swelling occurs, impeding venous return. The nature and etiology of these and other findings remain to be elucidated.

MECHANISMS OF LID, EXTRAOCULAR MUSCLE, AND OPTIC NERVE INVOLVEMENT IN THYROID EYE DISEASE

The protean nature of thyroid eye disease has resulted in many clinical misconceptions in the pathophysiology of extraocular muscle, lid, and optic nerve disorders. Some investigations have clarified the developments responsible for clinical signs and symptoms in thyroid eye disease.

Extraocular Muscle Disease

Although Naumann first noted the involvement of extraocular muscles in thyroid eye disease in 1853, the pathophysiologic mechanisms responsible for restrictive thyroid myopathy were not appreciated for many years.[217] As discussed earlier in this chapter, numerous investigators since 1898 have identified an inflammatory infiltrate and its sequelae in extraocular muscles.[75–79,83] Initially, most clinicians believed that the inability to elevate an eye was due to a paresis of the superior rectus rather than to tethering of the inferior rectus muscle.[218–220] Data from Dunnington and Berke on forced duction test results suggested that restrictive myopathy was responsible for many of the motility problems observed in thyroid eye disease.[221] Ridley, in a paper discussing thyroid ophthalmopathy, also supported the idea of restrictive myopathy, which has since been demonstrated by a number of clinical and electrophysiologic studies.[221–223] Jensen observed no changes in the electromyographic recordings of extraocular muscles in thyroid ophthalmopathy patients.[224] Metz studied 15 patients with stable thyroid eye disease, all of whom had limited upgaze. Electro-oculographic measurements of saccadic velocities were normal.[225] Feldon and Unsold used a more sensitive technique to measure eye muscle movements, observing that peak velocities decreased with more advanced extraocular muscle disease.[226] While the vast majority of thyroid-related diplopia is secondary to muscle tethering, some cases of paresis on an idiopathic basis or secondary to such other diseases as myasthenia gravis have been reported.[227]

Several issues remain unresolved regarding restrictive myopathy in thyroid eye disease. CT, MRI, and ultrasonography demonstrate more generalized extraocular muscle enlargement than can be appreciated clinically, yet examination generally reveals greater inferior and medial recti involvement.[228] The likelihood that upgaze will be the first affected eye movement in thyroid eye disease has not been satisfactorily explained; Kriss' idea that this muscle is involved more commonly because of its proximity to the lymphatic circulation appears too simple. Even the fact that vertical fusional amplitudes are less than horizontal ones does not explain why the inferior rectus, and not the superior rectus, is more commonly symptomatic. Finally, it is unclear why clinical oblique muscle involvement in the disease process is rare.

Eyelid Changes in Ophthalmopathy

Advances in other areas of ophthalmology research were analogous to the uneven development of understanding about extraocular muscle pathology. For instance, lid lag and stare were among the first recognized signs of thyroid eye disease, yet concepts regarding their pathophysiology remained obscure for many years.[229,230] Various investigations demonstrated that sympathetic stimulation and increased levels of thyroid hormone could produce lid retraction and stare, and that these eye signs resolved with amelioration of thyrotoxicosis.[3,28,30] Histologically, the findings in the levator are similar to extraocular muscles; there is minimal intramuscle cell inflammation, although one study showed cytomorphic evidence of muscle cell enlargement.[231–233] The latter findings may help to explain why the levator-superior rectus muscle complex is sometimes shown to be enlarged on coronal CT or MRI.[172] Proptosis is correlated with change in levator function, and this helps to explain why there is an increased tendency for these patients to develop levator disinsertions.[234]

Sympathetic stimulation of Müller's muscle is probably responsible for most of the medically reversible lid retraction in Graves' disease; it often improves after administration of sympatholytic agents.[235–237] Exophthalmos is another factor in lid retraction—increased orbital volume causes anterior displacement of the globe, which can also cause lid retraction and scleral show. A third mechanism responsible for eyelid retraction is inferior rectus fibrosis. The superior rectus-levator muscle complex must overcontract on attempted upgaze to counteract the fibrotic inferior rectus muscle, resulting in lid retraction. Despite this knowledge, it is usually impossible to delineate the relative roles of exophthalmos, compensatory levator overaction, and sympathetic overaction in lid retraction.[228,238] Occasionally a trial with sympatholytic agents is useful, although false-positive and false-negative results can occur.

As discussed in the therapy sections, varied surgical procedures have been developed to treat eyelid retraction.[239–247]

Optic Neuropathy

The first description of thyroid optic neuropathy was in 1921.[248] Although there were histologic studies of a few damaged nerves, they did not clarify the pathogenesis of the neuropathy.[248,249] Among the mechanisms postulated to cause optic neuropathy in thyroid eye disease were humoral, vascular, toxic, and miscellaneous factors.[250–252]

It is unclear why approximately 5% of thyroid eye disease patients develop optic neuropathy. As previously mentioned, MRI and CT have demonstrated that apical compression of the nerve by enlarged extraocular muscles results in this disease complication. As discussed in Chapter 5, recent CT and MRI studies have shown that increased extraocular muscle volume or area correlate with compressive optic neuropathy (Figure 6-8).[253,254] Probably the increased extraocular muscle volume is also responsible for increased orbital compliance that is observed in compressive neuropathy patients.[255] Moreover, in a few patients there appears to be inflammation of the optic nerve and its sheath. Some have theorized that optic neuropathy patients have shallow orbits, or that they lack the ability to self-decompress anteriorly. However, in one study, patients with optic neuropathy had significantly more proptosis than those who did not develop this complication.[256] In that study diabetic patients were more frequent in the neuropathy group (16%) versus others (2%).[256] It has not yet been determined prospectively which thyroid ophthalmopathy patients are at greatest risk for optic neuropathy, although older patients with enlarged extraocular muscles and limited motility are more likely to develop this complication.[257–262] An axial spin-lattice MRI (Figure 6-9) shows enlarged muscles producing unilateral optic nerve compression, while the contralateral nerve appears (and functions) in an uninvolved manner.

CONCLUSION

The inciting events in the development of thyroid ophthalmopathy remain unknown. Increasingly, data demonstrate immunologic alterations in thyroid eye disease; however, it remains unclear which of these alterations are pathogenically important or merely secondary epiphenomena. It is probable that these immune system abnormalities are significant, but a better understanding of the nature of the immunologic alterations responsible for Graves' disease development will be necessary before the relationship between ophthalmopathy and thyroid disease or the importance of immunologic alterations in thyroid eye disease can be fully understood.

While basic pathophysiologic mechanisms in ophthalmopathy await further study (see Chapters 8–13), improved understanding of lid retraction, restrictive myopathy, and optic neuropathy have led to more effective therapeutic approaches in the management of thyroid eye disease.

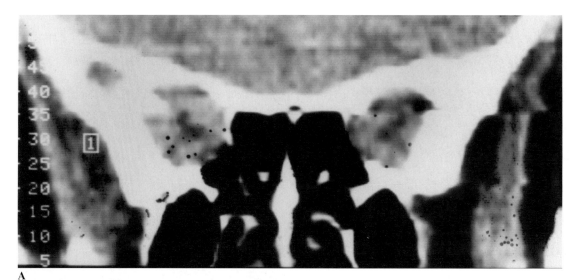

A

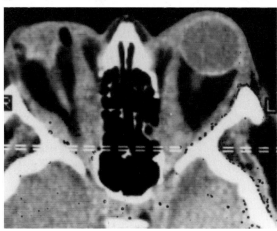

B

Figure 6-8. Computed tomography scans demonstrating compression of the apical portion of the optic nerve by enlarged recti muscles. A. Axial scan. B. Coronal reformation.

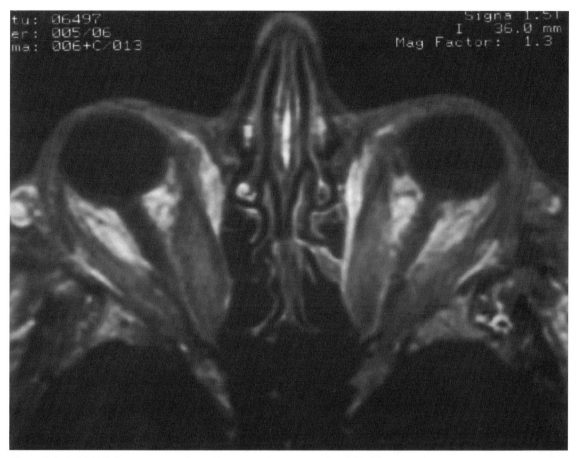

Figure 6-9. Axial MR shows compressive optic neuropathy worse on the right side.

REFERENCES

1. Burch HB, Wartofsky L. Graves' ophthalmopathy: current concepts regarding pathogenesis and management. Endocr Rev 1993;14:747.
2. Dobyns BM. Present concepts of the pathologic physiology of exophthalmos. J Clin Endocrinol Metab 1950;10:1202.
3. Werner SC. Ocular Manifestations in the Thyroid. In S Ingbar, S Werner (eds), The Thyroid. New York: Harper & Row, 1971;528.
4. Aranow H Jr, Day RM. Management of thyrotoxicosis in patients with ophthalmopathy: antithyroid regimen determined primarily by ocular manifestations. J Clin Endocrinol Metab 1965;25:1.
5. Kriss JP, McDougall IR, Donaldson SS. Graves' ophthalmopathy. In DT Krieger, CW Borden (eds), Theory in Endocrinology. Philadelphia: BC Decker, 1983.
6. Coleman DJ, Jack RL, Franzen LA, Werner SC. High resolution B-scan ultrasonography of the orbit. V. eye changes in Graves' disease. Arch Ophthalmol 1972;88:465.
7. Forrester JV, Sutherland JR, McDougall IR. Dysthyroid ophthalmopathy: orbital evaluation with B-scan ultrasonography. J Clin Endocrinol Metab 1977;45:221.
8. Shammas HJ, Minckler DS, Ogden C. Ultrasound in early thyroid orbitopathy. Arch Ophthalmol 1980;98:277.

9. Werner SC, Coleman DJ, Franzen LA. Ultrasonographic evidence of a consistent orbital involvement in Graves' disease. N Engl J Med 1974;290:1447.

10. Skalka HW. The use of ultrasonography in the diagnosis of endocrine orbitopathy. Neurol Ophthalmol 1980;1:109.

11. Gorman CA. Temporal relationship between onset of Graves' ophthalmopathy and diagnosis of thyrotoxicosis. Mayo Clin Proc 1983;58:1515.

12. Amino N, Yuasa T, Yabu Y, et al. Exophthalmos in autoimmune thyroid disease. J Clin Endocrinol Metab 1980;51:1232.

13. Wiersinga WM, Smit T, van der Gaag R, Koornneeff L. Clinical presentation of Graves' ophthalmopathy. Ophthalmic Res 1989;21:73.

14. Sattler H. Die Basedow'sche krankheit. Graefe-saemisch Handb Ges Augenh 1909;9:1.

15. Pequegnat EP, Mayberry WE, McConahey WM, Wyse EP. Large doses of radioiodide in Graves' disease: effect on ophthalmopathy and long-acting thyroid stimulator. Mayo Clin Proc 1967;42:802.

16. Rapoport B, Greenspan FS, Fietti S, Pepitone M. Clinical experience with a human thyroid cell bioassay for thyroid-stimulating immunoglobulin. J Clin Endocrinol Metab 1984;58:332.

17. Salvi M, Zhang ZG, Haegert D, et al. Patients with endocrine ophthalmopathy not associated with overt thyroid disease have multiple thyroid immunological abnormalities. J Clin Endocrinol Metab 1990;70:89.

18. Enzmann DR, Donaldson SS, Kriss JP. Appearance of Graves' disease on orbital computed tomography. J Comput Assist Tomogr 1979;3:815.

19. Von Basedow CA. Exophthalmos durch hypertrophie des zellgewebes in der augenhohle. Wchnschr F D Ges Heilk 1840;6:197.

20. Cooper W. On protrusions of eyes in connection with anemia, palpitation and goitre. Lancet 1849;1:55.

21. Jones CH, Cantab MB. On a case of proptosis, goitre, palpitation, etc. Lancet 1860;2:562.

22. Boddaert R. Recherches expérimentales sur la production de l'exophtalmie et la pathogenie de l'oedeme. Bull Acad R de Med de Belg 1891;5:690.

23. Thomson ES. Orbital edema in exophthalmic goitre. Am J Ophthalmol 1924;7:27.

24. Bernard C. Leçons sur la physiologie et la pathologie du système nerveux (Vols 1–2). Paris: JB Ballière et Fils, 1852;499.

25. Krauss W. Zur anatomie der glatten muskeln der menschlichen augenhohle nach untersuchungen am neugeborenen. I Arch F Augenh 1912;71:277.

26. McLean JM, Norton EWD. Unilateral lid retraction without exophthalmos. Arch Ophthalmol 1958;61:681.

27. Drescher EP, Benedict WL. Asymmetric exophthalmos. Arch Ophthalmol 1950;44:109.

28. Woods AC. The ocular changes of primary diffuse toxic goitre. Medicine (Baltimore) 1946;25:113.

29. Aird RB. Experimental exophthalmos and the associated myopathy induced by the thyrotropic hormone. Arch Ophthalmol 1940;24:1167.

30. Marine D. Studies on pathological physiology of exophthalmos of Graves' disease. Ann Intern Med 1938;12:443.

31. Plummer WA, Wilder RM. Etiology of exophthalmos. Arch Ophthalmol 1935;13:833.

32. Smelser GK. A comparative study of experimental and clinical exophthalmos. Am J Ophthalmol 1937;20:1189.

33. Sellers EA, Ferguson JKW. Exophthalmos in rats after prolonged administration of propylthiouracil. Endocrinology 1949;45:345.

34. Loeb L, Friedman H. Exophthalmos produced by injections of acid extract of anterior pituitary gland of cattle. Proc Soc Exp Biol Med 1932;29:648.

35. Marine D, Rosen SH. Exophthalmos in thyroidectomized guinea pigs by thyrotropic substance of anterior pituitary and the mechanism involved. Proc Soc Exp Biol Med 1933;30:901.

36. Wybar KC. The nature of endocrine exophthalmos. Bibl Ophthalmol 1957;49:119.

37. Cope CL. The anterior pituitary lobe in Graves' disease and in myxedema. QJM 1938;31:151.

38. Hertz S, Oastler EG. Assay of blood and urine for thyrotropic hormone in thyrotoxicosis and myxedema. Endocrinology 1936;20:520.

39. Robinson AR. Thyrotropic and antithyrotropic factors in some types of thyroid disease. Med J Aust 1941;1:349.

40. Starr P, Rawson RW. Estimation of thyrotropic hormone in human urine and blood in health and disease by the micrometric analysis of the response of the guinea pig thyroid. Proceedings of the American Society of Clinical Investigation. J Clin Invest 1937;16:657.

41. Means JH. The nature of Graves' disease with special reference to its ophthalmic component. Am J Med Sci 1944;207:1.

42. Collard HB, Mills FH, Rundle FF, Sharpey-Schaeffer EP. Thyrotropic hormone in blood. Clin Sci 1940;4:323.

43. Hertz S, Means JH, Williams RH. Graves' disease with dissociation of thyrotoxicosis and ophthalmopathy. West J Surg 1941;49:493.

44. Purves HD, Griesbach WE. Thyrotropic hormone in thyrotoxicosis, malignant exophthalmos and myxoedema. Br J Exp Pathol 1949;30:23.

45. Furth ED, Becker DV, Ray BS, Kane JW. Appearance of unilateral infiltrative exophthalmos of Graves' disease after successful treatment of this same process and the contralateral eye by apparently total surgical hypophysectomy. J Clin Endocrinol 1962;22:518.

46. Kourides IA, Weintraub BD, Ridgway EC, Maloof F. Pituitary secretion of free alpha and beta subunit of human thyrotropin in patients with thyroid disorders. J Clin Endocrinol Metab 1975;40:872.

47. Volpe R. The pathogenesis of Graves' disease: an overview. Clin Endocrinol Metab 1978;7:3.

48. Wall JR, Henderson J, Strakosch CR, Joyner DM. Graves' ophthalmopathy. Can Med Assoc J 1981;124:855.

49. Sergott RC, Glaser JS. Graves' ophthalmopathy. A clinical and immunologic review. Surv Ophthalmol 1981;26:1.

50. Volpe R. Suppressor T lymphocyte dysfunction is important in the pathogenesis of autoimmune thyroid disease: a perspective. Thyroid 1993;3:345.

51. Volpe R. Immunoregulation in autoimmune thyroid disease. Thyroid 1994;4:373.

52. Kohn LD, Shimura H, Shimura Y, et al. The thyrotropin receptor. Vitam Horm 1995;50:287.

53. Kohn LD, Winand RJ. Relationship of thyrotropin to exophthalmos-producing substance. Formation of an exophthalmos-producing substance by pepsin digestion of pituitary glycoproteins containing both thyrotropic and exophthalmogenic activity. J Biol Chem 1971;246:6570.

54. Kriss JP, Konishi J, Herman MM. Studies on the pathogenesis of Graves' ophthalmopathy. Recent Prog Horm Res 1975;31:533.

55. Thomas HM Jr. Exophthalmos in light of current anti-thyroid therapy. Am J Med 1951;11:581.

56. Burch FE. The exophthalmos of Graves' disease. Minn Med 1929;12:668.

57. Bedrossian EH. Unilateral thyrotropic exophthalmos. Am J Ophthalmol 1951;34:727.

58. Fischer C. Discussion of WR Parker. Double luxation of the eyeballs in a case of exophthalmic goiter. Trans Am Ophthalmol Soc 1921;19:134.

59. Gleason JE. Idiopathic myositis involving the extraocular muscles. Ophthalmic Res 1903;12:471.

60. Plummer WA, Wilder RM. Some observations on the etiology of exophthalmos in exophthalmic goiter. Proc Staff Meet Mayo Clin 1934;9:765.

61. Dayton GO Jr. The ocular changes in thyrotropic exophthalmos. Am J Ophthalmol 1953;36:1049.

62. Kronfeld PC. Die augenmuskeln bei hyperthyreoiditischem, die thyreoidektomie ueberdauerndem exophthalmus. Ber Zusammenkunft Dtsch Ophth Gesellsch Leipzig 1932;49:529.

63. Thomas HM Jr, Woods AC. Progressive exophthalmos following thyroidectomy. Bull Johns Hopkins Hosp 1936;59:99.

64. Friedenwald JS. Orbital myositis and choked disc in exophthalmic goitre. Ann Surg 1932;96:995.

65. Medine MM. Malignant exophthalmos. Am J Ophthalmol 1951;34:1587.

66. Hufnagel TJ, Hickey WF, Cobbs WH, et al. Immunohistochemical and ultrastructural studies on the exenterated orbit of a patient with Graves' disease. Ophthalmology 1984;91:1411.

67. Rundle FF, Pochin EE. Orbital tissues in thyrotoxicosis: a quantitative analysis relating to exophthalmos. Clin Sci 1944;5:51.

68. Enzmann D, Marshall WH Jr, Rosenthal AR, Kriss JP. Computed tomography in Graves' ophthalmopathy. Radiology 1976;118:615.

69. Trokel SL, Jakobiec FA. Correlation of CT scanning and pathologic features of ophthalmic Graves' disease. Ophthalmology 1981;88:553.

70. Feldon SE, Weiner JM. Clinical significance of extraocular muscle volumes in Graves' ophthalmopathy: a quantitative computed tomography study. Arch Ophthalmol 1982;100:1266.

71. Ringel SR, Wilson WB, Barden MT, Kaiser KK. Histochemistry of human extraocular muscles. Arch Ophthalmol 1978;96:1067.

72. Carry MR, Rignel SP, Starcevich JM. Mitochondrial morphometrics of histologically identified human extraocular muscle fibers. Anat Rec 1986;214:8.

73. Silcock AQ. Case of exophthalmic goiter. Trans Ophthalmol Soc UK 1886;6:103.

74. Dudgeon LS, Urquhart AL. Lymphorrages in the muscles in exophthalmic goitre. Brain 1926;49:182.

75. Askanazy M. Pathologische-anatomische beitrage zur kenntiss des morbus Basedowii, insbesondere über die dabei auftretende muskelerkrankung. D Arch Klin Med 1898;61:118.

76. Mulvany JH. The exophthalmos of hyperthyroidism. Am J Ophthalmol 1944;27:589.

77. Tengroth B. Histological studies of orbital tissues in a case of endocrine exophthalmos before and after remission. Acta Ophthalmol 1964;42:588.

78. Falconer MA, Alexander WS. Experiences with malignant exophthalmos; relationship of condition to thyrotoxicosis and to pituitary thyrotropic hormone. Br J Ophthalmol 1951;35:253.

79. Daicker B. Das gewebliche substrat der verdickten aussberen augenmuskeln bei der endokrinen orbitopathie. Klin Monatsbl Augenheilkd 1979;174:843.

80. Havard CWH. Progress in endocrine exophthalmos. Br Med J (English Abstract) 1979;1:1001.

81. Kroll HA, Kuwabara T. Dysthyroid ocular myopathy. Arch Ophthalmol 1966;76:244.

82. Daicker B. The histological substrate of the extraocular muscle thickening seen in dysthyroid orbitopathy. Klin Monatsbl Augenheilkd 1979;174:843.

83. Tallstedt ML, Norberg R. Immunohistochemical staining of normal and Graves' extraocular muscle. Invest Ophthalmol Vis Sci 1988;29:175.

84. Kiljanski JI, Nebes V, Wall JR. The ocular muscle cell is a target of the immune system in endocrine ophthalmopathy. Int Arch Allergy Immunol 1995;106:204.

85. Smelser GK, Ozanics V. Studies on the nature of exophthalmos-producing principle in pituitary extracts. Am J Ophthalmol 1954;38:107.

86. Riley FC Jr. Orbital pathology in Graves' disease. Mayo Clin Proc 1972;47:975.

87. Wegelius O, Asboe-Hansen G, Lamberg BA. Retrobulbar connective tissue changes in malignant exophthalmos. Acta Endocrinol (Copenh) 1957;25:452.

88. Ludwig AW, Boas NF, Soffer LJ. Role of mucopolysaccharides in the pathogenesis of experimental exophthalmos. Proc Soc Exp Biol Med 1950;73:137.

89. Forbes G, Gorman CA, Gehring D, Baker HL Jr. Computer analysis of orbital fat and muscle volumes in Graves' ophthalmopathy. AJNR Am J Neuroradiol 1983;4:737.

90. Char DH, Norman D. The use of computed tomography and ultrasonography in the evaluation of orbital masses. Surv Ophthalmol 1982;27:49.

91. Char DH. Advances in thyroid orbitopathy. Neuroophthal 1992;12:25.

92. Duke-Elder S. System of Ophthalmology (Vol 13, part 2). St. Louis: Mosby, 1974;935.

93. Trokel SL, Hilal SK. Recognition and differential diagnosis of enlarged extraocular muscles in computed tomography. Am J Ophthalmol 1979;87:503.

94. Perros P, Kendall-Taylor P. Pathogenetic mechanisms in thyroid-associated ophthalmopathy. J Intern Med 1992;231:205.

95. Kahaly G, Schuler M, Sewell AC, et al. Urinary glycosaminoglycans in Graves' ophthalmopathy. Clin Endocrinol 1990;33:35.

96. Frecker M, Stenszky V, Balazs C, et al. Genetic factors in Graves' ophthalmopathy. Clin Endocrinol 1986;25:479.

97. Farid NR. Immunogenetics of autoimmune thyroid disorders. Endocrinol Metab Clin North Am 1987;16:229.

98. Sergott RC, Felbert NT, Savino PJ, et al. Association of HLA antigen Bw35 with severe Graves' ophthalmopathy. Invest Ophthalmol Vis Sci 1983;24:124.

99. Todd JA, Acha-Orbea H, Bell JI, et al. A molecular basis for MHC class II-associated autoimmunity. Science 1988;240:1003.

100. Dong R-P, Kimura, A, Okubo, R, et al. HLA-ADPB1 loci confer susceptibility to Graves' disease. Hum Immunol 1992;35:165.

101. Weetman AP, So AK, Warner CA, et al. Immunogenetics of Graves' ophthalmopathy. Clin Endocrinol 1988;28:619.

102. Weetman AP, Zhang L, Webb S, Shine B. Analysis of HLA-DQB and HLA-DPB alleles in Graves' disease by oligonucleotide probing of enzymically amplified DNA. Clin Endocrinol 1990;33:65.

103. Kendall-Taylor P, Stephenson A, Stratton A, et al. Differentiation of autoimmune ophthalmopathy from Graves' hyperthyroidism by analysis of genetic markers. Clin Endocrinol 1988;28:601.

104. Singh VK, Yamaki K, Donoso LA, Shinohara T. Molecular mimicry. Yeast histone H3-induced experimental autoimmune uveitis. J Immunol 1989;142:1512.

105. Quaratino S, Thorpe CJ, Travers PJ, Londei M. Similar antigenic surfaces, rather than sequence homology, dictate T cell epitope molecular mimicry. Proc Natl Acad Sci U S A 1995;92:10398.

106. Elisei R, Weightman D, Kendall-Taylor P, et al. Muscle autoantigens in thyroid associated ophthalmopathy: The limits of molecular genetics. J Endocrinol Invest 1993;16:533.

107. Heufelder AE. Pathogenesis of Graves' ophthalmopathy: recent controversies and progress. Eur J Endocrinol 1995;132:532.

108. Heufelder AE, Bahn RS. Elevated expression in situ of selectin and immunoglobulin superfamily adhesion molecules in retroocular connective tissues from patients with Graves' ophthalmopathy. Clin Exp Immunol 1993;91:381.

109. Hart IR, McKenzie JM. Comparison of the effects of thyrotropin and the long-acting thyroid stimulator on guinea pig adipose. Endocrinology 1971;88:26.

110. Gill DL, Marshall NJ, Ekins RP. Binding of thyrotropin to receptors in fat tissue. Mol Cell Endocrinol 1978;10:89.

111. Doniach D. The pathogenesis of endocrine exophthalmos: a short review. Proc R Soc Med 1977;70:695.

112. Winand RJ, Kohn LD. The binding of ^{3}H-thyrotropin and ^{3}H labeled exophthalmogenic factor by plasma membranes of retro-orbital tissue. Proc Natl Acad Sci U S A 1972;69:1711.

113. Kohn LD, Winand RJ. Experimental exophthalmos. Alteration of normal hormone-receptor interactions in the pathogenesis of a disease. Isr J Med Sci 1974;10:1348.

114. Bolonkin D, Tate RL, Luber JH, et al. Experimental exophthalmos. Binding of thyrotropin and an exophthalmogenic factor derived from thyrotropin to retro-orbital tissue plasma membranes. J Biol Chem 1975;250:6516.

115. Winand RJ, Salmon J, Lambert PH. Characterization of the Exophthalmogenic Factor Isolated from the Serum of Patients with Malignant Exophthalmos. In K Fellinger, R Hofer (eds), Further Advances in Thyroid Research. Vienna, Austria: Verlag der Wiener Mediz Acad, 1971;583.

116. Winand RJ, Kohn LD. Stimulation of adenylate cyclase activity in retro-orbital tissue membranes by thyrotropin and an exophthalmogenic factor derived from thyrotropin. J Biol Chem 1975;250:6522.

117. Mullin BR, Levinson RE, Friedman A, et al. Delayed hypersensitivity in Graves' disease and exophthalmos: identification of thyroglobulin in normal human orbital muscle. Endocrinology 1977;100:351.

118. Ludgate M, Swillens S, Mercken L, Vassart G. Homology between thyroglobulin and acetylcholinesterase: an explanation for pathogenesis of Graves' ophthalmopathy? Lancet 1986;2:219.

119. Weetman AP, Tse CK, Randall WR, et al. Acetylcholinesterase antibodies and thyroid autoimmunity. Clin Exp Immunol 1988;71:96.

120. Hansson HA, Petruson B, Skottner A. Somatomedin C in pathogenesis of malignant exophthalmos of endocrine origin. Lancet 1986;1:218.

121. Jacobson DM. Acetylcholine receptor antibodies in patients with Graves' ophthalmopathy. J Neuroophthalmol 1995;13:166.

122. Francis T, Burch HB, Cai WY, et al. Lymphocytes express thyrotropin receptor specific mRNA as detected by the PCR technique. Thyroid 1991;1:223.

123. Heufelder AE, Bahn RS. Evidence for the presence of a functional TSH-receptor in retroocular fibroblasts from patients with Graves' ophthalmopathy. Exp Clin Endocrinol 1992;100:62.

124. Feliciello A, Porcellini A, Ciullo I, et al. Expression of thyrotropin receptor mRNA in healthy and Graves' disease retro-orbital tissue. Lancet 1993;342:337.

125. Paschke R, Elisei R, Vassart G, Ludgate M. Lack of evidence supporting the presence of mRNA for the TSH receptor in extraocular muscle. J Endocrinol Invest 1993;16:329.

126. Paschke R, Vassart G, Ludgate M. Current evidence for and against the TSH receptor being the common antigen in Graves' disease and thyroid associated ophthalmopathy. Clin Endocrinol 1995;42:565.

127. Perros P, Kendall-Taylor P. Demonstration of thyrotropin binding sites in orbital connective tissue: possible role in the pathogenesis of thyroid-associated ophthalmopathy. J Endocrinol Invest 1994;17:163.

128. Tonacchera M, Costagliola S, Cetani F, et al. Patient with monoclonal gamopathy, thyrotoxicosis, pretibial myxedema and thyroid-associated ophthalmopathy; demonstration of direct binding of autoantibodies to the thyrotropin receptor. Eur J Endocrinol 1996;134:97.

129. McLachlan SM, Bahn R, Rapoport B. Endocrine ophthalmopathy: a re-evaluation of the association with thyroid autoantibodies. Autoimmunity 1992;14:143.

130. Morris J, Hay ID, Nelson RE, Jiang NS. Clinical utility of thyrotropin receptor antibody assays: comparison of radio-receptor and bioassay methods. Mayo Clin Proc 1988;63:707.

131. Korducki JM, Loftus SJ, Bahn RS. Stimulation of glycosaminoglycan production in cultured human retroocular fibroblasts. Invest Ophthalmol Vis Sci 1992;33:2037.

132. Weetman AP. Minireview: extrathyroidal complications of Graves' disease. QJM 1988;86:2617.

133. Heufelder AE, Dutton CM, Sarkar G, et al. Detection of TSH receptor RNA in cultured fibroblasts from patients with Graves' ophthalmopathy and pretibial dermopathy. Thyroid 1993;3:297.

134. Mengistu M, Lukes YG, Nagy EV, et al. TSH receptor gene expression in retroocular fibroblasts. J Endocrinol Invest 1994;17:437.

135. Chang T-C, Wu S-L, Hsiao Y-L, et al. TSH and TSH receptor antibody-binding sites in fibroblasts of pretibial myxedema are related to the extracellular domain of entire TSH receptor. Clin Immunol Immunopathol 1994;71:113.

136. Endo T, Ohno M, Kotani S, et al. Thyrotropin receptor in non-thyroid tissues. Biochem Biophys Res Commun 1993;190:774.

137. Bahn RS, Dutton CM, Heufelder AE, Sarkar G. A genomic point mutation in the extracellular domain of the thyrotropin receptor in patients with Graves' ophthalmopathy. J Clin Endocrinol Metab 1994;78(2):256.

138. Bahn RS, Heufelder AE. Pathogenesis of Graves' ophthalmopathy. N Engl J Med 1993;329:1468.

139. Atkinson S, Holcombe M, Kendall-Taylor P. Ophthalmopathic immunoglobulin in patients with Graves' ophthalmopathy. Lancet 1984;2:374.

140. Faryna M, Nauman J, Gardas A. Measurement of autoantibodies against human eye muscle plasma membranes in Graves' ophthalmopathy. Br Med J 1985;290:191.

141. Kendall-Taylor P. The pathogenesis of Graves' ophthalmopathy. Clin Endocrinol Metab 1985;14:331-349.

142. Ahmann A, Baker JR Jr, Weetman AP, et al. Antibodies to porcine eye muscle in patients with Graves' ophthalmopathy: identification of serum immunoglobulins directed against unique determinants by immunoblotting and enzyme-linked immunosorbent assay. J Clin Endocrinol Metab 1987;64:454.

143. Nauman J, Faryna M, Gardas A. Humoral Immunity in Graves' ophthalmopathy. In HA Drexhage, WM Wiersinga (eds), The Thyroid and Autoimmunity. Amsterdam: Elsevier, 1986;248.

144. Kendall-Taylor P, Jones D, Atkinson S. The specificity of autoantibodies in Graves' disease. Acta Endocrinol 1987 (Suppl);281:330.

145. Adler G, Nauman J, Faryna M, et al. Humoral mediated immunity in Graves'-Basedow ophthalmopathy. Radiobiol Radiother 1987;28:570.

146. Kadlubowski M, Irvine WJ, Rowland AC. Anti-muscle antibodies in Graves' ophthalmopathy. J Clin Lab Immunol 1987;24:105.

147. Miller A, Sikorska H, Salvi M, Wall JR. Evaluation of an enzyme-linked immunosorbent assay for the measurement of autoantibodies against eye muscle membrane antigens in Graves' ophthalmopathy. Acta Endocrinol (Copenh) 1986;113:514.

148. Bjelkenkrantz K, Karlsson A, Mendel-Hartvig I, Totterman TH. Ophthalmopathic immunoglobulin not detected in patients with Graves' ophthalmopathy. Br Med J 1986;292:597.

149. Sikorska H, Wall JR. Failure to detect eye muscle membrane specific autoantibodies in Graves' ophthalmopathy. Br Med J 1985;291:604.

150. Banovac K, Levis S, Byrne F. A study of the binding of Graves' immunoglobulins to orbital antigens. J Endocrinol Invest 1988;11:483.

151. Mengistu M, Laryea E, Miller A, Wall JR. Clinical significance of a new autoantibody against a human eye muscle soluble antigen, detected by immunofluorescence. Clin Exp Immunol 1986;65:19.

152. Salvi M, Miller A, Wall JR. Human orbital tissue and thyroid membranes express a 64kDa protein which is recognized by autoantibodies in the serum of patients with thyroid-associated ophthalmopathy. FEBS Lett 1988;232:135.

153. Kodama K, Sikorska H, Bandy-Dafoe P, et al. Demonstration of a circulating autoantibody against a soluble eye-muscle antigen in Graves' ophthalmopathy. Lancet 1982;2:1353.

154. Metz HS, Woolf PD, Patton ML. Endocrine ophthalmopathy in adolescence. J Pediatr Ophthalmol Strabismus 1982;19:58.

155. Kuroki T, Ruf J, Whelan L, et al. Antithyroglobulin monoclonal and autoantibodies cross-react with an orbital connective tissue membrane antigen: a possible mechanism for the association of ophthalmopathy with autoimmune thyroid disorders. Clin Exp Immunol 1985;62:361.

156. Waring S, Kodama K, Sikorska H, Wall JR. TSH and orbital antibodies [letter to the editor]. Lancet 1983;2:224.

157. Takeda Y, Kriss JP. Radiometric measurement of thyroglobulin-antithyroglobulin immune complex in human serum. J Clin Endocrinol Metab 1977;44:46.

158. Kidd A, Okita N, Row VV, Volpe R. Immunologic aspects of Graves' and Hashimoto's diseases. Metabolism 1980;29:80.

159. Wang PW, Hiromatsu Y, Laryea E, et al. Immunologically mediated cytotoxicity against human eye muscle cells in Graves' ophthalmopathy. J Clin Endocrinol Metab 1986;63:316.

160. Cenmamo G, Bizzaro A, Castello G. T-lymphocyte-subsets in endocrine exophthalmos. Metab Pediatr Syst Ophthalmol 1985;8:43.

161. Felberg NT, Sergott RC, Savino PJ, et al. Lymphocyte subpopulations in Graves' ophthalmopathy. Arch Ophthalmol 1985;103:656.

162. Barsouk A, Wengrowicz S, Scalise D, et al. New assays for the measurement of serum antibodies reactive with eye muscle membrane antigens confirm their significance in thyroid-associated ophthalmopathy. Thyroid 1995;5:195.

163. Hiromatsu Y, Fukazawa H, How J, Wall JR. Antibody-dependent cell-mediated cytotoxicity against human eye muscle cells and orbital fibroblasts in Graves' ophthalmopathy—roles of class II MHC antigen expression and gamma-interferon action on effector target cells. Clin Exp Immunol 1987;70:593.

164. Wall JR, Trewin A, Joyner DM. Peripheral blood lymphocyte transformation in response to human thyroid fractions in patients with Graves' hyperthyroidism and ophthalmopathy. Acta Endocrinol (Copenh) 1980;93:419.

165. Wenzel B, Kotulla P, Wenzel KW, et al. Mitogenic response of peripheral blood lymphocytes from patients with Graves' disease incubated with solubilized thyroid cell membranes containing TSH receptor and with thyroglobulin. Immunobiology 1981;160:302.

166. Munro RE, Lamki L, Row VV, Volpe R. Cell-mediated immunity to the exophthalmos of Graves' disease as demonstrated by the migration of inhibition factor (MIF) test. J Clin Endocrinol Metab 1973;37:286.

167. Mahieu P, Winand R. Demonstration of delayed hypersensitivity to retrobulbar and thyroid tissues in human exophthalmos. J Clin Endocrinol Metab 1972;34:1090.

168. Winand R, Mahieu P. Prevention of malignant exophthalmos after treatment of thyrotoxicosis. Lancet 1973;1:1196.

169. Blau HM, Kaplan I, Tao TW, Kriss JP. Thyroglobulin-independent, cell mediated cytotoxicity of human eye muscle cells in tissue culture by lymphocytes of a patient with Graves' ophthalmopathy. Life Sci 1983;32:45.

170. Prummel MF, Wiersinga WM, Van der Gaag R, et al. Soluble IL-2 receptor levels in patients with Graves' ophthalmopathy. Clin Exp Immunol 1992;88:405.

171. Heufelder AE, Scriba PC. Characterization of adhesion receptors on cultured microvascular endothelial cells derived from the retro-orbital connective tissue of patients with Graves' ophthalmopathy. Eur J Endocrinol 1996;134:51.

172. Van Der Gaag R, Schmidt ED, Koornneef L. Retrobulbar histology and immunohistochemistry in endocrine ophthalmopathy. Dev Ophthalmol 1993;25:1.

173. Weetman AP, Cohen S, Gatter KC, et al. Immunohistochemical analysis of the retrobulbar tissues in Graves' ophthalmopathy. Clin Exp Immunol 1989;75:222.

174. DeCarli M, D'Elios MM, Mariotti S, et al. Cytolytic T cells with Th1-like cytokine profile predominate in retroorbital lymphocytic infiltrates of Graves' ophthalmopathy. J Clin Endocrinol Metab 1993;77:1120.

175. Grubeck-Loebenstein B, Trieb K, Sztankay A, et al. Retrobulbar T cells from patients with Graves' ophthalmopathy are CD8+ and specifically recognize autologous fibroblasts. J Clin Invest 1994;93:2738.

176. Kahaly G, Karger B. Endocrine ophthalmopathy: molecular, immunological and clinical aspects. Dev Ophthalmol 1993;25:1.

177. Jaume JC, Portolano S, Prummel MF, et al. Molecular cloning and characterization of genes for antibodies generated by orbital tissue-infiltrating B cells in Graves' ophthalmopathy. J Clin Endocrinol 1994;78:348.

178. Prummel MF, Chazenbalk G, Jaume JC, et al. Profile of lambda light chain variable region genes in Graves' orbital tissue. Mol Immun 1994;31:793.

179. Griffith AD, Malmqvist M, Marks JD, et al. Human anti-self antibodies with high specificity from phage display libraries. EMBO J 1993;12:725.

180. Hiromatsu Y, Fukazawa H, Guinard F, et al. A thyroid cytotoxic antibody that cross-reacts with an eye muscle cell surface antigen may be the cause of thyroid-associated ophthalmopathy. J Clin Endocrinol Metab 1988;67:565.

181. Boucher A, Bernard N, Zhang ZG, et al. Nature of 64kDa eye muscle and thyroid membrane proteins and their significance in thyroid-associated ophthalmopathy—an hypothesis. Autoimmunity 1994;16:79.

182. Dong Q, Ludgat M, Vassart G. Cloning and sequencing of a novel 64kDa autoantigen recognized by patients with autoimmune thyroid disease. J Clin Endocrinol Metab 1991;72:1375.

183. Kendler DL, Rootman J, Huber G, Davis T. A 64kDa membrane antigen is a recurrent epitope for natural autoantibodies in patients with Graves' thyroid and ophthalmic diseases. Clin Endocrinol 1991;35:539.

184. Ross PB, Koenig RJ, Arscott P, Ludgate M. Tissue specificity and serologic reactivity of an autoantigen associated with autoimmune thyroid disease. J Clin Endocrinol Metab 1993;77:433.

185. Bernard NF, Nygen TN, Tyutyuikov A, et al. Antibodies against 1D, a recombinant 64kDa membrane protein, are associated with ophthalmology in patients with thyroid autoimmunity. Clin Immunol Immunopathol 1994;70:225.

186. Schifferdecker E, Ketzler-Sasse U, Boehm BO, et al. Re-evaluation of eye muscle autoantibody determination in Graves' ophthalmopathy: failure to detect a specific antigen by use of enzyme-linked immunosorbent assay, indirect immunofluorescence, and immunoblotting techniques. Acta Endocrin 1989;121:643.

187. Wall JR, Hayes M, Scalise D, et al. Native gel electrophoresis and isoelectric focusing of a 64-kilodalton eye muscle protein shows that it is an important target for serum autoantibodies in patients with thyroid-associated ophthalmopathy and not expressed in other skeletal muscle. J Clin Endocrinol Metab 1995;80:1226.

188. Tandon N, Yan SL, Arnold K, et al. Immunoglobulin class and subclass distribution of eye muscle and fibroblast antibodies in patients with thyroid-associated ophthalmopathy. Clin Endocrinol 1994;40:629.

189. Wall JR, Triller H, Boucher A, et al. Antibodies reactive with an intracellular epitope of a recombinant 64kDa thyroid and eye muscle protein in patients with thyroid autoimmunity and ophthalmopathy. J Endocrinol Invest 1993;16:863.

190. Wall JR, Triller H, Chung F, et al. Cross-reactive antibodies in the serum of balb/c mice immunized with thyroid or eye muscle membranes. J Endocrinol Invest 1994;17:105.

191. Arnold K, Tandon N, McIntosh RS, et al. T cell responses to orbital antigens in thyroid-associated ophthalmopathy. Clin Exp Immunol 1994;96:329.

192. Foss AJE, Fisher EW, McDonald N, et al. The site of autoantigen and dysthyroid eye disease: the significant negative. Eye 1993;7:806.

193. Campbell RJ. Pathology of Graves' Ophthalmopathy. In CA Gorman, RA Waller, JA Dyer (eds), The Eye and Orbit in Thyroid Disease. New York: Raven, 1884;25.

194. De Bellis A, Bizzarro A, Gattoni A, et al. Behavior of soluble intercellular adhesion molecule-1 and endothelial-leukocyte adhesion molecule-1 concentrations in patients with Graves' disease with or without ophthalmopathy in patients with toxic adenoma. J Clin Endocrinol Metab 1995;80:2118.

194a. Klett ZG, Elner SG, Elner VM. Differential expression of immunoreactive HLA-DR and ICAM-1 in human cultured orbital fibroblasts. Ophthal Plast Reconstr Surg 1996;12:153.

195. Heufelder AE, Bahn RS. Detection and localization of cytokine immunoreactivity in retro-ocular connective tissue in Graves' ophthalmopathy. Eur J Clin Invest 1993;23:1.

196. Bahn RS. The fibroblast is the target cell in the connective tissue manifestations of Graves' disease. Int Arch Allergy Immunol 1995;106:213.

197. Heufelder AE, Bahn RS, Smith TJ. Regulation by glucocorticoids of interferon gamma induced HLA-DR antigen expression in cultured human orbital fibroblasts. Clin Endocrinol 1992;37:59.

198. Heufelder AE, Wenzel BE, Bahn RS. Glucocorticoids modulate the synthesis of expression of a 72-kDa heat shock protein culture in Graves' retro-ocular fibroblasts. Acta Endocrin 1993;128:41.

199. Heufelder AE, Bahn RS. Modulation of Graves' orbital fibroblast proliferation by cytokines and glucocorticoid receptor agonists. Invest Ophthalmol Vis Sci 1994;35:120.

200. Rotella CM, Alvarez F, Kohn LD, Toccafoni R. Graves' autoantibodies to extrathyroidal TSH receptor: their role in ophthalmopathy and pretibial myxedema. Acta Endocrinol 1987 (Suppl);281:344.

201. Sisson JC, Kothary P, Kirchick H. The effects of lymphocytes, sera, and long-acting thyroid stimulator from patients with Graves' disease on retrobulbar fibroblasts. J Clin Endocrinol Metab 1973;37:17.

202. Kahaly G, Hansen C, Beyer J, Winand R. Plasma glycosaminoglycans in endocrine ophthalmopathy. J Endocrinol Invest 1994;17:45.

203. Sisson JC. Stimulation of glucose utilization and glycosaminoglycan production by fibroblasts derived from retrobulbar tissue. Exp Eye Res 1971;12:285.

204. Rundle FF, Finlay-Jones LR, Noad KB. Malignant exophthalmos: a quantitative analysis of orbital tissues. Aust Ann Med 1953;2:128.

205. Imai Y, Odajima R, Inoue Y, Sisiba Y. Effect of growth factors on hyaluronate and proteoglycan synthesis by retroocular tissue fibroblasts of Graves' ophthalmopathy in culture. Acta Endocrinol 1992;126:541.

206. Bahn RS, Heufelder AE. Retroocular fibroblasts: important effector cells in Graves' ophthalmopathy. Thyroid 1992;2:89.

207. Metcalfe RA, Weetman AP. Stimulation of extraocular muscle fibroblasts by cytokines and hypoxia: possible role in thyroid-associated ophthalmopathy. Clin Endocrinol 1994;40:67.

208. Tellez M, Cooper J, Edmonds C. Graves' ophthalmopathy in relation to cigarette smoking and ethnic origin. Clin Endocrinol 1992;36:291.

209. Haag E, Asplund K. Is endocrine ophthalmopathy related to smoking? Br Med J 1987;295:634.

210. Balzas C, Stenszky V, Farid NR. Association between Graves' ophthalmopathy and smoking. Lancet 1990;336:74.

211. Shine B, Fells P, Edwards OM, Weetman AP. Association between Graves' ophthalmopathy and smoking. Lancet 1990;335:1261.

212. Bartalena L, Martino E, Marcocci C, et al. More on smoking habits and Graves' ophthalmopathy. J Endocrinol Invest 1989;12:733.

213. Nunnery WR, Martin RT, Heinz GW, Gavin TJ. The association of cigarette smoking with clinical subtypes of ophthalmic Graves' disease. Ophthal Plast Reconstr Surg 1993;9:77.

214. Winsa B, Mandahl A, Karlsson FA. Graves' disease, endocrine ophthalmopathy and smoking. Acta Endocrinol 1993;128:156.

214a. Pfeilschifter J, Zeigler R. Smoking and endocrine ophthalmopathy: impact of smoking severity and current vs. lifetime cigarette consumption. Clin Endocrinol 1996;45:477.

215. Hudson HL, Levin L, Feldon SE. Graves' exophthalmos unrelated to extraocular muscle enlargement. Superior rectus muscle inflammation may induce venous obstruction. Ophthalmology 1991;98:1495.

216. Benning H, Lieb W, Kahaly G, Grehn F. Color doppler ultrasound findings in patients with thyroid ophthalmopathology. Ophthalmology 1994;91:20.

217. Naumann M. Herzleiden mit anschwellung der schilddruese und exophthalmos. Dtsch Klin 1853;5:269.

218. Goldstein JE. Paresis of superior rectus muscle associated with thyroid dysfunction. Arch Ophthalmol 1964;72:5.

219. Brain WR. Exophthalmic ophthalmoplegia. Trans Ophthalmol Soc UK 1937;57:107.

220. Warner F. Ophthalmoplegia externa complicating the case of Graves' disease. Med Times Gaz 1882:540.

221. Schultz RO, Van Allen MW, Blodi FC. Endocrine ophthalmoplegia. With an electromyographic study of paretic extraocular muscles. Arch Ophthalmol 1960;63:217.

222. Scott WE, Thalacker JA. Diagnosis and treatment of thyroid myopathy. Ophthalmology 1981;88:493.

223. Reny A, Leclerc J, Raspiller A, Hartemann P. Les deficits moteurs oculopalpebraux au cours des dysthyroidies. Ann Endocrinol (Paris) 1971;32:64.

224. Jensen SF. Endocrine ophthalmoplegia. Acta Ophthalmol 1971;49:679.

225. Metz HS. Saccadic velocity studies in patients with endocrine ocular disease. Am J Ophthalmol 1977;84:695.

226. Feldon SE, Unsold R. Graves' ophthalmopathy evaluated by infrared eye-movement recordings. Arch Ophthalmol 1982;100:324.

227. Hermann JS. Paretic thyroid myopathy. Ophthalmology 1982;89:473.

228. Hamed LM, Lessner AM. Fixation duress in the pathogenesis of upper eye lid retraction in thyroid orbitopathy. A prospective study. Ophthalmology 1994;101:1608.

229. Pochin EE. Mechanism of lid retraction in Graves' disease. Clin Sci 1939;4:91.

230. Von Stellwag C. Ueber gewisse innervationsstoerungen bei der Basedow'schen krankheit. Wien Med Wochnschr 1869;14:737.

231. Kagoshima T, Hori S, Inou Y. Qualitative and quantitative analyses of Müller's muscle in dysthyroid ophthalmopathy. Jpn J Ophthalmol 1987;31:646.

232. Rootman J, Patel S, Berry K, Nugent R. Pathological and clinical study of Müller's muscle in Graves' ophthalmopathy. Can J Ophthalmol 1987;22:32.

233. Small RG. Enlargement of levator palpebrae superiorus muscle fibers in Graves' ophthalmopathy. Ophthalmology 1989;96:424.

234. Frueh BR, Garber FW, Musch DC. The effects of Graves' eye disease on levator muscle function. Ophthal Surg 1986;17:142.

235. Gay AJ, Wolkstein MA. Topical guanethidine therapy for endocrine lid retraction. Arch Ophthalmol 1966;76:364.

236. Cant JS, Lewis DR, Harrison MT. Treatment of dysthyroid ophthalmopathy with local guanethidine. Br J Ophthalmol 1969;53:233.

237. Eden KC, Trotter WR. Lid-retraction in toxic diffuse goitre. Lancet 1942;2:385.

238. Grove AS Jr. Upper eyelid retraction and Graves' disease. Ophthalmology 1981;88:499.

239. Henderson JW. Relief of eyelid retraction. A surgical procedure. Arch Ophthalmol 1965;74:205.

240. Harvey JT, Anderson RL. The aponeurotic approach to eyelid retraction. Ophthalmology 1981;88:513.

241. Putterman AM. Surgical treatment of the thyroid-related upper eyelid retraction. Graded Müller's muscle excision and levator recession. Ophthalmology 1981;88:507.

242. Baylis HI, Cies WA, Kamin DF. Correction of upper eyelid retraction. Am J Ophthalmol 1976;82:790.

243. Putterman AM, Urist MJ. A simplified levator palpebrae superioris muscle recession to treat over corrected blepharoptosis. Am J Ophthalmol 1974;77:358.

244. Chalfin J, Putterman AM. Müller's muscle excision and levator recession in retracted upper lid. Treatment of thyroid-related retraction. Arch Ophthalmol 1979;97:1487.

245. Crawford JS, Eisterbrook M. The use of bank sclera to correct lid retraction. Can J Ophthalmol 1976;11:309.

246. Buffam FV, Rootman J. Lid retraction—its diagnosis and treatment. Int Ophthalmol Clin 1978;118:75.

247. Flanagan JC. Retraction of the eyelid secondary to thyroid ophthalmopathy—its surgical correction with sclera and the fate of the graft. Trans Am Ophthalmol Soc 1980;78:657.

248. Naffziger H. Pathologic changes in the orbit in progressive exophthalmos. Arch Ophthalmol 1933;9:1.

249. Merrill HG, Oaks LW. Extreme bilateral exophthalmos: report of two cases with autopsy findings in one. Am J Ophthalmol 1933;16:231.

250. Paufique L, Guinet P, Papillon J. Le traitement de l'exophtalmie oedemateuse sans hyperthyroidie. Ann Ocul 1950;183:449.

251. Offret M-C, Offret G. L'exophthalmie maligne de la maladie de Basedow. Arch d'Ophtalmol 1945;5:429.

252. Wagener HP. Lesions of the optic nerve and exophthalmos of endocrine origin. Am J Med Sci 1956;232:226.

253. Hallin ES, Feldon SE. Graves' ophthalmopathy: II. Correlation of clinical signs with measures derived from computed tomography. Br J Ophthalmol 1988;72:678.

254. Barrett L, Glatt HJ, Burde RM, Gado MH. Optic nerve dysfunction in thyroid eye disease: CT. Radiology 1988;167:503.

255. Frueh BR, Musch DC, Grill R, et al. Orbital compliance in Graves' eye disease. Ophthalmology 1985;92:657.

256. Neigel JM, Rootman J, Belkin RI, et al. Dysthyroid optic neuropathy. The crowded orbital apex syndrome. Ophthalmology 1988;95:1515.

257. Winstanley J. Visual Field Defects in Dysthyroid Eye Disease and Their Management. In JS Cant (ed), Proceedings of the Second McKenzie Memorial Symposium. St. Louis: Mosby, 1972;230.

258. Igersheimer J. Visual changes in progressive exophthalmus. Arch Ophthalmol 955;53:94.

259. Henderson JW. Optic neuropathy of exophthalmic goiter (Graves' disease). Arch Ophthalmol 1958;59:471.

260. Hedges TR, Scheie HG. Visual field defects in exophthalmus associated with thyroid disease. Arch Ophthalmol 1955;54:885.

261. Gorman CA, Desanto LW, MacCarty CS, Riley FC. Optic neuropathy of Graves' disease: treatment by transantral or transfrontal orbital decompression. N Engl J Med 1974;290:70.

262. Feldon SE, Muramatsu S, Weiner JM. Clinical classification of Graves' ophthalmopathy. Identification of risk factors for optic neuropathy. Arch Ophthalmol 1984;102:1469.

7

Thyroid Eye Disease: Natural History and Response to Hyperthyroidism Treatment

The inciting events and factors responsible for the exacerbation or remission of thyroid eye disease remain enigmatic. Sattler reviewed the natural history of Graves' ophthalmopathy in the pretreatment era and noted that eye signs could occur before, at the same time, and after the diagnosis of hyperthyroidism.[1] Thyroid eye changes undergo apparently spontaneous exacerbations or remissions; more than 300 cases of improvement in untreated eyes were reported before 1960.[2] Different investigators have argued that surgical, radiotherapeutic, or medical treatments for thyrotoxicosis had no effect, improved, or worsened eye changes. This chapter discusses current therapy for systemic hyperthyroidism and its effect on the natural history of thyroid eye disease.

Modern treatment offers three main options for systemic treatment of hyperthyroidism: surgery, radioactive iodine, and anti-thyroid drugs. Surgery was the first proved treatment, the drug thiouracil was introduced in 1943, and radioactive iodine (RAI) was first used in clinical trials in 1944.[3]

DRUG THERAPY

Thionamides are the primary pharmacologic agents used in hyperthyroidism treatment. Most commonly used are propylthiouracil (PTU), methimazole (Tapazole), and a 3-carbethoxy derivative of methimazole, carbimazole, widely used in Great Britain.[4,5] These drugs block iodide organification and inhibit the coupling of iodotyrosines; PTU also inhibits the peripheral conversion of thyroxine (T_4) to triiodothyronine (T_3). In addition, these drugs have a number of immunoregulatory effects, including alterations of activated helper/inducer cells and cytotoxic/suppressor cells (increased) plus reduction of human leukocyte (HLA)-DR antigens on thyroid-infiltrating T cells and diminution in circulating thyroid-stimulating hormone receptor (TSHr) antibodies.[6–12]

The thionamides are given orally; PTU's initial dosage is 100–200 mg three times a day. An advantage of methimazole is that it is given once daily, usually at a starting dosage of 20 or 30 mg.[13] Thionamides do not influence release of thyroid hormones but do impair hormone synthesis, normally resulting in delayed clinical response. This latency period can range from 3 days to months, depending on such factors as the quantity of hormone stored in the thyroid colloid, the thyroid secretory rate, hyperthyroid severity, and the degree of medication-produced inhibition of hormone synthesis.[4,14] Improvement is usually noted rapidly, generally within weeks after the start of therapy, and metabolic parameters are restored to normal within 6 weeks. Patients with severe hyperthyroidism respond more slowly to treatment. Drug therapy duration is empiric, depending on the involution of the disease process. Most clinicians use these agents for at least 1 year, although carbimazole is often used for 2 or more years. Some prospective studies tend to show better long-term remission rates when agents are given for more than 1 year.[15,16]

PTU is often used as the first agent, especially when rapid control of severe thyrotoxicosis is necessary. Cooper and others have suggested that since methimazole (Tapazole) is less expensive, can be given once daily, and probably has lower morbidity, it may be a better first-line drug than PTU.[17] Medical therapy using PTU as the initial drug would be indicated in patients with thyroid storm, or those who are pregnant or lactating.

The patient's clinical status is probably the most important measure of therapeutic response, but there are some laboratory, histologic, and clinical parameters that sometimes help predict individual responses to any treatment. Patients who respond best to medical therapy have had hyperthyroidism for less than 1 year, their thyroid gland decreases in size during drug therapy, and thyroidal uptake of ^{131}iodine radioisotope (I) or ^{125}I is suppressed by the administration of thyroid hormone and an antithyroid drug.[18–20] Patients at higher risk for recurrence have larger thyroid glands, a family history of thyroid disease, and in some studies, the presence of ophthalmopathy.[21,22]

The choice of antithyroid therapy varies in different countries; these drugs are more popular with endocrinologists in Europe and Japan.[9,22] While some investigators thought that giving patients T_4 to avoid post-treatment hypothyroidism would decrease the relapse rate, recent studies have not borne out that hypothesis.[23–25]

The results of some immunologic tests have also been correlated with prognosis. Rapoport and coworkers noted that 12 patients with negative thyroid-stimulating immunoglobulins (TSIs) following antithyroid drug therapy remained in remission, while five of seven who were TSI-positive at that time had a rapid relapse.[26] Bliddal et al. noted that the TSH-binding inhibitory immunoglobulin (TBII) index, which measures one of the TSHr antibodies, also correlates with drug response when measured at cessation of drug therapy. Patients with TBII indices below 0.35 relapsed, while those above 1.00 remained in remission.[27] Similar data have been generated by others (see Chapter 3).[28,29] There is not uniform agreement on the prognostic accuracy of these studies. Schleusener and coworkers noted in a multicenter prospective trial that neither HLA-DR3 nor TSH antibodies were predictive for clinical course after medical therapy.[30] DeBruin and coworkers noted that the presence of HLA-Cw7 and the continued presence of serum antibodies were poor prognostic signs; ophthalmopathy did not correlate with drug response in that study.[31] Several other immunologic factors have also correlated with treatment response.[32–35] In a meta-analysis of 18 reports, Feldt-Rasmussen and colleagues noted the chance of relapse was 65% less if TSHr antibodies were absent.[34] Patients requiring longer than average courses of drug therapy have a generally higher incidence of disease recurrence; however, short-term antithyroid drug therapy with carbimazole has resulted in a failure rate of up to 88%.[4] Approximately one-third to one-half of patients treated with thionamides undergo complete remission.[5] After a single course of antithyroid drug therapy, the failure rate with various thionamides approaches 50–60%. Even with multiple courses of therapy, a 30–40% relapse rate is observed.[3,13,36,37]

Major advantages of the antithyroid agents are reversibility, a lower incidence of hypothyroidism than with surgery or irradiation, and a very low mortality risk. Major disadvantages include the need for long-term therapy, the high recurrence rate, and required serial evaluation. Adverse reactions to the newer thionamides are uncommon—a mild rash develops in less than 5% of cases; joint stiffness and drug fever are also rare; agranulocytosis and glomerulonephritis occur in less than 1% of patients.[13,38,39]

Antithyroid drugs are used in younger patients as a definitive treatment, in surgical patients to achieve a euthyroid state before thyroidectomy, and in patients before, during, and in the immediate post-treatment RAI period to control hyperthyroidism.[40] While some reports have observed that antithyroid drugs are useful with RAI, other reports have noted lower RAI efficacy if drugs are used before radiation.[41]

Most relapses after antithyroid drugs occur within the first 3–6 months after cessation of treatment. There probably is a lower incidence of successful medical therapy with the increased amount of dietary iodine.[42] Although less common in antithyroid medical therapy than in other treatment modalities, hypothyroidism is a major complication, developing in approximately one-third of patients followed for 20 years after treatment.[13,43,44]

Some adjunctive agents are useful with standard treatment modalities. Inorganic iodine (saturated solution KI, or Lugol's solution), which decreases gland hypervascularity and hyperplasia and inhibits hormone release, is often used with other drugs or before surgery in severe thyrotoxicosis, especially if there is an impending thyroid crisis. Similarly, beta-blocking agents (most commonly propranolol), which inhibit the sympathetic stimulation associated with thyrotoxicosis, or steroids that decrease the secretion of thyroid hormones and the peripheral conversion of T_4 to T_3, are often used in the management of severe Graves' disease.[31]

RADIOACTIVE IODINE THERAPY

RAI's role in the treatment of Graves' disease has been brought into question again by a study performed by Tallstedt and colleagues.[45,46] As discussed above, the first-line choice of Graves' disease therapy varies in different countries.[47]

RAI has been the treatment of choice in many adult patients older than 50, and produces disease control results comparable to surgical thyroidectomy. Major indications are moderately large glands or failure to respond to antithyroid drugs.[48] Major disadvantages of RAI therapy are the higher incidence of secondary hypothyroidism, variable response to radiation in different thyroid glands, the possible adverse effect on eye disease, and the possibility of germinal cell mutation in patients of reproductive age. Data regarding this latter issue are unclear; a study of 70,000 pregnancies in survivors of the Hiroshima and Nagasaki bombings showed no significant genetic defects among offspring.[13] Antithyroid therapy imparts roughly as much ^{131}I radiation to the gonads as does a barium enema study.[49,50] After 5 years, approximately 30% of patients treated with RAI become hypothyroid; at 10 years the incidence is 40–80%.[13,51]

Beierwaltes reported on the results of a cooperative trial of 22,000 patients treated with ^{131}I and 14,000 treated surgically.[52] The study revealed a 2.7% yearly cumulative incidence of hypothyroidism with ^{131}I and 1.8% with surgery.[52] Similar results have been reported by others.[53] None of those studies demonstrated an increased incidence of carcinoma in adult patients treated with RAI.[54,55]

RAI dosage varies. Most patients have received 100 µg/g estimated gland weight corrected for percent of uptake. Attempts to lower doses of radiation to the thyroid gland, and thus decrease the incidence of secondary hypothyroidism, have had an associated higher incidence of disease recurrence. Sridama and colleagues observed that even when compensation for gland size is used, it is almost impossible to achieve the goal of early hyperthyroidism control without late-developing hypothyroidism.[56–58]

THYROIDECTOMY

Surgery has the lowest incidence of recurrent hyperthyroidism—fewer than 10% of patients (more or less depending on the extent of thyroidectomy) require additional antithyroid treatment for relapse or recurrence. In one study of 55 patients, 90% were euthyroid at 4 years.[59] Postsurgical thyroid insufficiency is common; early studies reported hypothyroidism in 4–30% of surgical cases, while more recent data demonstrate development of this complication in as many as 43% of patients.[51] Most clinicians recommend thyroid surgery for the following patients: those who will not comply with medical therapy; those who are not available for follow-up evaluation; those who have contraindications (e.g., allergies, etc.) to medical therapy; or those who refuse [131]I. Patients in whom thyroid cancer cannot be ruled out otherwise should have surgery, as should young patients with very large goiters, patients with severe hyperthyroidism, patients whose cases require rapid disease control, or patients whose conditions persist after adequate medical treatment. The incidence of serious surgical complications is lower in institutions that handle a large volume of thyroid disease patients. For instance, hypoparathyroidism, vocal cord paralysis, and mortality have been reported in up to 4% of surgical cases, but in major centers surgical morbidity is less than 0.1%.[60,61]

In one study, preoperative ophthalmopathy was highly correlated with recurrence of hyperthyroidism ($p < 0.0001$) after subtotal thyroid resection.[62]

EFFECT OF THERAPY ON THYROID EYE DISEASE

Different studies have attempted to ascertain the effect of antithyroid therapies on thyroid eye disease, yet there remains a dearth of prospective randomized treatment trial data. As previously mentioned, the report by Sattler in the pretreatment era demonstrated that spontaneous exacerbations and remissions of eye disease occur at various times before and after the diagnosis of Graves' disease.[1] Despite the paucity of randomized trials, numerous generalizations regarding the course of eye findings in Graves' disease can be made. Usually eye findings occur within 6 months to 1 year of confirmed hyperthyroidism, although thyroid ophthalmopathy has been known to develop as long as 20 years after the initial diagnosis.[63] Hegele and Volpe reported a hyperthyroid patient without eye disease who relapsed 23 years after initial RAI therapy with both systemic and eye findings.[58]

Thyroid eye disease is usually a self-limited process, remitting spontaneously within 3 to 36 months;[64–67] less than 10% of patients develop serious long-term eye problems.[68–72] Calissendorff and coworkers reviewed 154 Swedish patients and noted that only 23% of hyperthyroid patients had moderate ophthalmopathy (class III or IV), and none in their series had class V or VI involvement.[73] Only 2–7% of thyroid eye patients develop severe, potentially vision-threatening orbitopathy; elderly men are at a greater risk to develop this complication. Correction of thyrotoxicosis through any therapeutic modality results in decreased lid retraction and stare. When lid position and levator function return to normal, it often gives the illusion that the proptosis is improved. In most studies, however, clinically significant exophthalmos rarely changes after it reaches its maximum. Extraocular muscle dysfunction is transient in a significant number of patients.

Hales and Rundle performed a natural history study. They reported on the changes in thyroid ophthalmopathy in 104 patients who had several evaluations during 13 years after initial examination.[69] In this group, eight patients had euthyroid ophthalmopathy, 59 had Graves' disease with associated ophthalmopathy, and 37 initially presented with hyperthyroidism without eye findings. In 44 hyperthyroid patients with eye findings, lid retraction disappeared in 25 (57%) without ancillary ocular treatment following correction of hyperthyroidism. This finding has also been noted by others.[3,74,75] In 70% of patients proptosis remained unchanged. The extraocular muscle problems remained stable in 50%, and improved (25%) or worsened (25%) in the other patients.

In a subgroup of 29 cases who presented with severe exophthalmos, lid retraction improved in 50%, explaining why eye findings appeared slight or absent in approximately half of the patients' follow-up examinations.[69] In this group, strabismus and proptosis were essentially unchanged.

Most subjects without eye findings 1 year after the diagnosis of Graves' disease did not develop them. Those with late-onset eye symptoms developed minimal ocular signs only; approximately 20% of this group developed only mild proptosis or extraocular muscle dysfunction.[69] Other investigators have reported similar findings, although severe disease necessitating orbital decompression or other surgical procedures does occur with euthyroid or Graves' ophthalmopathy.[76,77] In a longitudinal study of 120 thyroid eye disease patients, Bartley noted 89 required minimal ocular therapy, and some ophthalmic surgery was necessary in 20%.[78]

Hales and Rundle concluded that proptosis tends to remain stable once it reaches its maximum (in the first 1–2 years after diagnosis); a conclusion shared by many other researchers. Hamilton and coworkers noted that approximately 15% of hyperthyroid patients will have significant eye changes at onset (mainly proptosis and eyelid retraction); 1–5 years after systemic therapy, 10% of the population studied either continued to have or acquired serious eye problems.[71] In the study by Hamilton and colleagues, 27% of patients developed proptosis, 58% had increased proptosis, and 15% had no significant changes in exophthalmos during the course of the serial evaluations.[71] Overall, 91.8% of patients experienced improvement or disappearance of eye changes; 45.8% had no residual eye findings at the end of the study. Only five patients retained significant symptoms, and another 13 developed significant eye changes.[68] No statistically significant correlation between eye changes and the rapidity of disease control was observed. Eye changes worsened in 2.8% of 57 patients controlled within 4 months, but deterioration occurred in 8.4% of those in which disease was controlled more slowly. This observation contradicts the clinical impression held by some other researchers who have noted exacerbation of eye disease when patients were rapidly controlled.[79] In a more recent study using rapid control with carbimazole followed by T_4 supplementation, Peros and colleagues noted that 64% of 59 previously hyperthyroid patients had spontaneous improvement of their ophthalmic findings.[80] Hamilton et al. did not observe the correlation between eye disease and the development of myxedema noted in other studies but did note a connection between recalcitrant hyperthyroidism and worsening of eye disease.[71,81]

In contrast, more recent studies have concluded that post-treatment hypothyroidism is associated with exacerbation of ophthalmic findings.[82,83] In a study by Prummel and coworkers, an association between severity of hyperthyroidism before treatment and a greater degree of ocular involvement was noted.[82]

The condition of the euthyroid ophthalmopathy group reported by Hales and Rundle tended to improve over time.[68] At the final evaluation, only one of six patients still had lid retraction, ophthalmoplegia improved in four of five, and proptosis improved in three, disappeared in one, and increased and showed no change in two each. In general, patients with euthyroid ophthalmopathy tend to have a more benign ocular course than those with hyperthyroidism. Teng and coworkers reported a 3-year follow-up of 27 patients with ophthalmic Graves' disease in which there appeared to be improved eye findings associated with normal thyroid suppression tests.[84] Similarly, Franco followed 45 patients with euthyroid ophthalmopathy and noted that exophthalmos decreased in many and disappeared in 18%.[85] While many euthyroid ophthalmopathy patients eventually develop hyperthyroidism, no data demonstrate that this change correlates with eye disease.[86]

There is ongoing controversy over the effects of different types of antithyroid treatment on thyroid eye disease.[1,76,82,83,87–90] As previously mentioned, some investigators in the pre- and post-treatment era have found that eye changes do not appear to correlate with thyroid status.[1,76,87] In a 1958 review, McCullagh and coworkers noted that 64% of ophthalmopathy patients improved after RAI and 55% improved after surgery.[91,92] Other investigators have reported a worsening of eye findings in patients treated with RAI[93–96] and that surgical thyroidectomy was advantageous[81,90] or deleterious.[62,68,70,92] Similarly, the rate at which hyperthyroidism was controlled and the development of hypothyroidism were also believed to be important parameters by some investigators.

Dobyns studied 203 patients after thyroidectomy and noted that, while proptosis increased by at least 1.25 mm in 65% of cases, lid retraction and stare disappeared, giving the impression of improved eye findings.[97] He also noted that 56% of 359 patients with malignant exophthalmos were male, and if a subset of 65 patients who required enucleation or decompression were considered, 67% were men.

Hamilton and coworkers retrospectively studied the prevalence of thyroid ophthalmopathy in two eras: when surgical thyroidectomy prevailed and when RAI was the most prevalent treatment of Graves' disease at the Mayo Clinic.[67] They observed a 5.1% incidence of significant ophthalmopathy after RAI therapy versus 3.4% after surgical thyroidectomy, a difference that was not statistically significant. The study concluded that most eye changes stabilize with time. The clinical impression was that patients who became myxedematous after treatment and those who had recurrent hyperthyroidism were more likely to develop severe eye disease. Other studies have similarly shown no difference in eye disease as a function of systemic thyroid treatment type.[73] Barth and colleagues noted in a retrospective analysis of 89 patients treated with RAI that those with ocular findings before therapy had worse ophthalmic outcomes.[98] Werner studied 525 hyperthyroid patients, observing ophthalmopathy in 161. After RAI treatment, 7 of 71 with infiltrative ophthalmopathy and 1 of 90 with noninfiltrative ophthalmopathy developed progressive eye disease, none requiring decompression.[99]

Jones et al. studied 100 hyperthyroid patients treated 5 years previously with [131]I.[100] They detected a twofold increase in periorbital edema, but a 50% decrease in other eye signs except proptosis; only 3% of 367 patients treated 3–6 years previously had decreased proptosis.[100]

Bartalena and colleagues have presented some data on the use of concurrent corticosteroids in patients who receive RAI therapy.[101] They treated 26 patients with RAI alone and an equal number with RAI and systemic prednisone for 4 months. In patients without ophthalmic findings before therapy, none developed eye changes. In those with mild eye changes, the group that received steroids did better, but none of the patients had severe ophthalmopathy.[101] Controversy remains about the use of RAI and steroids with this treatment regimen.[88,102–104]

Tallstedt and coworkers performed a randomized study of 114 patients between 35 and 55 years old and noted significantly more ophthalmopathy in those treated with RAI (33%, 13 of 39 patients) compared with patients who had subtotal thyroidectomy or antithyroid medicine (10–16%).[46] A number of possible explanations might have led to inadvertent, spurious results in the Tallstedt study.[105] First, patients who received RAI had a higher incidence of smoking; there is an association between smoking and more severe eye disease.[106–111] Second, 18 of 39 patients that were given RAI required more than one dose of the ^{131}I isotope; in the 21 patients who required a single treatment, only one developed eye disease. More severe hyperthyroidism has an association with eye disease so that those patients who required additional RAI were at a greater risk of developing ophthalmopathy.[105,112] Third, the management after treatment of hyperthyroidism was different in the surgery, medicine, and ^{131}I groups. In the latter subset, patients did not receive thyroid replacement until they were hypothyroid in contrast to the other two groups who were treated with T_4. As discussed above, the hypothyroid state that developed in most of the RAI patients may have adversely affected the eye disease.

Grace and Weeks noted no change in patients' exophthalmometry readings after thyroidectomy.[113] Soley and colleagues noted that almost 50% of patients had increased proptosis after thyroidectomy; there was no significant difference in the data for patients treated surgically or with RAI.[114]

Sridama and De Groot retrospectively reviewed 506 patients. Thyroidectomy was used in 164, RAI in 241, and antithyroid drugs in 182. They found no difference in new eye disease or worsening of existing ophthalmopathy.[112] One potential problem with this study is that the patients had very long followup with a mean interval of 5 years; it is possible that this study design would not have detected an eye change that occurred shortly after treatment.

Barbosa et al. compared three treatment regimens in a retrospective study.[115] They observed that if the ophthalmopathy worsened after therapy, it usually did so within the first year. While the populations treated with surgery, drugs, or RAI were small and not identical, the researchers noted no significant differences. Four percent of RAI-treated patients developed severe eye changes compared with none of those treated medically and 7% treated surgically.[116]

A number of early investigators believed that subtotal thyroidectomy exacerbated eye changes. They hypothesized that eye changes could not occur without remaining functional thyroid tissue, and thus that the totality of the thyroidectomy was a major factor in their progress.[66,115,117] White, Katz, and others thought that total thyroidectomy prevented or resulted in regression of thyroid eye changes, but ophthalmic data in these studies were scanty.[90,115,117] Werner, Boyle, and Pequenet et al. attempted thyroid ablation with RAI or surgery in a very small series; all investigators noted that eye disease could progress despite complete thyroid ablation.[87,118,119] In contrast, Bauer and Katz treated 18 cases with large doses of RAI to totally ablate the thyroid and noted that all eye changes except proptosis improved.[120]

Intervals between the diagnosis of hyperthyroidism, the detection of eye symptoms, and the necessity for orbital decompression have been specified in several publications. Between 1933 and 1959, Bartels and Irie studied 116 patients who eventually required decompression.[121] Nine patients had eye findings before systemic hyperthyroidism, 48 had a simultaneous onset, 32 developed ocular manifestations after the diagnosis but before therapy, 22 had the onset of eye signs after treatment of Graves' disease, and five had ophthalmopathy not associated with hyperthyroidism. Sixty-eight patients (58%) developed exophthalmos within the first year of treatment.[121] The interval from the onset of progressive exophthalmos to orbital decompression ranged from 2 months to 19 years; 75% of cases were decompressed within 2 years of eye symptom onset.[121] In a similar study, Gorman reviewed the data on 194 patients scheduled for orbital decompression.[76] Twenty-nine (15%) had never been clinically hyperthyroid. In 81% of the hyperthyroid patients, the date of the first eye signs occurred within 18 months before or after the diagnosis of Graves' disease.[76] The hyperthyroid patients' median duration of eye symptoms before decompression was 23 months (range: 17 days to 37 years) compared to only 12 months in the euthyroid patients.

NATURAL HISTORY OF THYROID OPHTHALMOPATHY COMPONENTS

Four major thyroid eye problems may require ophthalmic intervention: eyelid retraction, proptosis, extraocular myopathy, and optic neuropathy. As previously mentioned, eyelid retraction spontaneously remits in as many as 50% of patients. In contrast, proptosis usually remains stationary, although reduced eyelid retraction can give the illusion of decreased exophthalmos. In one report, however, 11 of 27 patients with exophthalmometry readings greater than 19 mm had decreased readings on serial followup within 3–19 years, 13 patients remained unchanged, and three of 27 had increased proptosis.[122]

Dysthyroid ophthalmopathy is the most common cause of spontaneous diplopia in middle-aged or older patients. As discussed in Chapters 4 and 5, most patients with extraocular muscle involvement (class IV) thyroid eye disease present with other signs of Graves' ophthalmopathy; occasionally this is the presenting manifestation of thyroid eye disease.

One of the most important observations regarding thyroid extraocular myopathy is the high incidence of spontaneous remission. As shown by Hales and Rundle, as well as by Hamilton and coworkers, many patients have transient extraocular muscle disease.[69,71] Hamilton et al. observed that only eight of 27 patients who developed extraocular muscle problems after RAI therapy for systemic thyrotoxicosis required intervention. Usually these patients should be watched for several months before muscle surgery, especially if serial measurements demonstrate varying degrees of strabismus. As discussed in Chapters 6 and 13, surgical intervention before the extraocular muscle findings are stabilized can lead to any of a number of therapeutic misadventures.

It is difficult to predict the course of patients with thyroid optic neuropathy. As mentioned in Chapters 4–6, only recently have investigators (using magnetic resonance imaging [MRI] or computed tomography [CT]) been able to determine that apical compression by enlarged recti muscles causes this abnormality.[123] Retrobulbar neuritis, in association with thyroid eye disease, was first described in English language literature in 1921. Since then, authors have described its variable course.[124–129] Henderson pointed out that patients could undergo spontaneous regression, but many investigators have been loath to observe these patients because of the problem's vision-threatening nature.[67] Trobe and coworkers summarized the data from others' investigations of 32 untreated eyes—21% of these patients had a final visual acuity of 20/100 or worse and six had vision ranging from count-fingers to no light perception.[129]

No substantive data demonstrate an association of optic neuropathy with response to systemic treatment or degree of proptosis. As previously discussed (see Chapter 4), thyroid optic neuropathy develops often in eyes without marked proptosis, although usually these patients have some limitation of extraocular muscle movement and injection. The threat to vision with thyroid optic neuropathy usually mandates therapy for all except patients with mild visual impairment. The effects of radiation, steroids, and orbital decompression are discussed in the chapters on these therapeutic modalities.

At our institution, we continue to use RAI to ablate hyperthyroidism in most adult patients.[130] If the patient has eye changes before RAI, we treat them with systemic corticosteroids. Regardless of whether drugs or RAI are used, we closely monitor patients' thyroid status and do not allow them to become hypothyroid. As discussed in the following chapters, only a small minority of patients require either aggressive medical or surgical treatment for their thyroid eye findings.

REFERENCES

1. Sattler H. Die Basedow'sche krankheit. Graefe-Saemisch Handb der Ges Augenh 1909;9:1.
2. Jallut O, Galetti PM. L'exophtalmie maligne. Schweiz Med Wochenschr 1964;50:639.
3. Soley MH, Miller ER, Foreman N. Graves' disease: treatment with radioiodine (^{131}I). J Clin Endocrinol 1949;9:29.
4. Sugrue D, McEvoy J, Feely J, Drury MI. Hyperthyroidism in the land of Graves': results of treatment by surgery, radio-iodine and carbimazole. QJM 1980;49:51.
5. Solomon DH. Treatment: Antithyroid Drugs, Surgery, Radioidine, Selection of Therapy. In SC Werner, SH Ingbar (eds), The Thyroid. New York: Harper & Row, 1978;814.
6. Totterman TH, Karlsson FA, Bengtsson M, Mendel-Hartvig I. Induction of circling activated suppressor-like T cells by methimazole therapy for Graves' disease. N Engl J Med 1987;316:15.
7. Wartofsky L. Has the use of antithyroid drugs for Graves' disease become obsolete? Thyroid 1993;3:335.
8. Pinchera A, Liberti P, Martino E, et al. Effects of antithyroid therapy on the long-acting thyroid stimulator and the antithyroglobulin antibodies. J Clin Endocrinol 1969;29:231.
9. Walfish PG, Tseng KH. Intrathyroidal activated (Ia$^+$ T-lymphocyte CD$^+$ subsets) and B cells in Graves' hyperthyroidism respond rapidly to propylthiouracil therapy: demonstration using fine needle aspirates and two-color laser flow cytometry. Autoimmunity 1992;13:35.
10. Fenzi G, Hashizume K, Roudebush CP, DeGroot LJ. Changes in thyroid-stimulating immunoglobulins during antithyroid therapy. J Clin Endocrinol Metab 1979;48:572.
11. Teng CS, Yeung RTT. Changes in thyroid-stimulating activity in Graves' disease treated with antithyroid drug and its relationship to relapse: a prospective study. J Clin Endocrinol 1980;50:144.
12. McGregor AM, Petersen MM, McLachlan SM, et al. Carbimazole and the autoimmune response in Graves' disease. New Engl J Med 1980;303:302.
13. Klein I, Becker DV, Levey GS. Treatment of hyperthyroid disease. Ann Intern Med 1994;121:281.
14. Cooper DS. Antithyroid drugs. N Engl J Med 1984;311:1353.
15. Allannic H. Strategy for antithyroid drug therapy in Graves' disease. Horm Res 1987;26:146.
16. LeClere J. Antithyroid drugs. Horm Res 1987;26:154.

17. Cooper DS. Which antithyroid drug? Am J Med 1986;80:1165.

18. Solomon DH, Beck JC, Vander Laan WP, Astwood EB. Prognosis of hyperthyroidism treated by antithyroid drugs. JAMA 1953;152:201.

19. Alexander WD, McLarty, DG, Robertson J, et al. Prediction of the long-term results of antithyroid drug therapy for thyrotoxicosis. J Clin Endocrinol Metab 1970;30:540.

20. Saberi M, Sterling FH, Utiger RD. Reduction in extrathyroidal triiodothyronine production by propylthiouracil in man. J Clin Invest 1975;55:218.

21. Orgiazzi J. Management of Graves' hyperthyroidism. Endocrinol Metab Clin North Am 1987;16:365.

22. de Rave S, Goldschmidt HMJ, Bravenboer B, et al. Logistic multiple regression analysis of factors predicting recurrence of hyperthyroidism after medical treatment of toxic diffuse goitre. Neth J Med 1991;39:131.

23. Ladenson PW. Treatment of Graves' disease. N Engl J Med 1991;324:989.

24. Hashizume K, Ichikawa K, Sakurai A, et al. Administration of thyroxine in treated Graves' disease. Effects on the level of antibodies to thyroid-stimulating hormone receptors and on the risk of recurrence of hyperthyroidism. N Engl J Med 1991;324:947.

25. Wiersinga W. Immunosuppression of Graves' hypothyroidism—still an elusive goal. N Engl J Med 1996;334:265.

26. Rapoport B, Greenspan FS, Filetti S, Pepitone M. Clinical experience with a human thyroid cell bioassay for thyroid-stimulating immunoglobulin. J Clin Endocrinol Metab 1984;58:332.

27. Bliddal H, Kirkegaard C, Siersbaek-Nielsen K, Friis T. Prognostic value of thyrotropin binding inhibiting immunoglobulins (TB II) in long-term antithyroid treatment, ^{131}I therapy given in combination with carbimazole and in euthyroid ophthalmopathy. Acta Endocrinol (Copenh) 1981;98:364.

28. Teng CS, Yeung RTT, Khoo RKK, Alagaratnam TT. A prospective study of the changes in thyrotropin binding inhibitory immunoglobulins in Graves' disease treated by subtotal thyroidectomy or radioactive iodine. J Clin Endocrinol Metab 1980;50:1005.

29. McGregor AM, Rees Smith B, Hall R, et al. Prediction of relapse in hyperthyroid Graves' disease. Lancet 1980;1:1101.

30. Schleusener H, Schwander J, Holl G, et al. Do HLA-DR typing and measurement of TSH-receptor antibodies help in the prediction of the clinical course of Graves' thyrotoxicosis after antithyroid drug treatment? Acta Endocrinol (Copenh) 1987 (Suppl);281:318.

31. DeBruin TWA, Bolk JH, Bussemaker JK, et al. Graves' disease: immunological and immunogenetic indicators of relapse. Br Med J 1988;296:1292.

32. Fukazawa H, Yoshida K, Kaise N, et al. Intercellular adhesion molecule-1 (ICAM-1) in the sera of patients with Graves' disease: correlation with disease activity and treatment status. Thyroid 1995;5:373.

33. Celik I, Akalin S, Erbas T. Serum levels of interleukin 6 and tumor necrosis factor-alpha in hyperthyroid patients before and after propylthiouracil treatment. Eur J Endocrinol 1995;132(6):668.

34. Feldt-Rasmussen U, Schleusener H, Carayon P. Meta-analysis evaluation of the impact of thyrotropin receptor antibodies on long term remission after medical therapy of Graves' disease. J Clin Endocrinol Metab 1994;78:98.

35. Garcia-Mayor RV, Paramo C, Luna Cano R, et al. Antithyroid drug and Graves' hyperthyroidism. Significance of treatment duration and TRAb determination on lasting remission. J Endocrinol Invest 1992;15:815.

36. Collen RJ, Landaw EM, Kaplan SA, Lippe BM. Remission rates of children and adolescents with thyrotoxicosis treated with antithyroid drugs. Pediatrics 1980;65:550.

37. Slingerland DW, Burrows BA. Long-term antithyroid treatment in hyperthyroidism. JAMA 1979;242:2408.

38. Harada T, Shimaoka K, Mimura T, Ito K. Current treatment of Graves' disease. Surg Clin North Am 1987;67:299.

39. D'Cruz D, Chesser AMS, Lightowler C, et al. Case report: antineutrophil cytoplasmic antibody-positive crescentic glomerulonephritis associated with anti-thyroid drug treatment. Br J Rheumatol 1995;34:1090.

40. Dunn JT. Choice of therapy in young adults with hyperthyroidism of Graves' disease: a brief, case-directed poll of fifty-four thyroidologists. Ann Intern Med 1984;100:891.

41. Kung AW, Yau CC, Cheng AC. The action of methimazole and L-thyroxine in radioiodine therapy: a study on the incidence of hypothyroidism. Thyroid 1995;5:7.

42. Solomon BL, Evaul JE, Burman KD, Wartofsky L. Remission rates with antithyroid drug therapy: continuing influence of iodine intake. Ann Intern Med 1987;107:510.

43. Wilcox PH. Antithyroid treatment: a personal series. Postgrad Med J 1967;43:146.

44. Wood LC, Ingbar SH. Hypothyroidism as a late sequela in patients with Graves' disease treated with antithyroid drugs. J Clin Invest 1979;64:1429.

45. Cooper DS. Treatment of Thyrotoxicosis. In LE Braverman, RD Utiger (eds), The Thyroid (6th ed). Philadelphia: Lippincott, 1991;887.

46. Tallstedt L, Lundell G, Torring O, et al. Occurrence of ophthalmopathy after treatment for Graves' hyperthyroidism. N Engl J Med 1992;326:1733.

47. Wartofsky L, Glinoer D, Solomon B, et al. Differences and similarities in the diagnosis and treatment of Graves' disease in Europe, Japan and the United States. Thyroid 1991;1:129.

48. Hennemann G, Krenning EP, Sankaranarayanan K. Place of radioactive iodine in the treatment of thyrotoxicosis. Lancet 1986;2:1369.

49. Schull WJ, Otake M, Neel JV. Genetic effects of the atomic bombs: a reappraisal. Science 1981;213:1220.

50. Robertson JS, Gorman CA. Gonadal radiation dose and its genetic significance in radioiodine therapy of hyperthyroidism. J Nucl Med 1976;17:826.

51. Nofal MM, Beierwaltes WH, Patna ME. Treatment of hyperthyroidism with sodium iodine ^{131}I. JAMA 1966;197:605.

52. Beierwaltes WH. The treatment of hyperthyroidism with iodine-131. Semin Nucl Med 1978;8:95.

53. Douglas JG. The Vanderbilt experience with I^{131} treatment for Graves' disease. South Med J 1973;66:92.

54. Holm LE. Malignant Disease Following Iodine-131 Therapy in Sweden. In JD Boice, JF Fraumeni (eds), Progress in Cancer Research and Therapy. Radiation Carcinogenesis: Epidemiology and Biological Significance (Vol 26). New York: Raven, 1984:263.

55. Hoffman DA. Late Effects of I-131 Therapy in the United States. In JD Boice, JF Fraumeni (eds), Progress in Cancer Research and Therapy. Radiation Carcinogenesis: Epidemiology and Biological Significance (Vol 26). New York: Raven, 1984:273.

56. McDougall IR, Greig WR. ^{125}I therapy in Graves' disease: long-term results in 355 patients. Ann Intern Med 1976;85:720.

57. Sridama V, McCormick M, Kaplan EL, et al. Long-term follow-up study of compensated low-dose ^{131}I therapy for Graves' disease. N Engl J Med 1984;311:426.

58. Hegele RA, Volpe R. Relapse of Graves' disease 23 years after treatment with radioactive iodine (^{131}I). J Clin Lab Immunol 1985;18:103.

59. Bradley EL III, DiGirolamo M, Tarcot Y. Modified sub-total thyroidectomy in the management of Graves' disease. Surgery 1980;87:623.

60. Beahrs OH, Sakulsky SB. Surgical thyroidectomy in the management of exophthalmic goiter. Arch Surg 1968;96:512.

61. Cusick EL, Krukowski ZH, Matheson NA. Outcome of surgery for Graves' disease reexamined. Br J Surg 1987;74:780.

62. Winsa B, Rastad J, Akerstrom G, et al. Retrospective evaluation of subtotal and total thyroidectomy in Graves' disease with and without endocrine ophthalmopathy. Eur J Endocrinol 1995;132:406.

63. Brain R. Pathogenesis and treatment of endocrine exophthalmos. Lancet 1959;1:109.

64. Duke-Elder S. System of Ophthalmology (Vol 13, part 2). St. Louis: Mosby, 1974;935.

65. Wall JR, Henderson J, Strakosch CR, Joyner DM. Graves' ophthalmopathy. Can Med Assoc J 1981;124:855.

66. Falconer MA, Alexander WS. Experiences with malignant exophthalmos: relationship of the condition to thyrotoxicosis and to the pituitary thyrotropic hormone. Br J Ophthalmol 1951;35:253.

67. Henderson JW. Optic neuropathy of exophthalmic goiter (Graves' disease). Arch Ophthalmol 1958;59:471.

68. Hamilton RD, Mayberry WE, McConahey WM, Hanson KC. Ophthalmopathy of Graves' disease: a comparison between patients treated surgically and patients treated with radioiodide. Mayo Clin Proc 1967;42:812.

69. Hales IB, Rundle FF. Ocular changes in Graves' disease. QJM 1960;29:113.

70. Thomas HM Jr, Woods AC. Progressive exophthalmos following thyroidectomy. Bull Johns Hopkins Hosp 1936;59:99.

71. Hamilton HE, Schultz RO, DeGowin EL. The endocrine eye lesion in hyperthyroidism. Arch Intern Med 1960;105:675.

72. Aron-Rosa D, Perez R, Abitbol Y. Malignant exophthalmos after iodine-131 treatment. Med Probl Ophthalmol 1975;14:432.

73. Calissendorff BM, Soderstrom M, Alveryd A. Ophthalmopathy and hyperthyroidism: a comparison between patients receiving different antithyroid treatments. Acta Ophthalmologica 1986;64:698.

74. Eden KC, Trotter WR. Lid-retraction in toxic diffuse goiter. Lancet 1942;2:385.

75. Bothman L. Endocrine in ophthalmology: with reports of cases of exophthalmos and cataracts following thyroidectomy. IMJ 1942;65:226.

76. Gorman CA. Temporal relationship between onset of Graves' ophthalmopathy and diagnosis of thyrotoxicosis. Mayo Clin Proc 1983;58:515.

77. Aranow H Jr, Day RM. Management of thyrotoxicosis in patients with ophthalmopathy: antithyroid regimen determined primarily by ocular manifestations. J Clin Endocrinol 1965;25:1.

78. Bartley GB. Epidemiologic characteristics and clinical course of ophthalmopathy associated with autoimmune thyroid disease in Olmstead County, Minnesota. Trans Am Ophthalmol Soc 1994;92:477.

79. Barbosa J, Wong E, Doe RP. Ophthalmopathy in Graves' disease. Arch Intern Med 1972;130:111.

80. Perros P, Crombie AL, Kendall-Taylor P. Natural history of thyroid associated ophthalmopathy. Clin Endocrinol 1995;42:45.

81. Havard CWH. Progressive endocrine exophthalmos. Br J Med 1979;1:1001.

82. Prummel MF, Wiersinga WM, Mourits MP, et al. Effect of abnormal thyroid function on severity of Graves' ophthalmopathy. Arch Intern Med 1990;150:1098.

83. Tallstedt L, Lundell G, Blomgren H, Bring J. Does early administration of thyroxine reduce the development of Graves' ophthalmopathy after radioiodine treatment? Eur J Endocrinol 1994;130:494.

84. Teng CS, Yeo PPB. Ophthalmic Graves' disease: natural history and detailed thyroid function studies. Br Med J 1977;1:273.

85. Franco PS, Hershman JM, Haigler ED Jr, Pittman JA Jr. Response to thyrotropin-releasing hormone compared with thyroid suppression tests in euthyroid Graves' disease. Metabolism 1973;22:1357.

86. Tamai H, Nakagawa T, Ohsako N, et al. Changes in thyroid functions in patients with euthyroid Graves' disease. J Clin Endocrinol Metab 1980;50:108.

87. Pequegnat EPP, Mayberry WE, McConahey WM, Wise EP. Large doses of radioiodide in Graves' disease: effect on ophthalmopathy and long-acting thyroid stimulator. Mayo Clin Proc 1967;42:802.

88. Pinchera A, Bartalena L, Marcocci C. Therapeutic controversies. Radioiodine may be bad for Graves' ophthalmopathy, but .... J Clin Endocrinol Metab 1995;80:342.

89. Marcocci C, Bartalena L, Bogazzi F, et al. Relationship between Graves' ophthalmopathy and type of treatment of Graves' hyperthyroidism. Thyroid 1992;2:171.

90. Catz B. Controversies in the Management of Graves' Ophthalmopathy. In SA Falk (ed), Thyroid Disease: Endocrinology, Surgery, Nuclear Medicine and Radiotherapy. New York: Raven, 1990;275.

91. McCullagh EP, Clamen M, Gardner WJ, et al. Exophthalmos of Graves': a summary of the present status of therapy. Ann Intern Med 1958;48:445.

92. Sloan LW. Surgical treatment of hyperthyroidism. N Y State J Med 1951;51:2897.

93. Kriss JP, Konishi J, Herman M. Studies on the pathogenesis of Graves' ophthalmopathy (with some related observations regarding therapy). Recent Prog Horm Res 1975;31:533.

94. Naffziger HC, Jones OW Jr. Surgical treatment of progressive exophthalmos following thyroidectomy. JAMA 1932;99:638.

95. Hetzel BS, Mason EL, Wang HK. Studies of serum long-acting thyroid stimulator (LATS) in relation to exophthalmos after therapy for thyrotoxicosis. Australas Ann Med 1968;17:307.

96. Donaldson SS, Bagshaw MA, Kriss JP. Supervoltage orbital radiotherapy for Graves' ophthalmopathy. J Clin Endocrinol Metab 1973;37:276.

97. Dobyns BM. Present concepts of the pathologic physiology of exophthalmos. J Clin Endocrinol Metab 1950;10:1202.

98. Barth A, Probst P, Burgi H. Identification of a subgroup of Graves' disease patients at higher risk for severe ophthalmopathy after radioiodine. J Endocrinol Invest 1991;14:209.

99. Werner SE, Coelho B, Quimby EH. Ten year results of I-131 therapy of hyperthyroidism. Bull N Y Acad Med 1957;33:783.

100. Jones DIR, Munro DS, Wilson GM. Observations on the course of exophthalmos after ^{131}I therapy. Proc R Soc Med 1969;62:15.

101. Bartalena L, Marcocci C, Bogazzi F, et al. Use of corticosteroids to prevent progression of Graves' ophthalmopathy after radioiodine therapy for hyperthyroidism. N Engl J Med 1989;321:1349.

102. Beck RW, DiLoreto DA. Treatment of Graves' ophthalmopathy. N Engl J Med 1990;322:1088.

103. Karlsson F, Westermark K, Dahlberg PA, et al. Ophthalmopathy and thyroid stimulation. Lancet 1989;2:691.

104. DeGroot LJ, Gorman CA, Pinchera A, et al. Radiation and Graves' ophthalmopathy. J Clin Endocrinol Metab 1995;80:339.

105. Mendlovic DB, Saeed-Zafar M. Ophthalmopathy after treatment for Graves' hyperthyroidism. N Engl J Med 1992;327:1320.

106. Tellez M, Cooper J, Edmonds C. Graves' ophthalmopathy in relation to cigarette smoking and ethnic origin. Clin Endocrinol 1992;36;291.

107. Balzas C, Stenszky V, Farid NR. Association between Graves' ophthalmopathy and smoking. Lancet 1990;336:74.

108. Bartalena L, Martino E, Marcocci C, et al. More on smoking habits and Graves' ophthalmopathy. J Endocrinol Invest 1989;12:733.

109. Shine B, Fells P, Edwards OM, Weetman AP. Association between Graves' ophthalmopathy and smoking. Lancet 1990;335:1261.

110. Winsa B, Mandahl A, Karlsson FA. Graves' disease, endocrine ophthalmopathy and smoking. Acta Endocrinol 1993;128:156.

111. Nunnery WR, Martin RT, Heinz GW, Gavin TJ. The association of cigarette smoking with clinical subtypes of ophthalmic Graves' disease. Ophthal Plast Reconstr Surg 1993;9:77.

112. Sridama V, DeGroot LJ. Treatment of Graves' disease and course of ophthalmopathy. Am J Med 1989;87:70.

113. Grace RV, Weeks C. Surgery of the thyroid in a large municipal hospital. Ann Surg 1941;113:496.

114. Soley MH. Exophthalmos in patients with various types of goiter. Arch Intern Med 1942;70:206.

115. White IL. Total thyroid ablation: a prerequisite to orbital decompression for Graves' disease ophthalmopathy. Laryngoscopy 1974;84:1869.

116. Barbosa J, Wong E, Doe RP. Ophthalmopathy of Graves' disease. Arch Intern Med 1972;130:111.

117. Catz B, Perzik SL. Subtotal vs. Surgical Ablation of the Thyroid, Malignant Exophthalmos and Its Relation to Remnant Thyroid. In C Cassona, M Adreoli (eds), Current Topics in Thyroid Research: Proceedings of the Fifth International Thyroid Conference. New York: Academic, 1965;1183.

118. Werner SE, Feind CR, Aida M. Graves' disease and total thyroidectomy. N Engl J Med 1967;276:132.

119. Boyle IT, Greig WR, Thomson JA, et al. Effect of thyroid ablation dysthyroid exophthalmos. Proc R Soc Med 1969;62:19.

120. Bauer FK, Catz B. Radioactive iodine therapy for progressive malignant exophthalmos. Acta Endocrinol (Copenh) 1966;51:15.

121. Bartels EC, Irie M. Thyroid Function in Patients with Progressive Exophthalmos: A Study of 117 Cases Requiring Orbital Decompression. In R Pittrivers (ed), Advanced Thyroid Research. New York: Pergamon, 1961;163.

122. Streeten DHP, Anderson GH Jr, Reed GF, Woo P. Prevalence, natural history, and surgical treatment of exophthalmos. Clin Endocrinol 1987;27:125.

123. Kennerdell JS, Rosenbaum AE, El-Hosby MH. Apical optic nerve compression of dysthyroid optic neuropathy on computed tomography. Arch Ophthalmol 1981;99:807.

124. Igersheimer J. Visual changes in progressive exophthalmos. Arch Ophthalmol 1955;53:94.

125. Hedges TR, Scheie HG. Visual field defects in exophthalmos associated with thyroid disease. Arch Ophthalmol 1955;54:845.

126. Day RM, Carroll FD. Corticosteroids in the treatment of optic nerve involvement associated with thyroid dysfunction. Arch Ophthalmol 1968;79:279.

127. Paufigue L, Guinet L, Papillon J. Le traitement de l'exophtalmie oedèmateuse sans hyperthyroidie. Ann Ocul 1950;183:449.

128. Offret M-C, Offret G. L'exophtalmie maligne de la maladie de Basedow. Arch d'Ophtalmol 1945;5:429.

129. Trobe JD, Glaser JS, Laflamme P. Dysthyroid optic neuropathy. Arch Ophthalmol 1978;96:1199.

130. Degroot LJ, Benjasuratwong Y. Evaluation of thyroid ablative therapy for ophthalmopathy of Graves' disease. Orbit 1996;15:187.

8

Thyroid Management: General Principles

Optimum management of thyroid ophthalmopathy depends on many variables. In determining the order and type of therapeutic approaches, the clinician must consider thyroid status, the stability, number, and severity of ocular signs, and the patient's general health and psychological status (Table 8-1).

The natural history of thyroid eye disease and its relationship to hyperthyroidism were reviewed in Chapter 7. Almost 90% of patients who develop ophthalmic complications of Graves' disease undergo spontaneous remission of most signs and symptoms within 3 years of systemic treatment. Onset is usually gradual—ophthalmic signs slowly increase and then abate as systemic hyperthyroidism is brought under control. Eyelid retraction, with resultant lid lag and stare, usually resolves when the hyperthyroid state is corrected. Unless corneal exposure or compressive optic neuropathy mandates intervention, surgery should not be contemplated in such cases for at least 6 months following the beginning of systemic therapy, and then only if the remaining eyelid retraction and/or the strabismus is stabilized. Many patients with extraocular muscle dysfunction improve without ocular therapy. It is therefore central to the discussion of eye disease management to know the patient's systemic thyroid status and to determine whether eye signs and symptoms are in an incipient, progressive, or regressive phase.

While patients with thyrotoxicosis often improve after systemic treatment, previously treated patients presenting with thyroid eye disease and minimal autonomous thyroid function rarely experience spontaneous ocular improvement after a second course of systemic antithyroid therapy. Indeed, the second or subsequent courses of systemic treatment do not appear to affect the progress of the eye disease over and above the baseline, although seemingly spontaneous exacerbations and remissions associated with thyroid ophthalmopathy may occur.

The nature of the patient's ocular symptoms are important in determining therapeutic options. Regardless of thyroid status or phase of ocular disease, such visually threatening problems as optic neuropathy or corneal damage secondary to exposure require rapid and effective treatment. Many ophthalmic problems should be watched or conservatively treated (symptomatically or with topical medicines) until they either stabilize or resolve. As an example, we have seen patients surgically treated for lid retraction or extraocular muscle problems before reaching a stable endpoint who then have an overcorrection after surgery.

Table 8-1. Therapeutic Options in Thyroid Eye Disease

Symptomatic maneuvers
    Sunglasses
    Sleep in supine position with head of bed elevated
    Occlusive goggles
Topical medications
    Artificial tears/ointment
    Alpha adrenergic blocking agents
Systemic drugs/procedures
    Diuretics
    Steroids
    Miscellaneous agents (metronidazole [Flagyl], etc.)
    Immunomodulators
        Cytotoxic agents
        Cyclosporine
    Plasmapheresis
Orbital radiation surgery
    Eyelid retraction
    Extraocular muscle restriction
    Orbital decompression

Many patients with thyroid ophthalmopathy require a series of planned sequential therapies. Some respond to nonsurgical therapies while others appear to fare best with combined medical and surgical treatment. Patients with specific thyroid ocular complications should only be managed with surgery.

Historically, less than 5% of all thyroid ophthalmopathy patients require surgical intervention. In a recent cohort incidence study of 120 patients with thyroid eye findings, 74% required no major ophthalmic treatment.[1] Patients older than 50 had a 2.6% greater chance of needing ocular surgery. At 5 years, an accumulative surgical probability is 24% in older patients and 12% in patients younger than 50.[1] Overall in that series, 8% required orbital decompression, 11% required strabismus surgery, and 13% required eyelid repair.

Orbital decompression and extraocular muscle surgery can markedly alter the shape and position of the eyelids. If either of these procedures is contemplated, eyelid surgery should be postponed. In addition, nationally more than 30% of patients require strabismus surgery after orbital decompression, and muscle surgery should be postponed until stabilization following that orbital procedure. Cosmetic repair of deformities in patients with thyroid ophthalmopathy is a major problem. It is crucial to determine all patients' psychological states and perceptions of the major unacceptable components of their appearance, then fully inform them about the potential complications of suggested therapies. Many thyroid ophthalmopathy patients are emotionally labile and have unrealistic concepts of what can be done to improve their appearance. It is important, therefore, to stress that no current therapy can arrest the underlying disease process and that ocular findings can recur after any form of therapy. Furthermore, it is absolutely vital, especially in patients with severe ophthalmopathy, to stress that multiple procedures will probably be necessary to manage eyelid retraction, proptosis, and myopathy. Finally, it is also necessary to delineate possible complications and tradeoffs that each repair approach entails.

Treatment of diplopia must be planned very carefully. Thyroid ophthalmopathy is the most common cause of diplopia in middle-aged or elderly patients. If the symptoms are intermittent or episodic, it is important to confirm the correct diagnosis; conditions such as myasthenia gravis can coexist with thyroid disease. Moreover, many intermittent thyroid diplopia problems resolve spontaneously. Patients with early thyroid eye disease or with an acute or subacute onset of severe inflammation or double vision often improve with steroid treatment.

The definitive management of most chronic thyroid myopathies is surgical. While prisms can be useful in some patients (those with very small vertical or horizontal deviations) they are not generally satisfactory. I wait until the patient's eye muscle measurements are stable for at least 3 months before intervening surgically. As mentioned above, if the patient is a likely candidate for decompression and extraocular muscle surgery, strabismus repair is deferred until after decompression (see Chapter 12).

Therapy for thyroid optic neuropathy is controversial; some investigators advocate steroids or other medications, others radiation, and others immediate orbital decompression. There is almost universal agreement, however, that most of these patients with marked vision decrease require rapid intervention. I favor steroids and radiation followed by decompression if those two therapies are not effective. Immunomodulation with cytotoxic agents or cyclosporine has been less effective in my hands and can have significant morbidity. Cyclosporine is probably indicated instead of irradiation in patients who do not have access to centers with radiation expertise or if the latter technique had not been efficacious.

The remainder of this book is divided into chapters on different aspects of treatment. Chapter 9 covers medical therapy, including the use of topical adrenergic blocking agents (guanethidine sulfate, thymoxamine, etc.), steroids, cytotoxic agents, plasmapheresis, and immunomodulatory agents. Chapter 10 discusses radiation therapy. Chapter 11 describes various techniques of lid surgery. The indications, advantages, disadvantages, and complications of orbital decompression are covered in Chapter 12, along with techniques of orbital decompression surgery. Treatment of extraocular muscle dysfunction is discussed in Chapter 13.

REFERENCE

1. Bartley GB, Fatourechi V, Kadrmas EF, et al. The treatment of Graves' ophthalmopathy in an incidence cohort. Am J Ophthalmol 1996;121:200.

9

Medical Therapy of Thyroid Ophthalmopathy

Systemic and topical medications have been used to treat thyroid ophthalmopathy. Chapter 7 reviews data on the effect of systemic thyroid therapy on eye disease. A rational approach to using nonsurgical therapies for thyroid orbitopathy is partially predicated on the acuteness and severity of disease and the relative efficacy and morbidity of treatments.

This chapter emphasizes the indications, efficacy, and complications that have been observed with medical therapies and summarizes the comparative data available on these agents in thyroid eye disease. There have been a few trials comparing radiation and corticosteroids, and they are discussed mainly here, but also in Chapter 10.

SYMPTOMATIC THERAPIES

Some maneuvers can increase patient comfort, especially for transient eye symptoms. For instance, many clinicians have observed that patients who sleep in a prone position have more problems with eye symptoms than those who sleep supine. A change in sleep position and elevation of the head of the bed can decrease periorbital and lid edema. While others have advocated the use of diuretics to treat periorbital and lid edema, I and others have not found this procedure beneficial.[1]

The gritty, foreign-body sensation many patients develop with thyroid ocular involvement is often alleviated with nonprescription eye drops. While the different tear preparations all have staunch advocates, I have not found one kind of artificial tear superior to another. We generally give patients office samples of four or five preparations and let them choose the one that gives the greatest relief. Allergic reaction to the preservatives in the medications can develop in patients who use artificial tears chronically. Such patients improve with preservative-free tear substitutes.

Finally, the photophobia often presenting in thyroid eye disease can be alleviated with sunglasses in many cases.

TOPICAL THERAPY WITH ADRENERGIC BLOCKING AGENTS

As discussed in Chapter 6, many factors are important in the pathophysiology of thyroid eyelid retraction. The probable mechanism for most early eyelid retraction, the type that often spontaneously resolves with correction of hyperthyroidism, is the increased alpha-adrenergic tone affecting Müller's muscle.[2] It is often impossible to determine how much upper eyelid retraction is secondary to increased adrenergic stimuli versus fibrosis of the levator, the inferior rectus muscle, or both. In patients with recent onset eyelid retraction, especially those who do not have significantly greater intraocular pressure in upgaze as compared with primary position, a trial with topical alpha-adrenergic blocking agents is reasonable. A number of different topical and systemic drugs, including reserpine, propranolol, bethanidine sulfate, guanethidine sulfate, and thymoxamine have been shown to have an effect on eyelid retraction.[3–5]

Most investigations have used topical guanethidine sulfate drops to alleviate lid retraction. This agent depletes the sympathetic storage sites and eventually produces a chemical sympathectomy. Preliminary studies with a 10% solution had a significant incidence of superficial punctate keratitis.[6] In an early short-term trial of 14 patients, Sneddon and Turner noted good results with guanethidine.[7] Cant and Lewis studied 81 patients to determine the efficacy of guanethidine. They observed a good response with 2% and 5% drops using various regimens from three times daily to less than once daily in all but one case. They recommended starting at 5% solution three times daily and, once a good lid position was obtained, decreasing the drops to daily or alternate-day application. To achieve a permanent effect, medication, often at a reduced dosage, usually has to be continued in perpetuity. Cant and Lewis noted that only seven of 77 patients maintained normal lid position after drops were stopped.[8]

In a separate study, Cartlidge and coworkers noted that the ptosis produced by a 5% solution was approximately 1.5 mm, and most patients reverted to the previous degree of eyelid retraction shortly after the drug was discontinued.[9] Similarly, Martin and Jay noted that 12 of 19 patients treated with guanethidine drops had some improvement in eyelid position, although three patients had to stop drops because of conjunctival vessel dilation.[10] In a follow-up to their original study, Cant and Lewis investigated the morbidity of various concentrations of guanethidine drops. Almost all patients experienced miosis and dilation of conjunctival vessels secondary to the pharmacologic effect of the drug. In most cases (60 patients), the conjunctival flush was acceptable. Three subjects developed intense vasocongestion. Fourteen patients had discomfort and burning on instillation of drops. Two of 10 patients on a 10% solution developed superficial punctate keratitis, which was only partially alleviated when the percentage dose was decreased. None of the 25 patients on 2% drops twice daily developed this complication. Four subjects had unilateral ptosis. Results do not improve using other agents with a mechanism of action similar to that of guanethidine.[3,11,12]

Major problems with these agents are their local toxicity, unpredictable response (in amount of associated ptosis produced and in effectiveness for individual patients), and limited long-term efficacy. While cardiovascular or respiratory effects can develop when adrenergic blockers are given systemically, they appear to be avoided by use of eye drops.

In general, the use of adrenergic blocking agents is limited to three clinical situations. First, the drugs are helpful in treating lid retraction in patients undergoing treatment for systemic hyperthyroidism. They often provide transient relief until the possibility of spontaneous correction or need for surgical intervention can be determined. Second, we have found that many patients with subacute eyelid retraction (<6 months) do very well with this agent, especially if the intraocular pressure does not rise more than 5 mm on upgaze, although some other investigators have not noted such positive results. Figures 9-1 through 9-4 demonstrate two patients who had excellent

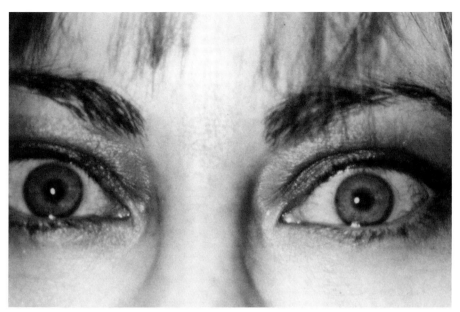

Figure 9-1. Eyelid retraction during hyperthyroidism.

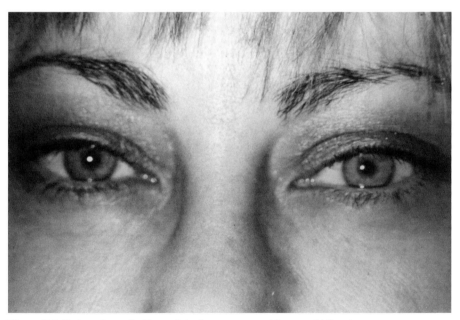

Figure 9-2. Patient shown in Figure 9-1 after treatment with guanethidine drops.

results on long-term therapy. We have our pharmacist make a 2% solution of guanethidine drops. Usually a beneficial effect is observed in the first 72 hours after treatment is started. Rarely, patients find the conjunctival irritation too great for the benefit received and stop these medications independently. In my experience and that of others, the incidence of complications that lead to cessation of therapy with 2% guanethidine

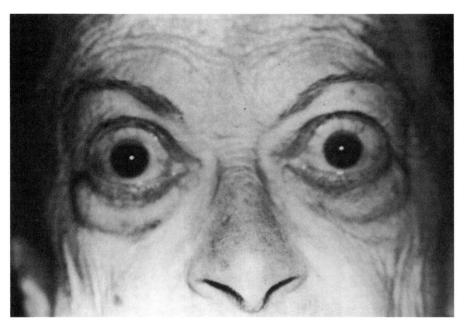

Figure 9-3. Eyelid retraction in euthyroid patient (treatment of Graves' disease more than 20 years ago, with 6-month history of stare).

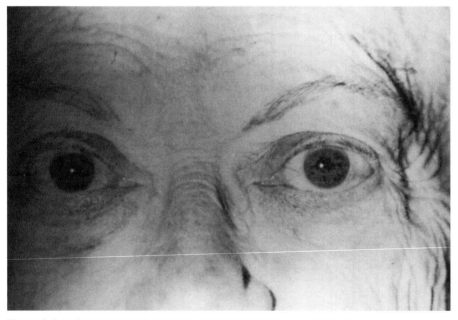

Figure 9-4. Patient shown in Figure 9-3 1 week after starting guanethidine drops.

drops is very small.[13,14] A minority of patients use these agents for topical sympathec-tomy, have an excellent response, and can discontinue them in 6–9 months with their eyelids reverting to a normal position. A third use has been to attempt to delineate the relative role of sympathetic effects (Müller's muscle) in producing eyelid retraction in patients before surgical therapy. I have not found this last use of any value in deter-mining the need for surgical treatment (see Chapter 11). Guanethidine drops are not commercially available. A pharmacist can make a 2% solution from the antihyperten-sion tablet, and several pharmacies do this for our patients.

STEROID THERAPY

In the early 1950s, there were scattered reports of steroids being used to treat thyroid eye disease.[15–26] In 1953, Kinsell et al. noted improvement in nine patients.[27] Many workers noted poor responses; evaluated retrospectively, most of these treatment fail-ures were due to low dosage or poor patient selection.

In 1963, Brown and coworkers reported one of the largest early trials of steroids in thyroid ophthalmopathy treatment.[28] They treated 19 of 101 patients—those with the most severe infiltrative ophthalmopathies—with systemic steroids. Eight had de-creased vision pretreatment, four had papilledema, and 11 had progressive proptosis or ophthalmoplegia. In this study, symptoms, chemosis, and injection decreased in the first 24–48 hours after starting either of two levels of oral prednisone therapy (35–45 mg or 60–80 mg). In six of eight patients with presumed optic neuropathy, visual acuity improved dramatically; the other two had mildly increased vision. Duc-tions improved in 10 of 19 patients within 1 week of treatment onset, and proptosis decreased in nine patients during the same interval. These authors used systemic steroids for a mean of 10 months and noted that eight of 19 patients (42%) relapsed when medication was tapered or discontinued. While five of these eight patients re-sponded to resumed and increased steroid doses, four patients eventually required orbital decompression. Eleven patients (58%) had some side effects, including ulcer, acne, Cushingoid changes, osteoporosis, and psychosis.[28]

In 1966, Werner published findings on two patients who responded to high-dose (100–140 mg daily) prednisone, making the point that some patients who do not re-spond to lower dosages do respond at this drug level.[29] There is no firm guideline to systemic steroid dosage in thyroid orbitopathy. Most authors recommend 40–80 mg of oral prednisone daily for 4 weeks, then gradual tapering of the dosage by 5 mg per day every week or two.[30–33] Many patients do develop disease exacerbation when the prednisone dosage is decreased to less than 30 mg daily.[30,33] Most clinicians try not to keep patients on these agents for more than six months.

The mechanism of steroid effect in thyroid orbitopathy is uncertain. Anti-inflammatory and immunomodulatory actions are probably most important, but steroids can also decrease mucopolysaccharide production by orbital fibro-blasts.[34,35] As discussed in Chapter 6, steroids have also been shown to modulate other cytokines and receptors on orbital fibroblasts.

Currently in my orbital unit, systemic steroids are used in five general groups of thyroid ophthalmopathy patients. First, this treatment is excellent for patients pre-senting with acute symptomatic inflammatory disease. The patient in Figures 9-5 and 9-6 is a typical example of this steroid usage. She initially presented with rapid onset of proptosis, periorbital edema, and ophthalmoplegia without a history of thy-roid disease. An axial computed tomography (CT) image revealed the typical

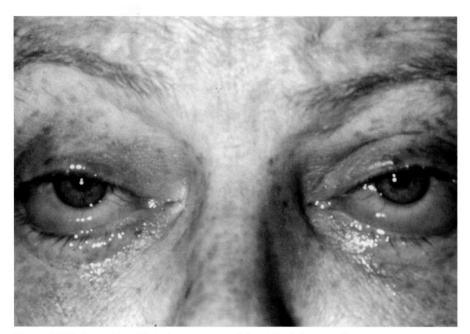

Figure 9-5. Patient with a relatively acute onset of thyroid ophthalmopathy.

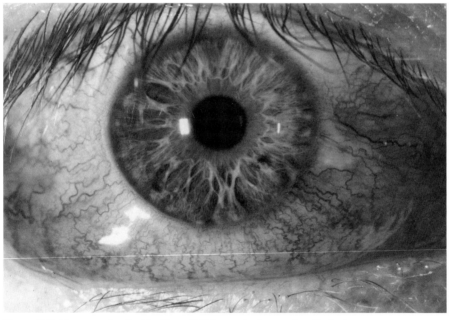

Figure 9-6. Close-up of patient in Figure 9-5 demonstrating conjunctival edema.

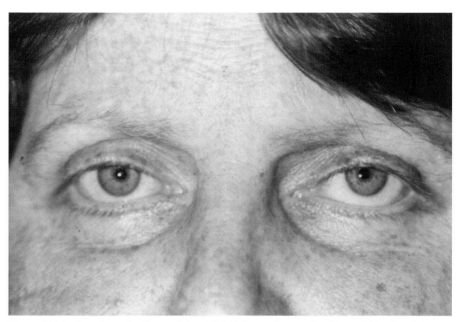

Figure 9-7. Patient shown in Figures 9-5 and 9-6 72 hours after starting 80 mg daily of prednisone.

changes of thyroid ophthalmopathy; the nontendinous portions of the muscles were involved without demonstrable fat or vascular orbital changes. The patient was placed on 80 mg of prednisone daily and had almost total resolution within 72 hours (Figure 9-7). Figures 9-8 and 9-9 show another patient with complete resolution of symptoms on 100 mg of oral prednisone daily for 10 days.

The second group of patients treated with steroids are those who develop thyroid optic neuropathy with relatively mild visual loss (visual acuities ≥20/80). Several investigators have reported favorable steroid response in these situations.[36–38] In a series of 10 patients, Day and Carroll noted that, in all cases, vision improved 2–37 days from the start of treatment. They also observed that many patients had to be maintained on high-dose steroids, since lowering intake resulted in decreased visual acuity.[39] Similarly, Ponzo and Tomsak observed that 13 of 16 eyes with thyroid optic neuropathy improved on steroids; however, eight relapsed at a later date.[36] In contrast, Gorman and colleagues noted that 14 of 18 optic neuropathy patients failed to respond to corticosteroid therapy.[40] I and my colleagues have not observed steroid therapy to have a permanent effect on most cases of thyroid optic neuropathy, although a small minority will involute and not require further therapy. As shown in Figures 9-8 and 9-9, this patient with thyroid optic neuropathy and best corrected visual acuity of 20/80 was examined and had a marked visual field defect (Figure 9-10). One week later on 100 mg oral prednisone daily the visual field results markedly improved (Figure 9-11). Corticosteroids were stopped 4 days later, and he has not developed recurrent optic neuropathy. Most thyroid optic neuropathy patients have ultimately been treated with radiation alone, radiation plus steroids, or radiation and orbital decompression.

The third group of patients treated with systemic steroids are those with recent (<6 months) onset of severe thyroid ophthalmopathy with predominantly inflammatory soft-tissue signs. In the fourth group are those few patients who, despite orbital

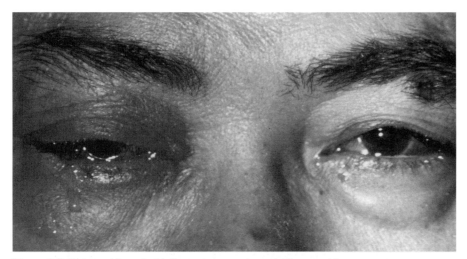

Figure 9-8. Patient with marked inflammatory symptoms before steroids.

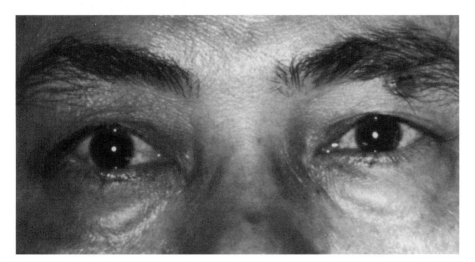

Figure 9-9. Patient shown in Figure 9-8 after 1 week of 100 mg oral prednisone daily.

radiation (see Chapter 10) and surgical decompression, require continuous steroids or steroids plus other immunomodulatory agents to control disease progression. As discussed in Chapter 7, patients with severe ocular findings at the time of presentation with systemic hyperthyroidism are treated with oral steroids during and after radioactive iodine therapy. Finally, these drugs are used preoperatively and intraoperatively on all patients undergoing orbital decompression. An important caveat to emphasize is that some patients received corticosteroids to manage their thyroid immune abnormality, which is not discussed here.

Overall, response to steroids is a function of disease duration, the inflammatory component, and type of eye involvement. Generally, patients with a short disease course, with marked inflammation, and mainly soft-tissue signs do well with steroids. Patients with chronic disease, little or no inflammation, and predominantly stable strabismus or proptosis and its sequelae (e.g., corneal exposure, etc.) usually do not respond to steroids. As discussed in Chapter 12, many patients who eventually have

Figure 9-10. Left visual field in patient shown in Figures 9-8 and 9-9 with 20/80 visual acuity and thyroid optic neuropathy.

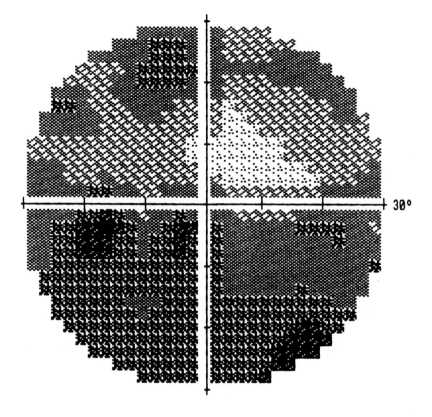

Figure 9-11. Patient's visual field (see Figure 9-10) after a 1-week course of 100 mg daily of oral prednisone.

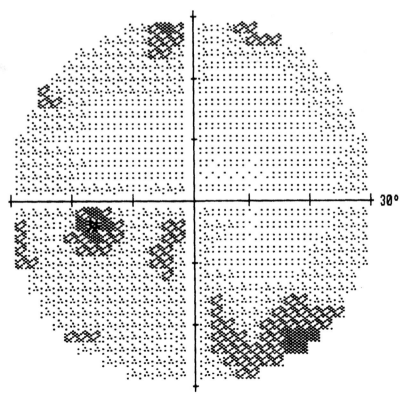

Table 9-1. Complications of Corticosteroid Therapy

 1. Pituitary-adrenal suppression
 2. Infection
 3. Cataract
 4. Systemic hypertension
 5. Osteoporosis
 6. Renal lithiasis
 7. Diabetes
 8. Ecchymoses
 9. Phlebitis
10. Hirsutism
11. Reactivation of chronic diseases (tuberculosis, etc.)
12. Psychosis

orbital decompression have been on long-term steroids and failed or developed systemic morbidity. In most series the response rate has been approximately 65%.[40a]

In my experience, 100 mg of oral prednisone daily is optimal if steroids are effective in a given case. We have seen patients fail at lower doses, then respond to 100 mg daily. In contrast, I have not seen improved response at higher corticosteroid doses.

Almost all patients on long-term systemic steroid therapy develop significant side effects, and this has lead us to markedly limit the duration of this therapy, or switch to irradiation or immunomodulation. If irradiation or immunomodulatory agents are used, a patient's initial steroid dosage is maintained, then gradually tapered, starting 2 weeks after the completion of radiation therapy, or after the known latency for effect with a given immunomodulatory or cytotoxic drug. Dosage reduction must be gradual to avoid life-threatening complications in long-term (>2 weeks) steroid users. Alternative day steroids do not seem to be effective in controlling active thyroid ophthalmopathy in any but rare cases.

Steroids are not needed in most thyroid orbitopathy patients who present to the ophthalmologist with thyroid eye disease of more than 1 year's duration; especially if their signs and symptoms consist predominantly of fibrotic extraocular muscle involvement, proptosis, or eyelid retraction. Steroids mainly affect leukocyte infiltration, which occurs early in the disease course; it is doubtful that the drugs have much effect on the fibrotic changes of chronic disease.[41] This helps explain the many early reports that noted poor responses to steroid therapy. They resulted from treatment of patients with chronic disease.[42,43]

The duration of steroid therapy is controversial. I have chosen to alter my steroid usage from the conventional approach because of the significant complications of long-term steroids. As an alternative we treat patients with 100 mg daily of oral prednisone for 10 days, then abruptly stop treatment. There is almost uniform agreement that patients who benefit from steroids do so rapidly. Approximately 30% of patients treated with the above regimen appear to receive a relatively permanent effect. Undoubtedly, if patients were treated for longer periods of time, or drugs were tapered slowly, a somewhat higher response rate would be seen; however, the complication rate would also increase.[28,44] (A list of common steroid complications is shown in Table 9-1.) Since orbital radiation (see Chapter 10) appears to have less morbidity than long-term corticosteroid treatment, it is preferable for patients who have no response, partial resolution, or relapse after cessation of steroids. The use of immunomodulatory agents is discussed below.

Other steroid treatment options are available. Some authors have tried pulse therapy; the relative efficacy is uncertain.[40a, 45,46] In one study, an 80% response rate was noted, but the author pointed out that in most trials, early results are more promising.[40a] Local periocular steroids have also been used to treat thyroid eye disease.[37,47–54] I have tried a retrobulbar steroids approach with little apparent benefit beyond minor improvement in conjunctival signs.[47–50] Overall, approximately 60–70% of patients have had a good or excellent steroid response versus slightly less with radiation.[55]

In two Italian studies, 20 Gy of photon irradiation combined with systemic steroids (70–80 mg methylprednisolone daily) was compared with radiation plus repeated retrobulbar steroids (40 mg methylprednisolone acetate). The former treatment was significantly more effective than the latter at reducing the ophthalmic index.[52,56] A measurable effect on extraocular muscles was noted in 17 of 27 patients treated with radiation and systemic steroids compared with eight of 28 with radiation plus retrobulbar steroids. Overall, the ophthalmic index decreased to 2.6 in the former versus 3.5 in the latter group ($p < 0.02$).[52]

These authors expanded their trial and assigned 20 patients to 20 Gy of radiation alone or radiation with steroids. The corticosteroids were delivered at 100 mg of prednisone daily for 7 days, then gradually tapered during 6 months. Patients were evaluated 6–9 months after treatment.[57] The patient group that received radiation and steroids did better; however, there were some dissimilarities between the two groups (the combined group had a shorter duration of ophthalmopathy), and the difference in treatment response was not significant.[57] The authors thought that 69% of the combined group had an excellent or good response compared with 38% in the group that received only radiation. Most of the patients in the combined group developed Cushingoid features. Prummel and colleagues performed a double-masked trial of a 3-month course of oral corticosteroids plus sham radiation versus 20 Gy of radiation alone.[58] They determined therapeutic response with a modified NO SPECS classification (see Chapter 4) at 6 months. Both groups had an equal response rate of approximately 50%, with the greatest effect on soft-tissue findings and motility improvements. There were more side effects with prednisone, and these authors concluded that radiation was therefore the treatment of choice.[58] Some authors have used pulse intravenous corticosteroids with variable results.[59,60]

IMMUNOSUPPRESSIVE THERAPY: CYTOTOXIC AGENTS, CYCLOSPORINE, AND PLASMAPHERESIS

Some investigators have reported on the use of various cytotoxic agents, including methotrexate, azathioprine, and cyclophosphamide, with generally good or equivocal results.[61–69] In some cases, a combination of cytotoxic agents plus radiation have been used, making it difficult to discern the relative efficacy of each modality.[70] Two prospective studies have been reported on cyclosporine in thyroid eye disease.[71,72] Prummel and colleagues compared a 3-month course of prednisone (60 mg/day for 2 weeks, then tapered) with cyclosporine (7.5 mg/kg/day) in 36 patients. The steroid-treated patients did significantly better than those who received cyclosporine (11 of 18 versus 4 of 18 responders). At 1 year, almost 50% required surgery or radiation.[71] Kahaly and colleagues compared relatively long-term systemic prednisone alone versus prednisone with moderately high-dose (5.0–7.5 mg/kg/day) cyclosporine for 1 year.[72] The combined group did better than the patients who received only steroids in terms of a more rapid onset of remission and its maintenance.[72] In general it appears that the best candidates for steroid therapy—namely, those with inflammatory

Table 9-2. Common Complications of Immunomodulatory Agents (Cytotoxic Drugs)

1. Bone marrow suppression
2. Increased infection
3. Carcinogenesis
4. Hepatotoxicity (azathioprine, chlorambucil, methotrexate)
5. Azoospermia (chlorambucil)
6. Hemorrhagic cystitis (cyclophosphamide)
7. Gastrointestinal disturbance (methotrexate, azathioprine)
8. Rash/fever (azathioprine, chlorambucil, methotrexate)
9. Hepatic or renal toxicity (cyclosporine)

signs of recent onset—respond well to cytotoxic or immunomodulatory drugs.[73] Wall et al. noted diminished congestion in all patients treated with cyclophosphamide. Proptosis decreased in three of 24 individuals, and extraocular muscle function improved in 11 of 20 patients.[63] It is puzzling to me why cytotoxic agents have been effective in a few patients with long-standing diplopia; I have not observed any positive benefit in this group of patients.

Plasmapheresis has been successfully used to treat many autoimmune diseases, but its efficacy has only been stringently demonstrated in a few syndromes, including hyperviscosity syndrome, cold antibody hemolytic anemia, post-transfusion purpura, myasthenia gravis, Refsum's syndrome, and Goodpasture's syndrome.[74] How this therapeutic modality works is unclear; clearance of immune complexes, toxic plasma proteins, specific serum factors, and unknown substances have all been postulated.

The use of plasmapheresis in thyroid eye disease has mirrored the problems observed in assessing responses in most other diseases. As discussed in Chapters 2 and 6, the concept of immune complex involvement in the pathophysiology of thyroid eye disease is attractive but unproved. There has been little evidence of elevated circulating levels of antigen-antibody complexes. Dandona and colleagues first reported a partial, short-term effect in a thyroid ophthalmopathy patient treated with plasmapheresis and azathioprine.[75] Other investigators did not observe similar favorable effects, and later Dandona and coworkers also noted equivocal results.[76–80] Kelly et al. reported on the immunologic and clinical parameters in 18 Graves' ophthalmopathy patients treated with plasmapheresis.[81] In that study, 13 patients also received azathioprine, and these authors found no significant changes in immunologic, clinical, or radiologic (CT and quantitative A-scan) evidence of thyroid ophthalmopathy.[81] Glinoer and coworkers reported on 11 patients who received multiple plasmapheresis sessions with systemic prednisone and azathioprine.[81–84] They noted that this form of treatment did not seem to affect corneal or extraocular muscle dysfunction but appeared to diminish soft-tissue findings. Overall, eight of 11 patients had long-term remissions, although it is impossible to discern how much of the therapeutic effect was due to steroids, cytotoxic drugs, or plasmapheresis. Major complications of cytotoxic drug treatment are listed in Table 9-2.

As discussed above, cyclosporine is an immunosuppressive agent that preferentially affects the activation of the T-inducer subset by several mechanisms, including blocking interleukin-2 induction. Promising results have been reported in renal transplantation and therapy for some autoimmune diseases, including some posterior uveitides.[85–91] Weetman and colleagues studied one chronic and one acute thyroid ophthalmopathy patient treated with cyclosporine. Of particular interest among the positive responses observed clinically and quantitatively were changed thyroid antibody lev-

Figure 9-12. Axial computed tomographies show change in extraocular muscle thickness after treatment with systemic cyclosporine. (Reprinted with permission from C Utech, KG Wulle, N Panitz, et al. Immunosuppressive treatment of Graves' ophthalmopathy with cyclosporine A. Transplant Proc 1988;20:173.)

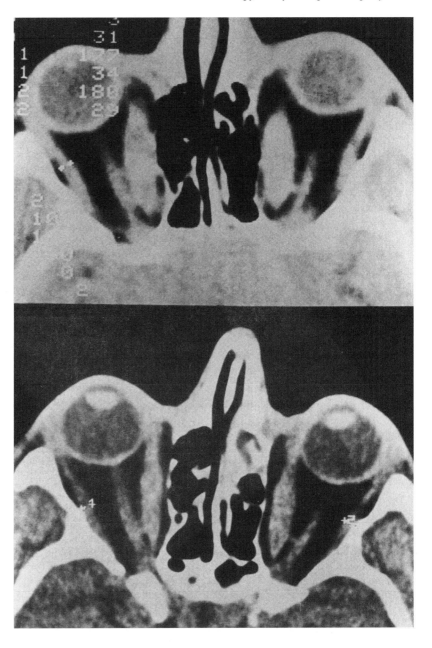

els.[92] Utech and coworkers studied 10 patients who had previously been treated with prednisone, radiation, or plasmapheresis; in six there was decreased extraocular muscle thickness on CT, and in seven there was subjective improvement.[93] Figure 9-12 shows CT examinations before and after cyclosporine therapy that show marked diminution of extraocular muscle swelling. When this group reviewed their own and others' data they found that approximately 40% of patients had sufficient treatment complications (Table 9-3) to require dose reduction or therapy cessation.[93–95]

Some investigators have theorized that combination steroid and cyclosporine therapy is more effective than either treatment alone, although the relative contribution and role of steroids (additive, synergistic, inductive, etc.) is not clear.[71,72,93,96] Ka-

Table 9-3. Complications of Cyclosporine Therapy

1. Renal insufficiency
2. Gastrointestinal disturbances
3. Paresthesias and central nervous system toxicity
4. Stomatitis/gingivitis
5. Systemic hypertension
6. Abnormal liver enzyme levels
7. Infections
8. Systemic myopathies
9. Hypertrichosis
10. Anemia
11. ?Lymphoma

haly and coworkers studied 48 patients with class III-V disease who were randomized on the basis of year of birth to prednisone or prednisone plus cyclosporine. They thought that improvement was significantly greater in the combined therapy group. Relapses occurred in eight of 20 of the former and only one of 20 of the combined group.[72] As discussed previously, prospective studies showed better results with combined therapy.[71,72]

Case reports have been published, some with positive, some with negative results, and often patients have had to stop cyclosporine because of toxicity.[97–99] Witte and coworkers treated 13 patients with class IV-VI disease during 4–7 months. In one patient, disease progressed despite therapy, and there was no apparent effect on proptosis, vision, or extraocular muscle thickness.[100] While subjective symptoms appeared to improve in that study, objective findings did not; other investigators have also noted little effect with this drug.[101,102] Similarly, others have noted limited efficacy of this agent.[99,103] A major problem with cyclosporine is that the measurement of serum levels can be inaccurate, and therefore some of the problems may have been due to relying too much on cyclosporine dosage (generally 10 mg/kg/day) rather than actual drug levels.[104]

Toxic side effects of most forms of immunomodulation (see Table 9-2) mitigate against their use, except in patients who have not responded to conventional therapy (steroids, radiation, or surgery) and who have vision-threatening complications of thyroid eye disease. It is likely that once the pathophysiology and role of immunologic abnormalities in thyroid ophthalmopathy are better delineated, newer, specific, less toxic immunomodulatory agents will become available and will play a larger role in the management of thyroid eye disease.[105,106] I use cyclosporine in patients intractable to other nonsurgical therapies, in patients who would be excellent candidates for orbital radiation but because of distance from a superb radiation oncology center are not, or in patients with visual loss that failed both radiation and orbital decompression.

Monitoring patients after various forms of medical treatment can be difficult. Horomatsu and others have used the differences between fibrosis and inflammation on T_1-weighted and T_2-weighted magnetic resonance (MR) scans to attempt to identify optimal candidates for medical treatment and monitor therapeutic response.[107] These workers used relatively thick sections and a low-strength magnet but were able to predict treatment response using short inversion recovery time signal intensities from the extraocular muscles.[107]

In a small study, somatostatin was less effective than corticosteroids.[107a] Other immunomodulatory agents are also being investigated. Ciamexon inhibits expression of human leukocyte (HLA)-DR antigens, an important component of the antigen recognition pathway. A few patients have been treated with this agent, and early results have been positive.[108,109]

There have been a few reports of positive results with other immunomodulatory agents.[109–111] Bromocriptine binds to dopamine receptors and its effects include decreased prolactin levels, inhibition of thyroid-stimulating hormones, and an anti-T lymphocyte action. Approximately 25 patients with thyroid orbitopathy have been treated with this agent.[109–113] The follow-up on these patients was limited, but bromocriptine response has occurred in cases that have failed systemic steroids, orbital radiation, or orbital decompression. Generally, patients have received approximately 2.5 mg three times daily for several months. Harden and coworkers noted that seven of 12 patients with endocrine exophthalmos treated with 400 mg of metronidazole three times a day displayed subjective improvement; however, the disease recurred when therapy was stopped.[114] An alternative autoimmune therapy approach is to treat with a monoclonal antibody toward ICAM-1, a cytokine active in thyroid orbitopathy. Although this treatment has been tried in rheumatoid arthritis, there are no data in thyroid eye disease.[114a]

In the Chinese literature there is an interesting report using the upper Tianzhu and Gengchi acupoints to treat thyroid extraocular muscle problems with acupuncture showing approximately 70% good results.[115] In another acupuncture study, the results were negative.[116] Similarly, in a randomized trial, Venalot was no better than placebo for thyroid disease.[117]

CONCLUSION

Many signs and symptoms of thyroid eye disease are transient; spontaneous remission does occur with control of the systemic manifestations of thyrotoxicosis or as part of the natural evolution of thyroid ophthalmopathy. Because of this, in patients with recent onset of thyroid ophthalmopathy, medical rather than surgical therapy is indicated.

As many as 50% of patients with thyroid eyelid retraction improve spontaneously. In these cases, topical drops are often sufficient for control, and only a minority of patients eventually requires surgery.

In patients with a severe inflammatory component; usually those who have relatively recent onset of eyelid retraction, proptosis, and conjunctival edema; short-course, high-dose, systemic steroid therapy is often effective. Most patients relapse when steroids are withdrawn or tapered. I and my coworkers generally use steroids to stabilize or control the eye disease, and, as discussed in Chapter 10, rely on low-dose radiation for long-term control of most of these cases.

Systemic steroids are also indicated in recent onset ophthalmoplegia and mild (visual acuity ≥20/80) optic neuropathy. Some patients obtain complete remission; the amount of fibrosis is probably a factor in those who have only a partial response. In patients with thyroid optic neuropathy, visual acuity often can be stabilized until definitive alternative therapy (radiation or surgery) is undertaken. The morbidity associated with chronic systemic steroid administration is well known; most patients develop Cushingoid changes, and, especially in older females, osteoporotic complications are common. While there are theoretic complications associated with radiation, these seem less significant than those observed with long-term steroid administration. As described, in some centers a combination of oral prednisone and radiation have shown better results than radiation alone.

It appears that most patients who respond well to immunosuppressive agents also respond to steroids or irradiation. The morbidity associated with cytotoxic agents is greater than that with steroids or irradiation. Carcinogenesis is a real, not theoretic, complication with some of these agents. Other life-threatening side effects have also been described. I prefer not to use these immunomodulatory therapies unless there are visually threatening complications that are unresponsive to standard modalities.

REFERENCES

1. Gorman CA. The presentation and management of endocrine ophthalmopathy. Clin Endocrinol Metab 1978;7:67.
2. Buffam FV, Rootman J. Lid retraction—its diagnosis and treatment. Int Ophthalmol Clin 1978;18:75.
3. Dixon RS, Anderson RL, Hatt MU. The use of thymoxamine in eyelid retraction. Arch Ophthalmol 1979;97:2147.
4. Pau H. Sympathikolyse durch lokale konjunktivale opilonapplikation am auge. Klin Monatsbl Augenheilkd 1955;126:171.
5. Waldstein SS, West GH, Lee WY, et al. Guanethidine in hyperthyroidism. JAMA 1964;189:609.
6. Gay AJ, Wolkstein MA. Topical guanethidine therapy for endocrine lid retraction. Arch Ophthalmol 1966;76:364.
7. Sneddon JM, Turner P. Adrenergic blockade and the eye signs of thyrotoxicosis. Lancet 1966;2:525.
8. Cant JS, Lewis DR, Harrison MT. Treatment of dysthyroid ophthalmopathy with local guanethidine. Br J Ophthalmol 1969;53:233.
9. Cartlidge NE, Crombie A, Anderson J, Hall R. Critical study of 5 percent guanethidine in ocular manifestations of Graves' disease. Br Med J 1969;4:645.
10. Martin B, Jay B. Use of guanethidine eye drops in dysthyroid lid retraction. Proc R Soc Med 1969;62:18.
11. Cant JS, Lewis DR. Unwanted pharmacological effects of local guanethidine in the treatment of dysthyroid upper lid protraction. Br J Ophthalmol 1969;53:239.
12. Skinner SW, Miller JE. Permanent improvement of thyroid-related upper eyelid retraction from bethanidine. Am J Ophthalmol 1969;67:764.
13. Wright P. Adverse reactions to guanethidine eye drops. Br J Ophthalmol 1987;71:323.
14. Haddad HM. Lid retraction with a guanethidine solution. Arch Ophthalmol 1989;107:169.
15. Lederer J, Hambresin L. Effet de l'adrenocorticotrophine dans un cas d'exophtalmie maligne Basedowian. Ann Endocrinol (Paris) 1950;11:634.
16. Fitzgerald JR, Bellows JG, Donegan JM, et al. Early clinical results of ACTH and cortisone in treatment of ocular diseases. Arch Ophthalmol 1951;45:320.
17. Scheie HG, Tyner GS, Buesseler JA, Alfano JE. Adrenocorticotropic hormone (ACTH) and cortisone in ophthalmology; report of cases. Arch Ophthalmol 1951;45:301.
18. Chandler GN, Hartfall SJ. Cortisone and ACTH in exophthalmic ophthalmoplegia. Lancet 1952;1:847.
19. Rubin IA, Billet E. Treatment of malignant exophthalmos with ACTH and cortisone. N Y State J Med 1954;54:2991.
20. Panel Appointed by the Medical Research Council. Cortisone in exophthalmos: report on a therapeutic trial of cortisone and corticotrophin (ACTH) in exophthalmos and exophthalmic ophthalmoplegia. Lancet 1955;1:6.
21. Leftwich P. Adrenal steroid hormone therapy in malignant exophthalmos: report of a case. S Afr Med J 1956;30:309.
22. Decourt J, Doumic JM, Michard JP, Louchart J. Action de la cortisone et de l'ACTH sur les exoptalmies Basedowiennes oedemateuses. Etudes de 15 observations. Sem Hop Paris 1956;32:186.

23. Dowlatabadi H, Linke A, Scheer KE. Die Behandlung des malignen exophthalmus mit prednisone. Acta Endocrinol (Copenh) 1958;29:442.

24. Salssa RM. Effects of cortisone and ACTH in certain endocrine conditions. Mayo Clinic Proc Staff Med 1950;25:497.

25. Woods AC. The present status of ACTH and cortisone in clinical ophthalmology. Am J Ophthalmol 1951;34:945.

26. Campos PC. Recession of malignant exophthalmos with deltacortone. J Philippine Med Assoc 1956;32:653.

27. Kinsell LW, Partridge JW, Foreman N. The use of ACTH and cortisone in the treatment and in the differential diagnosis of malignant exophthalmos: a preliminary report. Ann Intern Med 1953;38:913.

28. Brown J, Coburn JW, Wigod RA, et al. Adrenal steroid therapy of severe infiltrative ophthalmopathy of Graves' disease. Am J Med 1983;34:786.

29. Werner SC. Prednisone in and emergency treatment of malignant exophthalmos. Lancet 1966;2:1004.

30. Sergott RC. Oculocutaneous manifestations of thyroid disease. Int Ophthalmol Clin 1985;25:117.

31. Bahn RS, Gorman CA. Choice of therapy and criteria for assessing treatment outcome in thyroid-associated ophthalmopathy. Endocrinol Metab Clin North Am 1987;16:391.

32. Wiersinga WM, Smit T, Schuster-Uittenhoeve ALJ, et al. Therapeutic outcome of prednisone medication and of orbital irradiation in patients with Graves' ophthalmopathy. Ophthalmologica 1988;197:75.

33. Van Ouwerkerk VM, Wijngaarde R, Hennemann G, et al. Radiotherapy of severe ophthalmic Graves' disease. J Endocrinol Invest 1985;8:241.

34. Sergott RC, Felberg NT, Savino PJ, et al. Graves' ophthalmopathy—immunologic parameters related to corticosteroid therapy. Invest Ophthalmol Vis Sci 1981;20:173.

35. Sisson JC, Vanderburg JA. Lymphocyte-retrobulbar fibroblast interaction: mechanisms by which stimulation occurs and inhibition of stimulation. Invest Ophthalmol Vis Sci 1972;11:15.

36. Panzo GJ, Tomsak RL. A retrospective review of 26 cases of dysthyroid optic neuropathy. Am J Ophthalmol 1983;96:190.

37. Trobe JD, Glaser JS, Laflamme P. Dysthyroid optic neuropathy. Arch Ophthalmol 1978;96:1199.

38. Igersheimer J. Visual changes in progressive exophthalmus. Arch Ophthalmol 1955;53:94.

39. Day RM, Carroll FD. Corticosteroids in the treatment of optic nerve involvement associated with thyroid dysfunction. Arch Ophthalmol 1968;79:279.

40. Gorman CA, DeSanto LW, MacCarty CS, Riley FC. Optic neuropathy of Graves' disease: treatment by transantral or transfrontal orbital decompression. N Engl J Med 1974;290:70.

40a. Wiersinga WM. Advances in medical therapy of thyroid associated ophthalmopathy. Orbit 1996;15:177.

41. Clayman HM. Glucocorticoids I. Anti-inflammatory mechanisms. Hosp Pract (Off Ed) 1983;18:123.

42. Mulherin JL Jr, Temple TE Jr, Cundey DW. Glucocorticoid treatment of progressive infiltrative ophthalmopathy. South Med J 1972;65:77.

43. Bartalena L, Marcocci C, Chiovato L, et al. Orbital cobalt irradiation combined with systemic corticosteroids for Graves' ophthalmopathy: comparison with systemic corticosteroids alone. J Clin Endocrinol Metab 1983;56:1139.

44. De Santos LW. The total rehabilitation of Graves' ophthalmopathy. Laryngoscope 1980;90:1652.

45. Nagayama Y, Izumi M, Kiriyama T, et al. Treatment of Graves' ophthalmopathy with high-dose intravenous methylprednisolone pulse therapy. Acta Endocrinol (Copenh) 1987;116:513.

46. Guy JR, Jr, Fagien S, Donovan JP, Rubin ML. Methylprednisolone pulse therapy in severe dysthyroid optic neuropathy. Ophthalmology 1989;96:1048.

47. Gebertt S. Depot-methylprednisolone for subconjunctival and retrobulbar injections. Lancet 1961;2:344.

48. Garber MI. Methylprednisolone in the treatment of exophthalmos. Lancet 1966;1:958.

49. Haddad HM. Pathogenesis and treatment of endocrine exophthalmos. Int Surg 1973;58:482.

50. Jacobson DH, Gorman CA. Diagnosis and management of endocrine ophthalmopathy. Med Clin North Am 1985;69:973.

51. Brovet-Zupancic J, Moravec-Berger DR. Experience with treatment of endocrine ophthalmopathy. Radiobiol Radiother 1987;28:557.

52. Marcocci C, Bartalena L, Panicucci M, et al. Orbital cobalt irradiation combined with retrobulbar or systemic corticosteroids for Graves' ophthalmopathy: a comparative study. Clin Endocrinol 1987;27:33.

53. Thomas ID, Hart JK. Retrobulbar repository corticosteroid therapy in thyroid ophthalmopathy. Med J Aust 1974;2:484.

54. Yamamoto K, Saito K, Takai T, Yoshida S. Diagnosis of exophthalmos using orbital ultrasonography and treatment of malignant exophthalmos with steroid therapy, orbital radiation therapy, and plasmapheresis. Prog Clin Biol Res 1983;116:189.

55. Wiersinga WM. Immunosuppression in Endocrine Ophthalmopathy: Why and When. In G Kahaly (ed), Endocrine Ophthalmopathy, Molecular, Immunological and Clinical Aspects. Dev Ophthalmol 1993;25:120.

56. Pinchera A, Marcocci C, Bartalena L, et al. Orbital cobalt radiotherapy and systemic or retrobulbar corticosteroids for Graves' ophthalmopathy. Horm Res 1987;26:171.

57. Marcocci C, Bartalena L, Bogazzi F, et al. Orbital radiotherapy combined with high dose systemic glucocorticoids for Graves' ophthalmopathy is more effective than radiotherapy alone: results of a prospective randomized study. J Endocrinol Invest 1991;14:853.

58. Prummel MF, Morits MP, Bland L, et al. Randomized double-blind trial of prednisone versus radiotherapy in Graves' ophthalmopathy. Lancet 1993;342:949.

59. Kendall-Taylor P, Crombie AL, Stephenson AM, et al. Intravenous methylprednisolone in the treatment of Graves' ophthalmopathy. Br Med J 1988;297:1574.

60. Mori S, Yoshikawa N, Horimoto M, et al. Thyroid stimulating antibody in sera of Graves' ophthalmopathy patients as a possible marker for predicting the efficacy of methylprednisolone pulse therapy. Endocr J 1995;42:441.

61. Winand R, Mahieu R. Prevention of malignant exophthalmos after treatment of thyrotoxicosis. Lancet 1973;1:1196.

62. Burrow GN, Mitchell MS, Howard RO, Morrow LB. Immunosuppressive therapy for the eye changes of Graves' disease. J Clin Endocrinol 1970;31:307.

63. Wall JR, Strakosch CR, Fang SL, et al. Thyroid binding antibodies and other immunological abnormalities in patients with Graves' ophthalmopathy: effect of treatment with cyclophosphamide. Clin Endocrinol (Oxf) 1979;10:79.

64. Bigos ST, Nisula BC, Daniels GH, et al. Cyclophosphamide in the management of advanced Graves' ophthalmopathy. A preliminary report. Ann Intern Med 1979;90:921.

65. Werner SC. Immunosuppression in the Management of the Active Severe Eye Changes of Graves' Disease. In WJ Irvine (ed), Thyrotoxicosis. Baltimore: Williams & Wilkins, 1967;238.

66. Dyer JA. The oculorotatory muscles in Graves' disease. Trans Am Ophthalmol Soc 1976;74:425.

67. Wall JR, Henderson J, Strakosch CR, Joyner PM. Graves' ophthalmopathy. Can Med Assoc J 1981;124:855.

68. Peters O, Schreuer R, Vanhaelst L. Endocrine ophthalmopathy and asymptomatic atrophic thyroiditis. An unusual association. Acta Clin Belg 1985;40:17.

69. Perros P, Weightman DR, Crombie AL, Kendall-Taylor P. Azathioprine in the treatment of thyroid-associated ophthalmopathy. Acta Endocrinol (Copenh) 1990;122:8.

70. Teoh R, Woo J. Combined irradiation and low-dose cyclophosphamide in the treatment of Graves' ophthalmopathy. Postgrad Med J 1987;63:777.

71. Prummel MF, Mourits MP, Berghout A, et al. Prednisone and cyclosporine in the treatment of severe Graves' ophthalmopathy. N Engl J Med 1989;321:1353.

72. Kahaly G, Schrezenmeir J, Kruse U, et al. Cyclosporine and prednisone in treatment of Graves' ophthalmopathy: a controlled, randomized, prospective study. Eur J Clin Invest 1986;16:415.

73. Kahaly G, Yuan JP, Krause U, et al. Cyclosporin and thyroid-stimulating immunoglobulins in endocrine orbitopathy. Res Exp Med (Berl) 1989;189:355.

74. Shumak KH, Rock GA. Therapeutic plasma exchange. N Engl J Med 1984;310:762.

75. Dandona P, Marshall NJ, Bidey SP, et al. Successful treatment of exophthalmos and pretibial myxedema with plasmapheresis. Br Med J 1979;1:374.

76. Lewis RA, Slater N, Croft DN. Exophthalmos and pretibial myxedema not responding to plasmapheresis. Br Med J 1979;2:390.

77. Dandona P, Marshall NJ, Bidey SP, et al. Exophthalmos and pretibial myxedema not responding to plasmapheresis. Br Med J 1979;2:667.

78. Sawers JS, Irvine WJ, Toft AD, et al. Plasma exchange in conjunction with immunosuppressive drug therapy in the treatment of endocrine exophthalmos. J Clin Lab Immunol 1981;6:245.

79. Bourdiol M, Arne J-L, Maillard P, et al. Ophtalmopathie Basedowienne et plasmapherese. Bull Soc Ophtalmol France 1987;4:467.

80. Atabay C, Schrooyen M, Zhang Z-G, et al. Use of eye muscle antibody measurements to monitor response to plasmapheresis in patients with thyroid-associated ophthalmology. J Endocrinol Invest 1993;16:669.

81. Kelly W, Longson D, Smithard D, et al. An evaluation of plasma exchange for Graves' ophthalmopathy. Clin Endocrinol (Oxf) 1983;18:485.

82. Glinoer D, Schrooyen M. Plasma exchange therapy for severe Graves' ophthalmopathy. Horm Res 1987;26:184.

83. Glinoer D, Etienne-Decerf J, Schrooyen M, et al. Beneficial effects of intensive plasma exchange followed by immunosuppressive therapy in severe Graves' ophthalmopathy. Acta Endocrinol (Copenh) 1986;111:30.

84. Glinoer D. Traitement de l'exophtalmie severe par l'utilisation de l'echange plasmatique intensif. Rev Med Brux 1986;7:379.

85. Maraguchi A, Butler JL, Kehrl JH, et al. Selective suppression of an early step in human B cell activation by cyclosporin A. J Exp Med 1983;158:690.

86. LeGrue SJ, Friedman AW, Kahan BD. Binding of cyclosporin by human lymphocytes and phospholipid vesicles. J Immunol 1983;131:712.

87. Nussenblatt RB, Palestine AG, Chang CC. Cyclosporin A therapy in the treatment of intraocular inflammatory disease resistant to systemic corticosteroids and cytotoxic agents. Am J Ophthalmol 1983;96:275.

88. Yocum DE, Klippel JH, Wilder RL, et al. Cyclosporin A in severe treatment-refractory rheumatoid arthritis. Ann Intern Med 1988;109:863.

89. Yazdanbakhsh K, Choi JW, Li Y, et al. Cyclosporin A blocks apoptosis by inhibiting the DNA binding activity of the transcription factor Nur77. Proc Natl Acad Sci U S A 1995;92:437.

90. Pearson PA, Jaffe GJ, Martin DF, et al. Evaluation of a delivery system providing long-term release of cyclosporine. Arch Ophthalmol 1996;114:311.

91. Vitale AT, Rodriguez A, Foster CS. Low-dose cyclosporin A therapy in treating chronic, noninfectious uveitis. Ophthalmology 1996;103:365.

92. Weetman AP, McGregor AM, Hall R. Methimazole inhibits thyroid autoantibody production by an action on accessory cells. Clin Immunol Immunopathol 1983;28:39.

93. Utech C, Wulle KG, Bieler EU, et al. Treatment of severe Graves' ophthalmopathy with cyclosporin A. Acta Endocrinol (Copenh) 1985;110:493.

94. Utech C, Wulle KG, Panitz N, Kiefer H. Immunosuppressive treatment of Graves' ophthalmopathy with cyclosporine A. Transplant Proc 1988;20:173.

95. Pickardt CR. Cyclosporin A-Behandlung bei endokriner Orbitopathie. Internist (Berl) 1985;26:582.

96. Weissel M, Zielinski CC, Hauff W, Till P. Combined therapy with cyclosporin A and cortisone in Basedow endocrine orbitopathy: successful use in compressive optic neuropathy. Acta Med Austriaca 1993;20(1-2):9.

97. Bako G, Forizs E, Herczeg L, et al. Treatment of malignant Graves' ophthalmopathy with cyclosporin-A—a case report. Radiobiol Radiother 1987;28:574.

98. Gyula B, Erzsebet F, Laszlo H, et al. Sulyos endocrin ophthalmopathia kezelese Cyclosporin-A-val. Orv Hetil 1987;105:1017.

99. Gayno JP, Strauch G. Cyclosporine and Graves' ophthalmopathy. Horm Res 1987;26:190.

100. Witte A, Landgraf R, Markl A, et al. Treatment of Graves' ophthalmopathy with cyclosporin A. Clin Wochenschr 1985;63:1000.

101. Brabant G, Peter H, Becker H, et al. Cyclosporin in infiltrative eye disease. Lancet 1:1984;515.

102. Howlett TA, Lawton NF, Pells P, Besser GM. Deterioration of severe Graves' ophthalmopathy during cyclosporin treatment. Lancet 1984;2:1101.

103. Kvetny J, Frandsen HE, Johnsen T, et al. Treatment of Graves' ophthalmopathy with cyclosporin A. Acta Med Scand 1986;20:189.

104. Shaw LM. Cyclosporine monitoring. Clin Chem 1989;35:5.

105. Dweyer JM, Benson EM, Currie JN, O'Day J. Intravenously Administered IgG for the Treatment of Thyroid Eye Disease. In P Imbach (ed), Immunotherapy with Intravenous Immunoglobulins. London: Academic, 1991;387.

106. Antonelli A, Saracino A, Alberti B, et al. High-dose intravenous immunoglobulin treatment in Graves' ophthalmopathy. Acta Endocrinol (Copenh) 1992;126:13.

107. Hiromatsu Y, Kojima K, Ishisaka N, et al. The role of magnetic resonance imaging in thyroid-associated ophthalmopathy: its predictive value for therapeutic outcome in immunosuppressive therapy. Thyroid 1992;2:299.

107a. Kung AWC, Michon J, Tai KS, Chan FL. The effect of somatostatin versus corticosteroids in the treatment of Graves' ophthalmopathy. Thyroid 1996;6:381.

108. Utech C, Wulle KG, Pfannenstiel P, Adam W. Ciamexon-treatment in endocrine ophthalmopathy. Acta Endocrinol 1987 (Suppl);281:342.

109. Kolodziej-Maciejewska H, Reterski Z. Positive effect of bromocriptine treatment in Graves' disease orbitopathy. Exp Clin Endocrinol 1985;86:241.

110. Roehrich H, Dackis CA, Gold MS. Bromocriptine. Med Res Rev 1987;7:243.

111. Rennie DP, Wright J, McGregor AM, et al. An immunotoxin of ricin A chain conjugated to thyroglobulin selectively suppresses the anti-thyroglobulin autoantibody response. Lancet 1982;2:1338.

112. Kazeev KN, Zinkevich IV, Karaseva GI, Kostareva LN. Short-term results of parlodel therapy of patients with diffuse toxic goiter complicated by endocrine ophthalmopathy. Probl Endokrinol (Mosk) 1987;33:3.

113. Lopatynsky MO, Krohel GB. Bromocriptine therapy for thyroid ophthalmopathy. Am J Ophthalmol 1989;107:680.

114. Harden RM, Chisholm CJS, Cant JS. The effect of metronidazole on thyroid function and exophthalmos in man. Metabolism 1967;16:890.

114a. Oppenheimer MN, Lipsky PE. Adhesion molecules as targets for the treatment of autoimmune diseases. Clin Immun Immunopathol 1996;79:203.

115. Zesen W, Shubai J, Zutong Z. The effect of acupuncture in 40 cases of endocrinic ophthalmopathy. J Tradit Chin Med 1985;5:19.

116. Rogvi-Hansen B, Perrild H, Christensen T, et al. Acupuncture in the treatment of Graves' ophthalmopathy. A blinded randomized study. Acta Endocrinologica 1991;124:143.

117. Frank K, Ding G, Raue F, Ziegler R. Can the routine treatment of Graves' orbitopathy be efficiently supplemented by the administration of Venalot? Dev Ophthalmol 1989;20:127.

10

Radiation Therapy for Thyroid Eye Disease

Many different ionizing radiation energies and delivery systems have been used to treat human diseases, including thyroid ophthalmopathy. Radiation can be delivered as waves, x- and gamma-rays, or particles. The current measure of radiation dose is the gray (Gy). One gray equals 100 radiation absorbed doses (rads); 100 energy units (ergs) absorbed by 1 g of absorbing material is a rad. Most early radiation therapy, no longer used in thyroid eye disease, was delivered by low (85–140 kiloelectron volt [keV]) voltage or orthovoltage (180–400 keV) machines. These low-energy, poorly focused modalities deposited most of the radiation at the skin surface and had preferential bone absorption. Today's preferred megavoltage (4 or 6 megaelectron volt [MeV]) machines produce a photon beam that is well collimated, sharply defined, and skin sparing with a maximum dose at least 0.5 cm from the skin surface. Regardless of delivery method, most radiation treatments are given in fractionated daily doses to decrease morbidity to normal structures.[1–3] Figure 10-1 shows the relationship of maximum dose and distance from skin with various types of ionizing radiation beams.

Radiation therapy has been used since 1913, with varying success, to treat thyroid eye disease.[4–11] The rationale for early treatments was to irradiate the pituitary gland, decreasing the production of pathogenic factors thought to be responsible for exophthalmos. Most of these efforts, dependent on poorly collimated equipment, low radiation doses and low-energy beams, had poor results except when the posterior portion of the orbit was deliberately or inadvertently included in the radiation field.[12–15]

In 1950, Dobyns reviewed the literature and noted that 13 of 37 thyroid ophthalmopathy patients treated with radiation improved.[16] A few reports of orthovoltage irradiation of the orbit also documented good results. Jones treated 29 cases and observed clinical improvement in the majority, especially those with severe disease.[17] Similarly, Gedda and Lindgren observed good results in 10 of 16 patients receiving pituitary and orbital irradiation.[18] Using an analogous technique, Blahut and coworkers noted that patients with less than 6 months' history of orbital disease had a better response to therapy than those with long-standing disease—eight of eight versus two of five patients.[19] Beierwaltes also noted that patients with thyroid eye disease of more than 1 year's duration responded poorly to treatment, while those with disease duration of less than 1 year generally did well.[20]

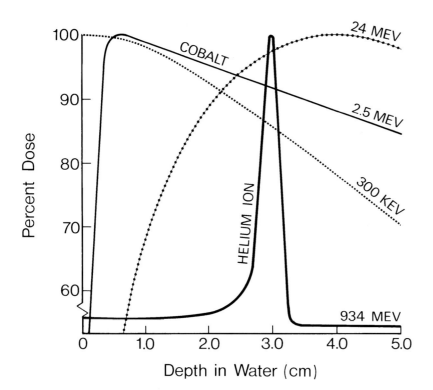

Figure 10-1. Schematic representation of depth dose curves for different forms of radiation.

In 1973, Donaldson and coworkers reported their initial results with 4-MeV linear accelerator irradiation.[21] They used a 4×5 cm field angled 5 degrees posteriorly to avoid the contralateral lens. The anterior border of the field was positioned just posterior to the lateral canthus to avoid the ipsilateral lens. The posterior field border was located just anterior to the sella turcica, and the vertical borders were planned to encompass the orbit and spare contiguous structures—sinuses and the central nervous system. (This treatment field is schematically shown in Figure 10-2.) Twenty-three patients were treated with ten 2-Gy fractions for a total of 20 Gy (2,000 rads). Transient edema was noted after the first week of treatment but subsided rapidly, and most patients showed improvement during the 2 weeks after radiation. Some continued to improve for as long as 1 year after the treatment course. Overall, approximately 65% of patients had an excellent or good response to radiation; those with rapid disease progression had the best results. Patients with chronic disease or those with long-standing ophthalmoplegia, minimal proptosis, or relatively few soft-tissue signs responded poorly. Poor response to systemic steroids did not influence radiation efficacy, and nine of 12 patients treated after steroid therapy had a good response to treatment.[21]

More recently, Donaldson and colleagues have modified their treatment with a beam-splitting technique that improves dose distribution to the extraocular muscles.[22] One hundred twenty-one patients were reported who have been treated and followed for more than 1 year. Eighty have received only radiation therapy; 67% of these patients have had a good or excellent response, 10% had no response, and in 2% thyroid eye disease has progressed. Forty-one patients have had extraocular muscle or lid surgery after irradiation; 81% of this latter group have had a good to ex-

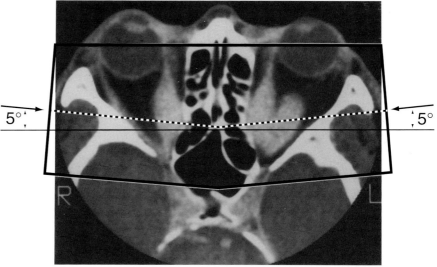

A

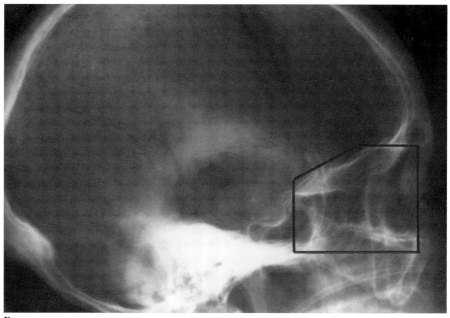

B

Figure 10-2. Axial (A) and lateral (B) schematic superimpositions of radiation treatment fields used for therapy of thyroid ophthalmopathy.

cellent response to treatment. Similar results have been reported by others; generally soft-tissue signs display the most improvement after radiation therapy.[22–24]

From 1964 to 1974, Ravin and coworkers treated 37 thyroid ophthalmopathy patients with 10 Gy (1,000 rads).[25] Muscle function in patients with muscle abnormalities did not return to normal; visual function improved in all nine patients with optic neuropathy, although one later required decompression.[25] Covington et al. also noted

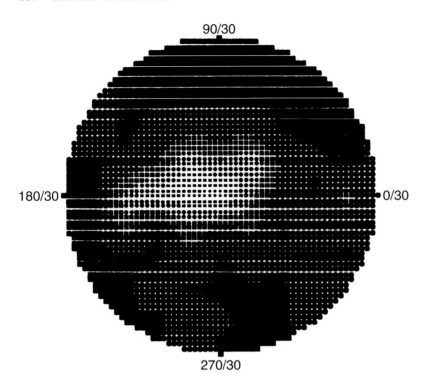

90/30

180/30

0/30

270/30

Figure 10-3. Preradiation visual field in a patient with thyroid optic neuropathy. Darker gray tones indicate areas of field loss.

an excellent response to radiation in patients with thyroid optic neuropathy.[26] Teng and colleagues noted less favorable results than Donaldson's using a similar treatment technique; however, their patients had milder and more chronic disease.[27] Only 25% of their cases (five patients) had persistent benefit; however, the vast majority had long-standing disease before treatment.

Bartalena and coworkers studied the relative therapeutic efficacy of steroids, radiation, and combined modalities in 48 patients with Graves' ophthalmopathy. Their study tended to bear out their predecessors' work: patients with symptoms of less than 2 years' duration fared better than those with more chronic disease, and the maximum efficacy was observed in those with disease onset of less than 1 year. Variation of modalities revealed that patients treated with steroids alone did not benefit as much as those who also received radiation. Using a clinical scoring system proposed by Donaldson (see Chapter 4), they noted that the therapeutic response difference between patients treated only with steroids and those who received steroids and radiation was statistically significant with a p value of less than 0.005. In the combined treatment group, 75% had an excellent or good response to radiation.[28]

Of the thyroid ophthalmopathy patients the authors reported from the University of California, San Francisco (UCSF), 62 had sufficient follow-up for meaningful evaluation.[29] This group received approximately 20 Gy to the midplane with approximately the same field parameters as those proposed by Donaldson et al.[22] Results have generally paralleled those reported by others, although a few thyroid optic neuropathy patients treated with radiation had only transient responses before developing progressive disease. Serial visual field changes document this course in one such patient (Figures 10-3 through 10-5). In four of 14 cases, recurrent or progressive compressive optic neuropathy necessitated surgical decompression within 5 months after comple-

Figure 10-4. Figure 10-3 patient's visual field 1 month after completion of radiation therapy. Note improvement.

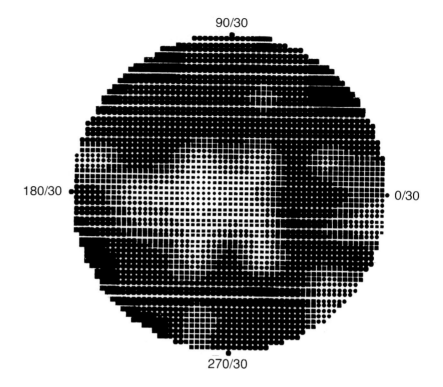

Figure 10-5. Same patients as in Figures 10-3 and 10-4: increased visual field loss 3 months after radiation therapy before surgical orbital decompression.

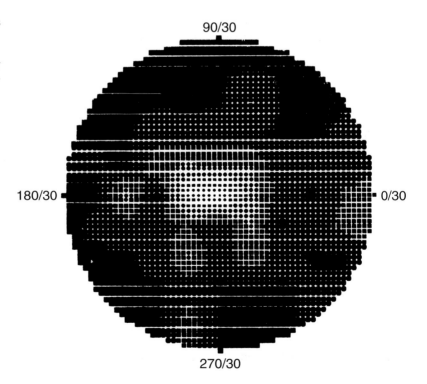

tion of radiation therapy in our report.[29] In contrast, some patients who have been surgically decompressed for thyroid optic neuropathy have later required irradiation for recurrent disease. Five of 11 patients decompressed in one series because thyroid optic neuropathy required postsurgical radiation to obtain an optimal visual result.[24] There have also been some anecdotal reports of patients who have required reinstitution of steroids after unsuccessful radiation or decompression.

Other groups have reported on radiation results. The majority of patients have previously been treated unsuccessfully with steroids (poor effect or unacceptable systemic morbidity) before irradiation. As examples, in a series from the University of California at Los Angeles (UCLA), 20 of 29 patients had been on systemic corticosteroids before irradiation.[30] Most of the results have mirrored previously discussed data.[30–34] In the UCLA study, 48% of all patients noted improvement after treatment, with soft-tissue changes ameliorated in 78%; as others have noted, only 24% had improvement in extraocular muscle function.[30] Five patients in that study deteriorated despite radiotherapy and required other therapies. Olivotto and coworkers reported on 32 patients; 19 of 28 (68%) patients had a good or excellent response; four patients recurred and three of the latter patients had orbital decompressions.[31] Hartemann and colleagues noted that 77% of 62 irradiated patients had a favorable response.[35]

Sandler and coworkers reviewed 35 thyroid orbitopathy patients irradiated with 20 Gy of fractionated photons.[36] Twenty-eight of 35 had received corticosteroids and relapsed or had disease progression. Radiation was effective in 71%; 14 patients required strabismus or lid surgery after radiation.[36] These authors believed that patients with a longer interval between disease onset and radiation did better, and those who failed did so quickly. Those conclusions are disputed by several other investigators, including our group.

Several groups have performed phase II dose-seeking studies. Pfluger and colleagues treated 17 cases with 10 Gy and 16 with 16 Gy fractionated photon radiation and noted better results with 16 Gy.[37] Kahaly and colleagues noted in a small study that alterations in fraction size 1 Gy weekly for 20 weeks versus 2 Gy daily for 10 days achieved comparable results.[37a]

In the largest series reported to date, the group at Stanford reported on 311 irradiated patients.[38] They did not find that the 69 patients who received 30 Gy had better results compared to others treated to 20 Gy.[38] Overall in this large study, proptosis improved in 51%, motility improved in 61%, and corneal exposure in 77%. Overall, 61% of patients had a good or excellent response to radiation.[38] Poor prognostic findings were patients with euthyroid orbitopathy, older patients, and males. After completion of radiation, 76% of patients on corticosteroids could stop them; 91 of 311 patients (29%) required ophthalmic surgery after completion of radiation. Kazin, Trokel, and Moore reported on 54 irradiated thyroid eye disease patients who received 20 Gy of fractionated photons.[39] Their results differed from ours in that 95% of their compressive optic neuropathy patients improved and only one of 29 required subsequent decompression.[39] Marcocci and colleagues from Pisa also have noted no better response to 30 as compared to 20 Gy.[40] This Italian group has conducted a number of steroid-radiation trials as discussed in Chapter 9. While some of their data suggested better response when a combination of steroids and radiation is used, if a Fisher's exact test is used to analyze that data, the difference between radiation alone and combined treatment is not significant.[40] Two other recent reports also show variable response to radiation alone.[41–42]

All of the series, which encompass results from approximately 1,000 patients treated in several centers, show that about 65% of patients have a good or excellent radiation response when soft-tissue signs of inflammation are present. Radiation has minimal efficacy in patients with extensive fibrosis.

Several investigators have attempted to use imaging or spectroscopy to distinguish inflammatory from fibrotic disease.[43,44] Just and colleagues noted short T_2 relaxation times are characteristic of edema on magnetic resonance imaging (MRI) while longer times suggest fibrosis. They studied irradiated patients and noted those with increased extraocular muscle T_2 times had more muscle shrinkage than those with normal T_2 values with an R value of 0.55.[44] Computed tomography (CT) examination will also demonstrate muscle shrinkage after successful radiation; however, it does not have predictive value.[45]

Dr. Donaldson and I have recently reviewed post-treatment complications at Stanford and UCSF and found no cases of radiation retinopathy (unpublished observations). There have been a few cases of isolated reports of radiation retinopathy; some are clearly due to technical treatment errors; a few we cannot explain.[46–50] In one series reported from Washington state, patients were inadvertently treated with double fraction size and dose; this radiation was equivalent to at least 2.5 times the recommended dose of 20 Gy.[49] I have seen two additional patients in whom that treatment error was made with similarly disastrous results. The development of radiation retinopathy at a 20 Gy fractionated dose level should be extremely rare. We do not recommend radiation in patients who may be at risk for radiation retinopathy for other reasons, such as those with coexistent diabetic retinopathy, patients who have had prior head radiation, or those on systemic chemotherapy. A few patients with diabetic changes have been irradiated without problem.[38] The bilateral blindness that can occur with poor radiation technique emphasizes my point that this treatment should only be used in centers with sufficient expertise and experience.

Some groups have continued to study the role of combined radiation and steroid therapy. Wiersinga and coworkers observed that 66% of patients had a favorable response to therapy, and approximately one-third did not respond.[34] Van Ouwerkerk et al. noted that vision usually improved after radiation plus steroids. They observed gradual diminution of proptosis; from 2 to 4½ years after therapy exophthalmos significantly decreased ($p < 0.001$).[32] As discussed in Chapter 9, an Italian group has noted that radiation plus systemic steroids was more effective than radiation plus periocular steroids, although it is uncertain how much of an additive or synergistic effect steroids have in addition to irradiation.[40,51,52] Pinchera and colleagues found that treatment with combined oral steroids and radiation was efficacious in 72% of cases; that success rate does not appear to be significantly different from those series discussed above in which only radiation was used.[52] Pinchera's group further studied 24 patients randomized to systemic oral steroids alone or steroids plus 20 Gy of radiation. Both treatment groups showed improvement after therapy; however, the mean final ophthalmologic index was significantly better in the combined group ($p < 0.001$).[52]

As previously mentioned, I use steroids as the first nonsurgical therapy in almost all patients requiring treatment for thyroid optic neuropathy (better than 20/200 visual acuity), new-onset proptosis with marked inflammatory soft-tissue signs, or recent-onset symptomatic ophthalmoplegia. If patients have little or no therapeutic response to steroids, if they relapse, or if contraindications or side effects proscribe steroid therapy, they are treated with 10 fractions of photon megavoltage irradiation. Radiation is usually effective. Figures 10-6 and 10-7 show a patient with inflammatory orbital disease that had responded to steroids, relapsed,

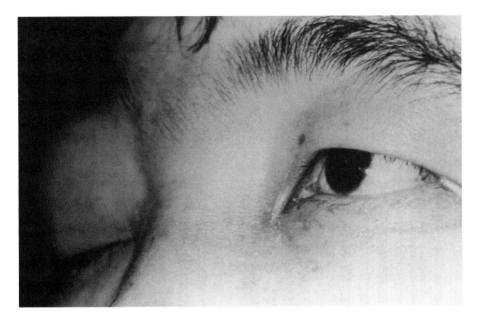

Figure 10-6. Patient with orbital pseudotumor after failure to respond to steroids. (Reprinted with permission from DH Char. Clinical Ocular Oncology [2nd ed]. Philadelphia: Lippincott-Raven, 1997.)

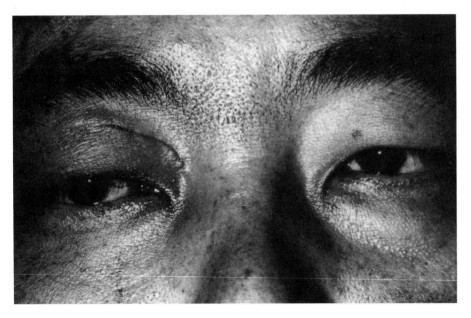

Figure 10-7. Patient shown in Figure 10-6 after 20 Gy of photon irradiation. (Reprinted with permission from DH Char. Clinical Ocular Oncology [2nd ed]. Philadelphia: Lippincott-Raven, 1997.)

then had a long-standing response to irradiation. Figure 10-8 shows a patient with orbitopathy associated with thyroid carcinoma after orbital irradiation (pretreatment photograph Figure 4-9). We have observed equivalent radiation results with orbital pseudotumor and thyroid eye disease.[53,54]

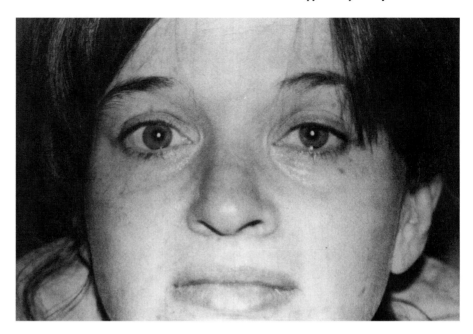

Figure 10-8. Patient with inflammatory orbititis after resection of papillary carcinoma of the thyroid (see Figure 4-9) and after 20 Gy of photon irradiation. She had a transient response to steroids and developed recurrent orbital inflammation.

As discussed above, most patients begin to respond within 2 weeks after the start of radiation treatment, although there is often transient increased chemosis and edema after the first week of therapy. Probably, patients irradiated because of orbital inflammation and/or visual loss should be continued on steroids during the initial phase of radiation to avoid exacerbation during the first 2 weeks of therapy. If the thyroid orbitopathy does not respond within 1 month after radiation therapy, it is not likely to do so later, although slow diminution of proptosis can continue for many years. Progressive field loss 4 weeks or more after radiation indicates the need for alternative treatment.

In patients whose disease progresses after radiation, surgical decompression, long-term steroids, or cyclosporine may be necessary. Generally, these few patients have also been steroid failures. If the major problem appears to be predominantly inflammatory in nature, then we usually use cyclosporine. In contrast, if the problem is continued or progressive proptosis with exposure, or marked decrease in visual acuity because of compressive neuropathy, then decompression is the treatment of choice.

In my experience, no serious morbidity has occurred with radiation therapy for thyroid ophthalmopathy. In a few series, one or two older patients have been noted by radiation therapists to have had cataracts, but I doubt this is radiation induced. We have not observed that complication in our patients, and the two cases do not give sufficient detail to ascertain whether they were radiation induced or senescent lens opacities.[30,51] While there is theoretic carcinogenic risk with any form of ionizing radiation, no thyroid ophthalmopathy patient has developed cancer after radiation to a cranial field.

CONCLUSION

I have found radiation therapy to have less morbidity than long-term steroids. In patients with severe acute or subacute inflammatory soft-tissue signs, recent onset of progressive proptosis, subacute or acute ophthalmoplegia, or vision loss, radiation therapy is often indicated after a short steroid course. The combination effect of these two modalities may be partially additive. Most patients with recent thyroid ophthalmopathy, especially those with marked inflammation, respond well to radiation, although occasional cases of thyroid optic neuropathy respond then relapse. All patients with optic nerve compression secondary to thyroid eye disease must be watched closely even if they have an initially favorable response to radiation. In my opinion, irradiation is contraindicated in patients having chronic thyroid eye disease with minimal or no inflammation, those with proptosis without inflammatory changes, or those with long-standing restrictive myopathy.

REFERENCES

1. Char DH. Radiation Therapy in the Management of Ocular and Adnexal Tumors. International Seminar in the Pharmacology of Ocular Surgery. Porvoo, Finland. In ML Sears, A Tarkkanen (eds), Surgical Pharmacology of the Eye. New York: Raven, 1985:523.
2. Merriam GR Jr, Szechter A, Focht EF. The effects of ionizing radiations on the eye. Front Radiat Ther Oncol 1970;6:346.
3. Hellman S. Principles and Practice of Oncology. In V DeVita (ed), Cancer. Philadelphia: Lippincott, 1982:103.
4. Juler FA. Acute purulent keratitis in exophthalmic goiter treated by repeated tarsorrhaphy resection of cervical sympathetics and x-rays: retention of vision in one eye. Trans Ophthalmol Soc UK 1913;33:58.
5. Burch FE. The exophthalmos of Graves' disease. Minn Med 1929;12:668.
6. Thomas HM, Woods AC. Progressive exophthalmos after thyroidectomy. Bull Johns Hopkins Hosp 1936;59:99.
7. Ginsburg S. Postoperative progressive exophthalmos with low basal metabolic rate. Ann Intern Med 1939;13:424.
8. Friedgood HB. Clinical applications of studies in experimentally induced exophthalmos of anterior pituitary origin. Clin Endocrinol (Oxf) 1941;1:804.
9. Mandeville FB. Roentgen therapy of orbital-pituitary portals for progressive exophthalmos following subtotal thyroidectomy. Radiology 1943;41:268.
10. Mann I. Exophthalmic ophthalmoplegia and its relation to thyrotoxicosis. Am J Ophthalmol 1946;29:654.
11. Detrait C. À propos d'un cas d'exophtalmie maligne. Acta Clin Belg 1947;2:240.
12. Papagni NL. La roentgenterapia degli esoftalmi endocrini. Radiol Med (Torino) 1959;45:542.
13. Lamberg BA. The thyro-hypophyseal syndrome. II. Roentgen irradiation of the pituitary region in the treatment of the hypophysial eye signs (including exophthalmos) after thyroidectomy. Acta Med Scand 1957;156:361.
14. McCullagh EP, Clamen M, Gardener WJ, et al. Exophthalmos of Graves' disease: a summary of present status of therapy. Ann Intern Med 1958;48:445.
15. Hermann K. Pituitary exophthalmos; assessment of methods of treatment. Br J Ophthalmol 1952;36:1.
16. Dobyns BM. Present concepts of pathologic physiology of exophthalmos. J Clin Endocrinol Metab 1950;10:1202.
17. Jones A. Orbital x-ray therapy of progressive exophthalmos. Br J Radiol 1951;24:637.
18. Gedda PO, Lindgren M. Pituitary and orbital roentgen therapy in the hyperophthalmopathic type of Grave's disease. Acta Radiol 1954;42:211.
19. Blahut RJ, Beierwaltes WH, Lampe I. Exophthalmos response during roentgen therapy. AJR Am J Roentgenol 1963;90:261.

20. Beierwaltes WH. X-ray treatment of malignant exophthalmos: a report on 28 cases. J Clin Endocrinol Metab 1950;13:1090.

21. Donaldson SS, Bagshaw MA, Kriss JP. Supervoltage orbital radiotherapy for Graves' ophthalmopathy. J Clin Endocrinol Metab 1973;37:276.

22. Kriss JP, McDougall IR, Donaldson SS. Graves' Ophthalmopathy. In DT Krieger, CW Bardin (eds), Therapy in Endocrinology. Philadelphia: BC Decker, 1983;104.

23. Brennan MW, Leone CR Jr, Janaki L. Radiation therapy for Graves' disease. Am J Ophthalmol 1983;96:195.

24. McCord CD Jr. Orbital decompression for Graves' disease. Exposure through lateral canthal and inferior fornix incision. Ophthalmology 1981;88:533.

25. Ravin JG, Sisson JC, Knapp WT. Orbital radiation for the ocular changes of Graves' disease. Am J Ophthalmol 1975;79:285.

26. Covington EE, Lobes L, Sudarsanam A. Radiation therapy for exophthalmos. Radiology 1977;122:797.

27. Teng CS, Crombie AL, Hall R, Ross WM. An evaluation of supervoltage orbital irradiation for Graves' ophthalmopathy. Clin Endocrinol (Oxf) 1980;13:545.

28. Bartalena L, Marcocci C, Chiovato L, et al. Orbital cobalt irradiation combined with systemic corticosteroids for Graves' ophthalmopathy: a comparison with systemic corticosteroids alone. J Clin Endocrinol Metab 1983;56:1139.

29. Hurbli T, Char DH, Weaver K, et al. Radiation therapy for thyroid ophthalmopathy. Am J Ophthalmol 1985;99:633.

30. Palmer D, Greenberg P, Cornell P, Parker RG. Radiation therapy for Graves' ophthalmopathy: a retrospective analysis. Int J Radiat Oncol Biol Phys 1987;13:1815.

31. Olivotto IA, Ludgate CM, Allen LH, Rootman J. Supervoltage radiotherapy for Graves' ophthalmopathy: CCABC technique and results. Int J Radiat Oncol Biol Phys 1985;11:2085.

32. Van Ouwerkerk BM, Wijngaarde R, Hennemann G, et al. Radiotherapy of severe ophthalmic Graves' disease. J Endocrinol Invest 1985;8:241.

33. Regnier R, Conreur L, Schrooyen M, et al. Utilité de l'irradiation des fonds orbitaires chez les patients souffrant d'exophtalmie maligne experiéncé de l'Institut Jules Bordet 1974-1983. Rev Med Brux 1986;7:419.

34. Wiersinga WM, Smit T, Schuster-Uittenhoeve ALJ, et al. Therapeutic outcome of prednisone medication and of orbital irradiation in patients with Graves' ophthalmopathy. Ophthalmologica 1988;197:75.

35. Hartemann P, LeClere J, Bey P, et al. Le traitement des ophtalmopathies thyroïdiennes par la radiothérapie orbitaire externe. Annales d'Endocrinologie (Paris) 1986;47:389.

36. Sandler HM, Rubenstein JH, Fowble BL, et al. Results of radiotherapy for thyroid ophthalmopathy. Int Radiation Oncology Biol Phys 1989;17:823.

37. Pfluger TH, Wendt TH, Toroutoglou N, et al. Retrobulbar bestrahlung bei endokriner ophthalmopathie: vergleich zwischen 10 und 16 Gy herddosis. Strahlenther Onkol 1990;166:673.

37a. Kahaly G, Roesler H, Lieb W, et al. Randomized trial comparing three protocols of orbital radiotherapy. Thyroid 1996;6(Supp):S-60.

38. Petersen IA, Kriss JP, McDougall IR, Donaldson SS. Prognostic factors in the radiotherapy of Graves' ophthalmopathy. Int J Radiat Oncol Biol Phys 1990;19:001.

39. Kazin M, Trokel S, Moore S. Treatment of acute Graves' orbitopathy. Ophthalmology 1991;98:1443.

40. Marcocci C, Bartalena L, Bruno-Bossio G, et al. Pinchera: orbital radiotherapy in the treatment of endocrine ophthalmopathy: when and why? Molecul Immunol Clin Aspects 1993;25:131.

41. Wilson WB, Prochova M. Radiotherapy for thyroid orbitopathy. Arch Ophthalmol 1995;113:1420.

42. Maalouf T, George JL, Angioi-Duprez C., et al. Effects of orbital radiotherapy on extraocular muscles in Graves' ophthalmopathy. Orbit 1995;15:25.

43. Winguth S, Kurhanewicz J, Wang ML, et al. ^{31}P magnetic resonance spectroscopy (MRS) of orbital myositis. Invest Ophthalmol Vis Sci 1991;32:2417.

44. Just M, Kahaly G, Higer HP, et al. Graves ophthalmopathy: role of MR imaging in radiation therapy. Radiology 1991;179:187.

45. Shah KJ, Dasher BG, Brooks B. Computed tomography of Graves' ophthalmopathy. Diagnosis, management and post-therapeutic evaluation. Clin Imaging 1989;13:58.

46. Miller ML, Goldberg SH, Bullock JA. Radiation retinopathy after standard radiotherapy for thyroid-related ophthalmopathy. Am J Ophthalmol 1991;112:600.

47. Parker RG, Withers HR. Radiation retinopathy. JAMA 1988;259:43.

48. Nikoskelainen E, Joensuu H. Retinopathy after irradiation for Graves' ophthalmopathy. Lancet 1989;2:690.

49. Kinyoun JL, Kalina RE, Brower SA, et al. Radiation retinopathy following orbital irradiation for Graves' ophthalmopathy. Arch Ophthalmol 1984;102:1473.

50. Kinyoun JL, Orcutt JC. Radiation retinopathy. JAMA 1987;258:610.

51. Marcocci C, Bartalena L, Panicucci M, et al. Orbital cobalt irradiation combined with retrobulbar or systemic corticosteroids for Graves' ophthalmopathy: a comparative study. Clinical Endocrinol 1987;27:33.

52. Pinchera A, Marcocci C, Bartalena L, et al. Orbital cobalt radiotherapy and systemic or retrobulbar corticosteroids for Graves' ophthalmopathy. Horm Res 1987;26:171.

53. Char DH. Clinical Ocular Oncology (2nd ed). Philadelphia: Lippincott-Raven, 1997.

54. Char DH, Miller T. Orbital pseudotumor: fine needle aspiration biopsy and response to therapy. Ophthalmology 1993;100:1702.

11

Surgical Management of Eyelid Retraction

Mechanisms of eyelid retraction are discussed in Chapter 6. These include increased sympathetic stimulation to Müller's muscle, fibrosis and adhesions of the upper and lower eyelid retractors, and, in the upper lid, increased tonus and overaction of the levator-superior rectus muscle complex secondary to fibrosis of the inferior rectus muscle. Levator inflammation and enlargement can occur with resultant retraction of the upper lid (Figure 11-1). Increased proptosis can also serve as a "wedge" to increase the size of the palpebral fissure.

The natural history of thyroid eye disease is discussed in Chapter 7. Usually, upper eyelid retraction is the most common lid manifestation of thyroid eye disease. Rarely, patients' upper eyelids may become ptotic as shown in Figure 11-2. As Frueh and others have demonstrated, disinsertion of the levator occurs earlier in thyroid orbitopathy patients than in normal patients.[1,2] As many as 50% of patients with eyelid retraction undergo resolution without ancillary treatment within the first year after antithyroid therapy.[3,4] Therefore, surgery should usually not be contemplated until the lid position is stable and retracted for at least 6 months to 1 year after diagnosis and treatment of hyperthyroidism. As discussed in Chapter 9, during this period many patients can be helped by sympatholytic topical therapy, although the results are not permanent and local drug toxicity, including corneal and conjunctival irritation, may be a problem. Measurement of the amount of eyelid retraction requiring correction is often difficult. Even when patients have "stable" retraction, eyelid position can vary from minute to minute depending on the patient's consciousness. As stated in Chapter 4, the average position for the upper eyelid is midway between the pupil and the limbus. When the concavity of the upper lid is at the limbus, retraction is 1–2 mm. Since intense concentration by the patient in an attempt to help the surgeon often alters lid position, it is advisable to estimate the amount of retraction by measuring the distance from the upper lid to the limbus and adding 1.5 mm.

There are two indications for surgery to correct eyelid retraction. The most common of these is cosmetic: symmetric or asymmetric "scleral show" is often sufficient to alter the patient's self-image or cause social embarrassment. A second indication is symptoms arising from increased ocular exposure, running the gamut from foreign body sensation to corneal ulcer.

Many surgical approaches for eyelid retraction have been advocated (Table 11-1). These include tarsorrhaphies, procedures on Müller's muscle, levator muscle, or both,

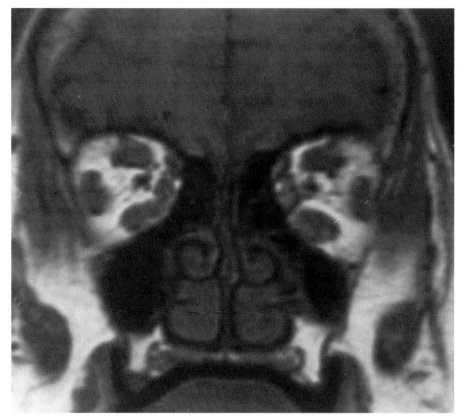

Figure 11-1. Coronal magnetic resonance imaging shows enlargement of most of the extraocular muscles with enlargement of the levator-superior rectus complex. Patient had retraction and lid lag.

and lower lid retractor surgery or the use of various spacers.[4–11] In 1934, Goldstein suggested en bloc recession of Müller's muscle and the levator by gradually deepening an incision in the upper border of the tarsus and allowing the isolated levator to retract; the levator and Müller's muscle were then sutured to the skin immediately caudad to the brow.[5] Schimek described two procedures: a slight modification of Goldstein's approach and a transverse tarsotomy. He achieved successful results in approximately 50% of cases treated with either of the two types of surgery.[12]

Blaskovics described a conjunctival levator-Müller's muscle disinsertion; up to 3 mm of correction was obtained with this procedure, although results were variable.[7] Moran advocated the use of local anesthesia and a skin incision to reach the levator, while Baylis suggested that a conjunctival approach was efficacious in mild retraction.[13,14] Henderson proposed a graded approach with severance of the insertion of Müller's muscle from the tarsus in mild cases, combined with levator disinsertion for more severe eyelid retraction.[15]

A number of authors have described the use of spacers, including collagen film, polytetrafluorethylene (Gortex), autologous fascia, tarsus, hard palate, periosteum, ear cartilage, and allogeneic bank sclera.[16–20] Some authors, including Crawford and Grove, have advocated modified levator surgery with marginal myotomies (Figure 11-3).[10] The results with that latter procedure have not been uniformly excellent.[21]

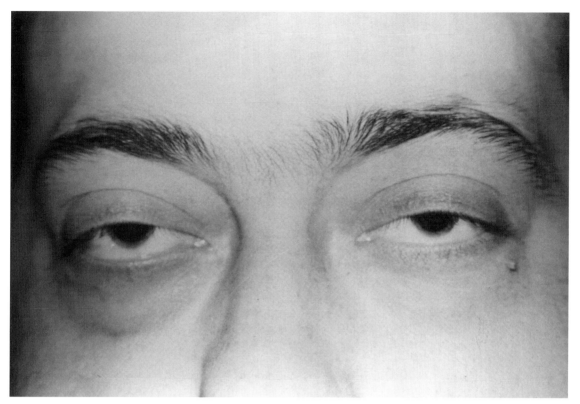

Figure 11-2. Ptosis in a patient who initially presented with eyelid retraction and developed bilateral levator disinsertions.

Table 11-1. Surgical Procedures to Repair Eyelid Retraction

1. Levator procedures
   a. Goldstein
   b. Modifications by others
   c. Proximal levator muscle
2. Müller's muscle procedure
   a. Blaskovics
   b. Modifications by others
3. Combination of Müller's muscle and levator procedures
   a. Henderson
   b. Modifications by others
4. Tarsorrhaphy
5. Spacing procedures
   a. Scleral grafts
   b. Autologous fascia or cartilage
   c. Processed collagen
   d. Tarsus
   e. Hard palate
   f. Periosteal grafts

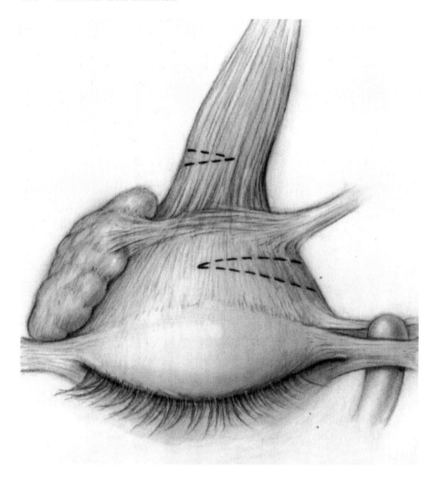

Figure 11-3. Levator marginal myotomies. (Adapted from JS Crawford, M Easterbrook. The use of bank sclera to correct lid retraction. Can J Ophthalmol 1976;11:309.)

ANATOMY OF EYELIDS

Several other publications discuss the anatomy of eyelids, so it is only briefly described here.[22] The levator palpebrae superioris is a specialized striated muscle that is approximately 50 mm in length—35 mm is muscular, and the lower 15 mm is an aponeurosis inserting into the anterior-inferior tarsus, the pretarsal orbicularis, and the skin to create the upper eyelid fold. Müller's muscle is a nonstriated sympathetically innervated smooth muscle arising from the levator approximately 10–15 mm superior to the tarsus and inserting into the superior edge of that structure.

In the inferior eyelid, three structures attach to the tarsus: the orbital septum, the capsulopalpebral fascia, and the inferior tarsal muscle. The capsulopalpebral fascia is an expansion of the suspensory Lockwood's ligament and is analogous to the levator of the upper eyelid; it extends posteriorly to cover the anterior surface of the inferior oblique, which lies between it and the inferior tarsal muscle. The inferior tarsal muscle is a sympathetically innervated structure comparable in function to Müller's muscle in the upper lids. The capsulopalpebral fascia and the inferior tarsal muscle interdigitate with the inferior rectus muscle fascia, which helps to explain the common occurrence of lower lid abnormalities after extensive inferior rectus recessions. Anatomies of the eyelids and orbit are shown schematically in Figures 11-4 and 11-5.

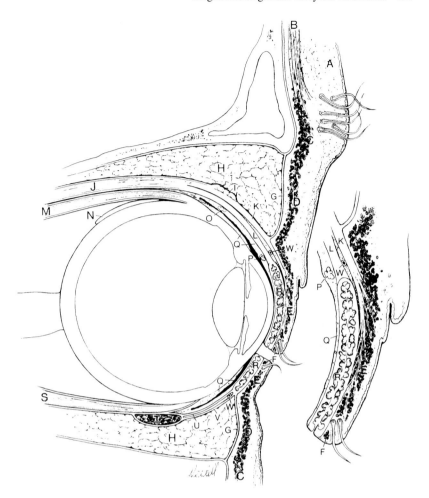

Figure 11-4. Normal eyelid anatomy. (Reprinted with permission from C Beard [ed]. Ptosis [3rd ed]. St. Louis: Mosby, 1982.)

CORRECTION OF UPPER EYELID RETRACTION

Goals of eyelid retraction surgery are to decrease exposure and improve cosmesis. The simplest early procedure, which was not originally devised for upper eyelid retraction, was the Berke levator tenotomy (Figures 11-6 through 11-8). In this approach, a superficial scratch incision was made with a scalpel just below the upper tarsal border, which was everted over a Desmarres retractor,[23] and then widened and deepened until its margins were approximately twice the desired amount of correction. After surgery, most clinicians use a Frost suture to pull down and stretch the upper eyelid for 5–10 days. Immediate and late results with this procedure were variable.

Baylis and colleagues modified this procedure slightly by making an incision in the upper border of the tarsus and deepening it until the vertical extent of the defect created was twice the correction desired in millimeters. The eyelid was then taped to the cheek for 4 days. The surgeons believed they could routinely correct approximately 2 mm of retraction with this technique. They observed that mild eyelid retraction could be managed by posterior recessions but thought that marked retraction was better treated through an anterior skin incision.[14]

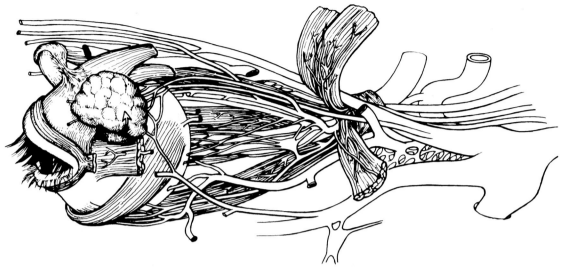

Figure 11-5. Normal orbital anatomy. (Reprinted with permission from C Beard, MH Quickert. Anatomy of the Orbit: A Dissection Manual [2nd ed]. Birmingham, AL: Aesculapius Publishing, 1969.)

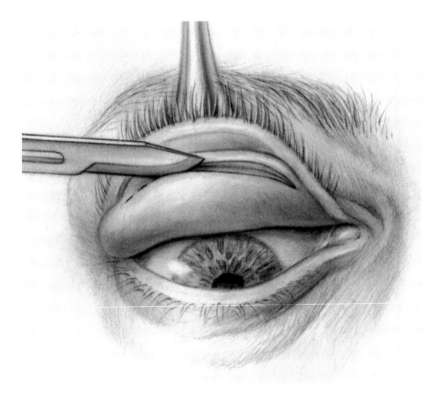

Figure 11-6. Schematic diagram of Berke tenotomy of levator. The upper eyelid is placed over a Desmarres retractor and a scratch incision is made.

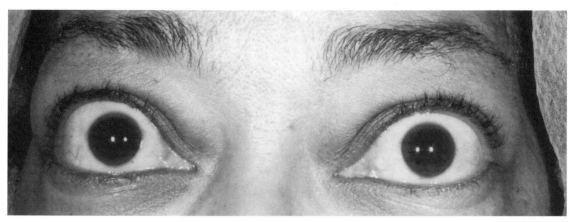

Figure 11-7. Patient before Berke tenotomy procedure. (Courtesy of Dr. Crowell Beard.)

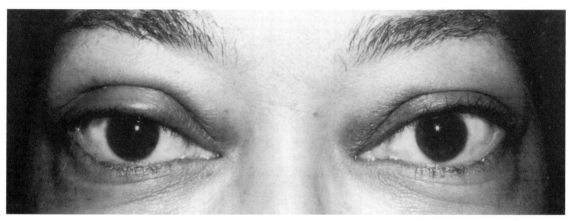

Figure 11-8. Patient after Berke tenotomy procedure, with a good result; the problem with this procedure was a lack of reproducibility. (Courtesy of Dr. Crowell Beard.)

Henderson's procedure consists of a graded Müller's muscle recession with posterior aponeurosis weakening if more eyelid lowering is required. This was the technique most used by ophthalmic surgeons until approximately 20 years ago.[15] Local infiltrative anesthesia without epinephrine is injected. The upper eyelid is everted over a Desmarres retractor and a buttonhole incision made with scissors through the conjunctiva at the upper border of the tarsus (Figure 11-9A).

A surgical plane is established between the conjunctiva and Müller's muscle by injection of balanced salt solution, use of a blunt spatula, or blunt dissection with a Stevens scissors. A blunt spatula is particularly useful for this purpose, but care must be taken; if the spatula is placed too superficially, a conjunctival laceration develops. In the correct location, the spatula easily separates the levator from Müller's muscle. It will not pass into this potential plane if it is inadvertently placed too deep and is in the levator complex. Müller's muscle is then detached from the upper border of the tarsus and is dissected free from the levator aponeurosis for approximately 10 mm (Figure 11-9B). A graded recession of Müller's muscle is performed, and the

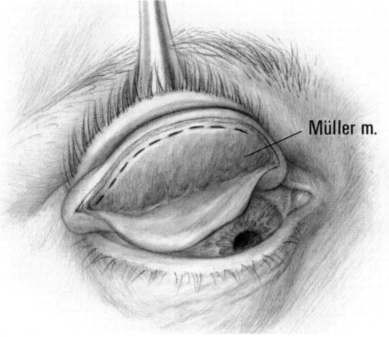

A

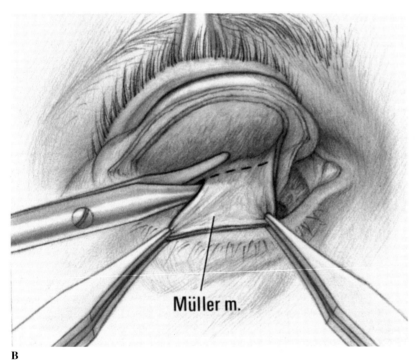

B

Figure 11-9. Schematic diagram of Henderson procedure (see text).

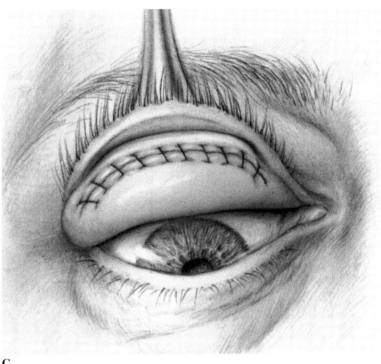

C

position of the lid is checked while the patient is in a sitting position. The incision is closed with an absorbable running suture (Figure 11-9C). Henderson observed that 2–3 mm of retraction could be corrected with this procedure. Tenzel modified the procedure slightly; other workers, including myself, have obtained less predictable results with a graded Müller's muscle recession.[24,25] In a series of 11 cases from Moorfields Eye Hospital, superior results were noted in 28%, 45% were improved, and results were poor in 28% of patients.[21] Beyer-Machule recommended obtaining a 30–40% overcorrection when the Frost suture is first removed; most of these patients will gradually return to a correct eyelid position within a month.[26] Upper eyelid massage three to four times a day is also recommended during that interval. As described by Henderson, if eyelid retraction is still present after the above surgical maneuver, a tenotomy of the levator aponeurosis is performed at the upper tarsal border. A Frost suture is then used to secure the upper eyelid, on maximal stretch, to the cheek for 24–72 hours. In the Moorfields experience with 30 patients, 62% had an excellent result, 27% were improved, and 11% had a poor outcome.[21]

The use of spacers, including allogeneic preserved eye bank scleral grafts, is described under lower eyelid procedures. While this technique can be used for upper eyelid surgery, and Beard believes it is useful in patients with severe upper eyelid retraction and exposure (C Beard. Personal communication with author, 1980), I and others have detected significant side effects that make this a less desirable approach.[27] The eyelids often become somewhat inflamed, red, and quite stiff. Occasionally, an inflammatory rejection reaction can develop. A graded approach usually combining an anterior procedure with extirpation of Müller's muscle, stretching and recession of the levator, and occasionally a lateral tarsorrhaphy, does not appear to produce as many complications. In my experience, these surgical procedures for upper eyelid retraction are cosmetically more acceptable than scleral grafts.

Putterman and colleagues have advocated a posterior graded recession of Müller's muscle and levator in thyroid eyelid retraction.[9,28] They believe that the major cause of upper eyelid retraction in most surgical candidates is a combination of Müller's muscle abnormalities plus increased activity of the levator-superior rectus complex forced to compensate for inferior rectus fibrosis.[29] They therefore concentrate their surgery on these two muscles and have modified previous procedures from Baylis, Henderson, Goldstein, and Blaskovics by performing a graded lowering of the upper eyelid. The upper lid is everted over a Desmarres retractor using a 4-0 silk traction suture through the middle of the upper lid margin. These authors use topical anesthesia to the conjunctiva followed by infiltration local anesthesia with 2% lidocaine (Xylocaine) and l:100,000 epinephrine. The conjunctiva is removed from the superior border of the tarsus, and a plane between it and Müller's muscle is established using blunt and sharp dissection. The lateral two-thirds of Müller's muscle is excised and allowed to retract; removal of the complete muscle produces nasal ptosis. The patient is placed in a sitting position, and if eyelid retraction is still present, the levator is incised and stripped layer by layer at the upper tarsal border until the desired lid height is obtained. The conjunctiva is reattached to the superior edge of the tarsus with a running 6-0 plain gut suture, with a Frost suture used for traction on the lid. In contrast to some techniques, this one aims for 1–2 mm of lid ptosis at the end of the procedure; the eyelid gradually rises over the first 3–4 weeks after surgery in most cases. As others have noted, eyelid massage is useful in correcting excess retraction. Putterman et al. have reported excellent results in 102 cases—less than a 10% incidence of complications, including nasal or complete ptosis, or residual eyelid retraction.[28] In a subsequent report, they noted 96% good results, and only seven of 156 patients required additional surgery.[30]

Harvey and Anderson used an anterior modification of this procedure, which I have found to be quite useful in most cases of upper eyelid retraction.[31] The anterior approach has at least three advantages. First, most patients have excess skin and subcutaneous changes as a sequela of orbital inflammation. Use of an anterior approach allows removal of those tissues and a better cosmetic effect. Second, an anterior approach allows better access to the lateral horn of the levator. Third, there is a clear delineation of lacrimal ductules so that they may be avoided.

It is best to perform this anterior procedure using infiltrative local anesthesia without epinephrine. While epinephrine improves hemostasis, Anderson and coworkers find that it sometimes causes artifacts in the measurements taken in the operating room; others disagree.[27] This technique is shown schematically in Figure 11-10. A skin incision is made in the upper lid crease, and scissors are used to carry the incision down to the levator (Figure 11-10A). Local anesthesia may be injected between the levator aponeurosis and Müller's muscle to enhance the separation of these structures. The levator is disinserted from the tarsus using scissors. First, the inferior edges of the levator aponeurosis are grasped and the horns cut, with care to avoid the lacrimal ductules (Figure 11-10B). Cutting the horns makes the levator much more mobile, facilitating the next step: tagging the inferior edges of the levator aponeurosis with three double-armed, 5.0 polyglactin 910 (Vicryl) sutures. Müller's muscle, identified by the peripheral arcade of vessels and its muscular fibers just superior to the tarsus, is extirpated from the underlying conjunctiva (Figure 11-10C). Small tears in the conjunctiva can occur during this procedure; it is not generally necessary to close them. It is important to remove virtually all of Müller's muscle in the area of recession. At this point in the procedure, the lid should be almost completely ptotic, or some Müller's muscle remains or the levator

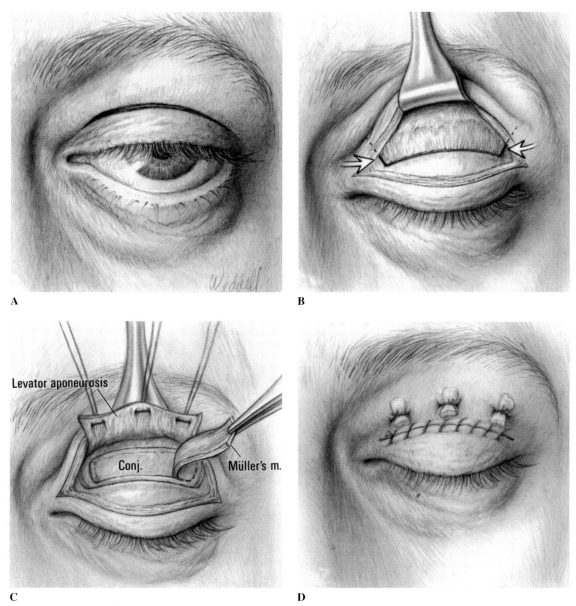

A

B

C

D

Figure 11-10. Schematic diagram of skin incision, graded levator recession, and Müller's muscle extirpation (see text).

has not been adequately dissected. The recessed levator aponeurosis is tied in its approximate final position with a bow knot, and the patient is placed in a sitting position. Unlike Putterman's procedure, this technique does not require overcorrection; the upper eyelid almost always remains where it was placed at the time of surgery. If levator position is correct, the sutures are tied, and the skin closed with a running 7-0 silk suture (Figure 11-10D). This procedure is shown in parasagittal schematic in Figure 11-10E. Typical cases with moderate to severe eyelid retraction are shown in Figures 11-11 through 11-16.

Figure 11-10. *(continued)*

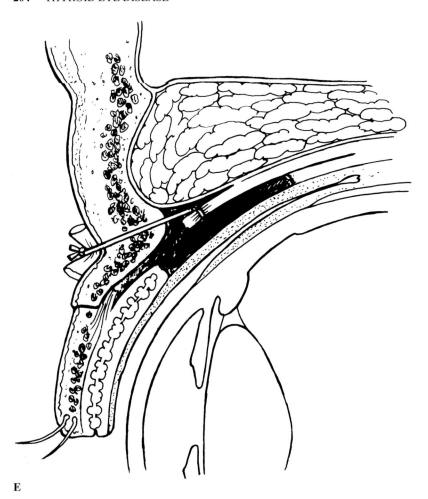

E

   While the above procedure is described as a graded recession of the levator, this is not completely accurate. There is little substantial material to which to suture the levator aponeurosis once it is disinserted from the tarsus, thus one actually does, at best, a small, medium, and large recession. While my results with this technique have been quite good, severing the levator's attachments to the skin, which creates the normal lid fold, does result in alteration or loss of the lid fold—patients must be warned of this possibility. An Italian report noted 75% success with a free levator recession without an attempt to grade its retroplacement.[32]

   Rarely, I have produced under- or overcorrection of upper eyelid retraction with this procedure. Figure 11-17 shows a patient with ptosis 1 year after surgery. In my experience, this is unusual and responds nicely to repositioning of the levator. There can be asymmetry between the medial and lateral aspect of the upper eyelid.[33] Early in a surgeon's experience with this technique, the lateral-nasal eyelid asymmetry can be attenuated with continued retraction laterally or relative ptosis nasally (Figure 11-18). Usually this is due to an inadequate incision into the lateral horn for fear of damaging lacrimal ductules. I have one case in which I believe this was not likely, and probably resulted from postoperative inflammation with premature release of the nasal eyelid sutures. This complication almost always requires a second procedure for correction.

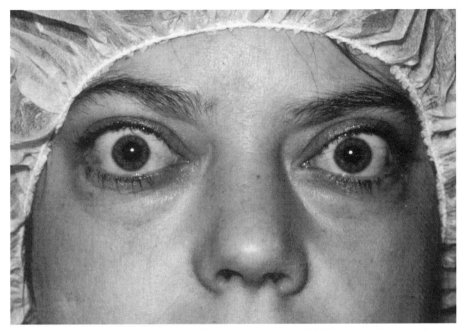

Figure 11-11. Patient before anterior graded levator recession and Müller's muscle extirpation.

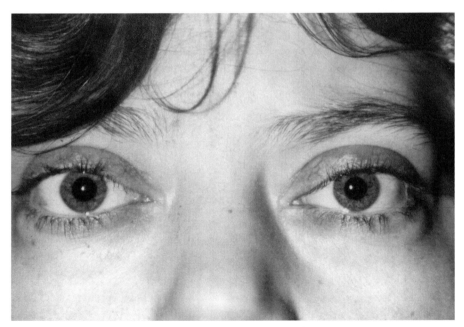

Figure 11-12. Same patient as in Figure 11-11 after surgery.

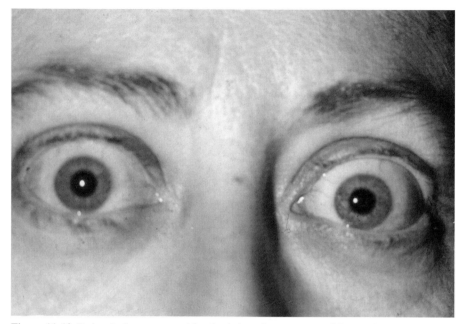

Figure 11-13. Patient before surgery with scleral show from upper eyelid retraction.

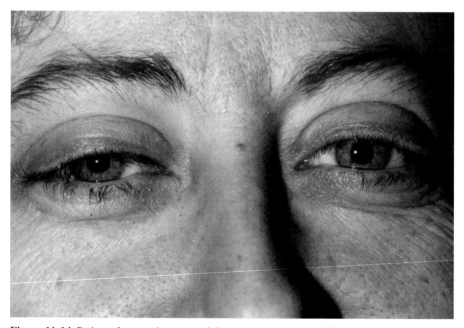

Figure 11-14. Patient after anterior approach levator recession and Müller's muscle extirpation with good result.

The problems, especially with nasal-lateral upper eyelid asymmetry, partially led Small to advocate a proximal upper eyelid levator procedure (Figure 11-19).[34] In that procedure, an incision in the upper eyelid is carried down to the superior transverse ligament. The latter structure is pulled down and the levator muscle superior to

Figure 11-15. Preoperative photograph of a patient with stable lid retraction.

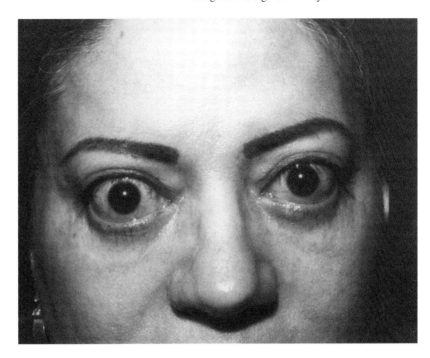

Figure 11-16. Three days after repair of lid retraction.

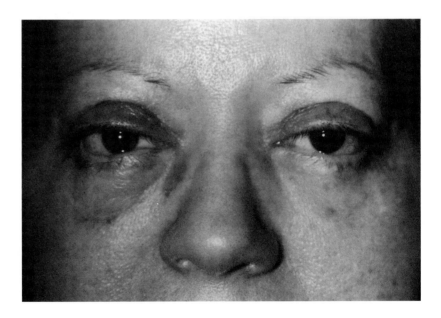

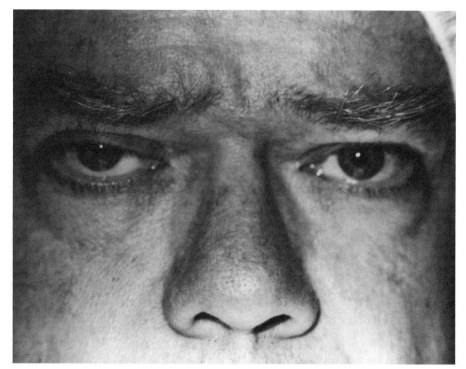

Figure 11-17. Ptosis occurring approximately 1 year after anterior graded levator recession and müllerectomy.

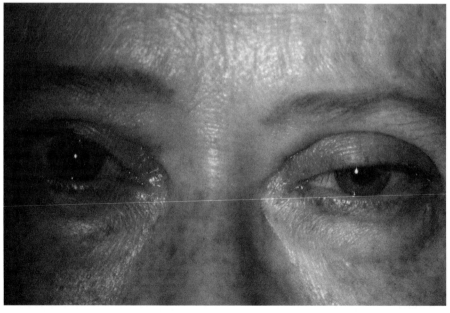

Figure 11-18. Marked asymmetry between the nasal and lateral portion of the upper eyelid after anterior graded levator recession.

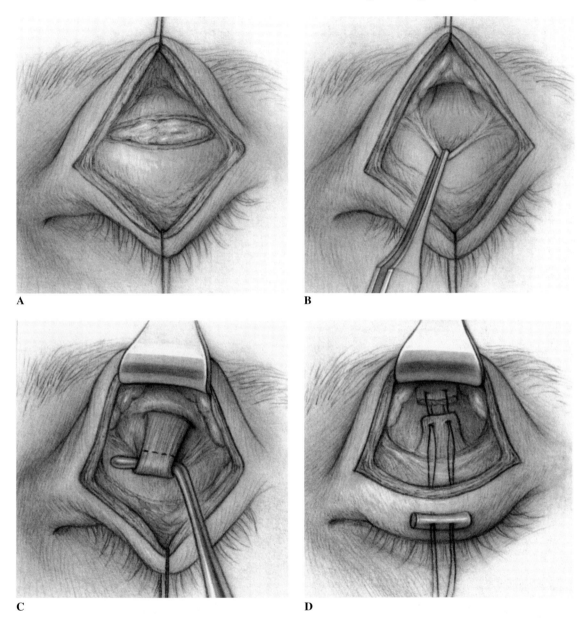

A   B

C   D

Figure 11-19. Schematic diagram of the proximal levator recession for upper eyelid retraction (see text).

it is grasped and recessed on an adjustable suture. The potential advantage of this approach is a more symmetric lowered upper eyelid. Small noted excellent results. In a recent report, he noted better results when adjustable sutures were used.[35]

Common complications of surgery to correct eyelid retraction are listed in Table 11-2. Over- or undercorrection of eyelid retraction should occur in less than 10% of cases, especially if the upper lid surgery is performed under local anesthesia, but occasional asymmetry will occur. Usually an upper lid that is still retracted can be lowered with vigorous massage or by everting it over a Desmarres retractor during the

Table 11-2. Complications of Surgical Correction of Eyelid Retraction

1. Undercorrection: total, lateral, or nasal
2. Overcorrection
3. Asymmetry
4. Extrusion, migration, or shrinkage of a scleral graft
5. Suture granuloma/pyogenic granuloma
6. Lid thickening and erythema (allogeneic scleral graft)
7. Corneal abrasion from sutures
8. Transection of lacrimal ductules
9. Transection of lacrimal canaliculus
10. Wound infection
11. Loss of eyelashes
12. Lid edema
13. Loss or alteration of lid fold
14. Cyst in scleral graft

first week after surgery. If one lid is overcorrected, it is best to wait at least 3 months after surgery before contemplating surgical repair.

As a general rule, extirpation of Müller's muscle alone reduces eyelid retraction by approximately 2 mm; severance of the levator aponeurosis from its attachments produces the remaining reduction in retraction. These procedures have produced successful results for patients with as much as 7 mm of upper eyelid retraction. As recently emphasized by Hamed and Lessner, repair of the fibrotic inferior rectus muscle sometimes results in marked improvement of upper eyelid retraction.[36]

CORRECTION OF LOWER EYELID RETRACTION

Correction of lower eyelid retraction is more difficult. Pathophysiologic mechanisms responsible for lower eyelid retraction are similar to those of the upper lid, but with significant additional components of gravity, inflammation, and fibrosis (secondary to contiguous inferior rectus myopathy) affecting the lower lid retractors. As discussed under extraocular muscle surgery (see Chapter 13), recession of only the inferior rectus can significantly alter the position of the lower eyelid; this is shown in Figures 13-2 and 13-3. Similarly, orbital decompression also can produce or exacerbate lower lid deformities, as well as increased inferior scleral show and, in association with decompression, an entropion (see Figure 12-8). The other major problem inherent in correction of lower eyelid retraction is a combination of aging and gravity. In the upper eyelid, gravity works to help the surgeon, while in the lower eyelid late sagging is the *bête noire* of all procedures.

Relatively minor amounts of inferior scleral show can be camouflaged with procedures analogous to those discussed above for upper eyelid retraction. However, these procedures are not routinely effective on lower eyelid retraction of more than 1–2 mm.

Use of allogeneic eye bank preserved scleral grafts was pioneered by Doctors Quickert and Beard at the University of California, San Francisco.[37] At the time a cornea is harvested for transplantation, the sclera is carefully cleaned of uveal tissue with a 4-in. by 4-in. gauze and cotton tip applicator. The sclera can be stored for as long as 1 year in 70% isopropyl alcohol without apparent deterioration. The evening before surgery, it is removed from this solution and placed in a sterile container with

Figure 11-20. Sagittal representation of dissection of conjunctiva and lower tarsus before placement of graft.

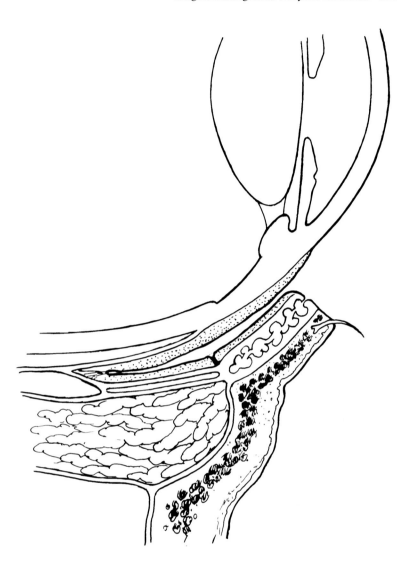

ophthalmic polymyxin B sulfate-bacitracin zinc-neomycin sulfate (Neosporin) solution. Other methods of sterilization and storage include radiation and freeze-drying.[38] While some investigators cite as a disadvantage the fact that alcohol preserved sclera is stiffer, it may not be a negative (see below).

When the sclera has been prepared, traction sutures are placed through the inferior tarsus and the lower eyelid everted over a Desmarres retractor. The conjunctiva is buttonholed and separated from the underlying retractors at the inferior border of the tarsus. After the lower eyelid retractors have been disinserted from the inferior tarsus using Stevens scissors, they are dissected and freed from the inferior rectus and inferior oblique muscles (Figure 11-20). Dissection must be sufficient to allow free mobilization of the inferior eyelid, so it can be pulled up to the superior orbital rim. Figure 11-21A shows, in parasagittal schematic section, placement of a spacer. Figure 11-21B shows the spacer sutured into place.

Several authors have advocated various ratios of vertical scleral graft dimensions because of shrinkage that occurs as a result of host reaction to a foreign

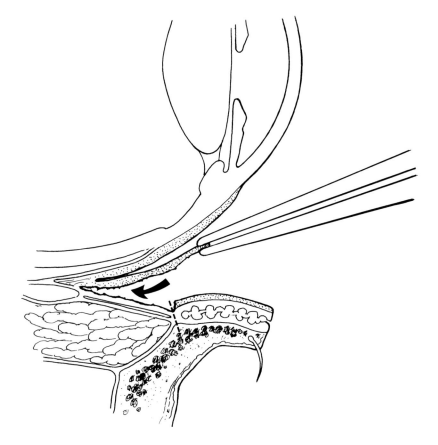

Figure 11-20. *(continued)*

graft.[8,25,27,39,40] I routinely use an elliptically shaped graft (Figure 11-21) of a vertical dimension approximately 2.5–3.0 times the number of millimeters the eyelid should be raised. A graft that is wider laterally than nasally is also advised, since sagging of the temporal portion of the lower eyelid is a common problem with symmetrical grafts. The graft is sutured between the lower edge of the tarsus and the cut edges of the retractors (Figure 11-22). We use several interrupted 5-0 chromic sutures brought through the eyelid and tied over cotton bolsters; a running 6-0 chromic suture is used to finish securing the graft. While some authors do not close the conjunctiva and observe gradual epithelialization over the bare graft, patients seem more comfortable if conjunctival closure is performed at the time of surgery. Since corneal abrasions secondary to suture knots can occur, we try to tie all sutures away from the center of the lid. A Frost suture is placed in the lower lid and taped onto the forehead for 48 hours. It is unusual to observe clinical evidence of a host reaction to foreign tissue. Patients are given an oral antibiotic four times a day for 1 week. When using this technique, we routinely overcorrect all cases (hence the 2–3 to 1 ratio of graft height to proposed correction) and start patients on a massage program 7 days after surgery.

Waller modified this procedure slightly by making an intratarsal incision 1.5 mm from the inferior edge of the tarsus.[27] An en bloc mobilization of the conjunctiva, tarsus, and retractors is made, and an ellipsoidal scleral graft larger in vertical width

Figure 11-21. Shape and size of spacer (usually scleral) graft.

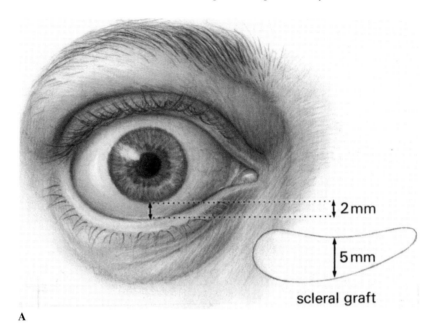

2mm

5mm

scleral graft

A

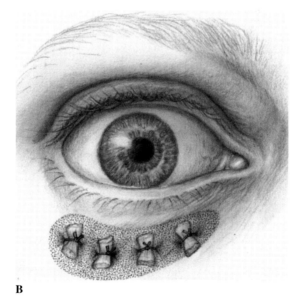

B

at its lateral side placed in the defect. He secured the graft with a running 6-0 plain gut and two double-armed 5-0 mattress sutures tied to bolsters over the skin. Graft epithelization occurred over 6–8 weeks.

Feldman and colleagues modified this procedure because of recurrent lower lid retraction.[41] They believe that the addition of a tarsorrhaphy and a lateral canthal suspension with a lateral strip may improve the results, although they reported these modifications in less than 10 cases.[41]

I and my colleagues have not been entirely pleased with the results of using eye-bank sclera to repair lower eyelid retraction. Most surgical complications are listed in

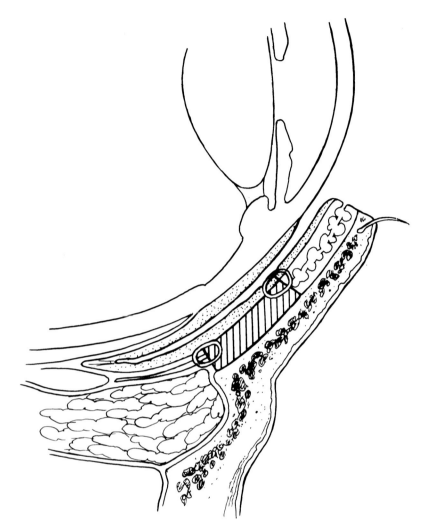

Figure 11-22. Schematic diagram of anterior and parasagittal placement of scleral grafts into the lower eyelid.

Table 11-2. Some patients who have a sufficient-size graft do not have adequate elevation of their lower eyelid, despite its mobility.

In unilateral cases, I prefer to use contralateral autologous upper eyelid tarsus to correct an ipsilateral lower eyelid retraction. Two examples in which this procedure was performed are shown in Figures 12-28 through 12-32. The contralateral upper eyelid is everted over a Desmarres retractor, and a proximal strip of tarsus with overlying conjunctiva is removed (Figure 11-23). This is sutured into the lower lid at the proximal edge of the lower tarsus (Figure 11-24). I have found this to be a useful procedure that minimizes the inflammation and bogginess often observed after allogeneic scleral grafts. I have used approximately 1.5 to 1 ratio of tarsus to the amount of retraction I wish to correct. While a number of complications have been described with the use of tarsal-conjunctival grafts to repair full thickness eyelid defects, I have not observed any serious complications in this setting.[42]

Gardner and colleagues reported on the use of this procedure in 38 patients with lower eyelid retraction. They used mainly 3.5 mm of vertical graft height and observed good results in 80% of cases.[43]

Figure 11-23. Schematic diagram (A) and photograph (B) of a procedure to harvest tarsus from the contralateral upper eyelid.

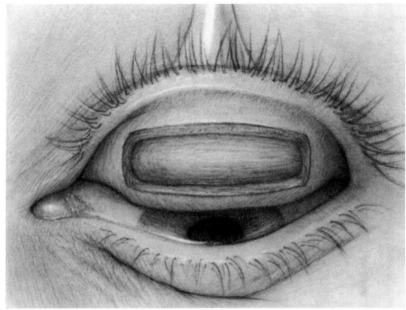

A

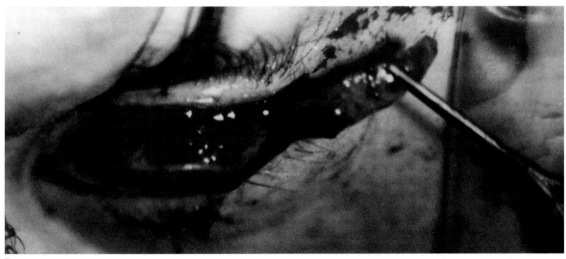

B

Another procedure we have used that does not require artificial or allogeneic material is an ear cartilage graft.[44] The procedure for obtaining an ear cartilage graft is relatively straightforward. As shown schematically in Figure 11-25, the pinna is brought forward, and the posterior ear skin is incised with a scalpel along the posterior rim of the helix to expose the cartilage in the scaphoid area, which is flat (Figure 11-25A). The dermis must be carefully scraped away from the underlying cartilage; failure to remove all dermis can result in cyst formation in the lower eyelid. The cartilage is then cut and care is taken not to damage the underside and anterior ear dermis (Figure 11-25B). A large enough piece of cartilage can often be obtained from one ear to perform bilateral lower eyelid repairs if only moderate retraction is present, and the ear has the usual amount of flat cartilage. Rarely, the ear cartilage

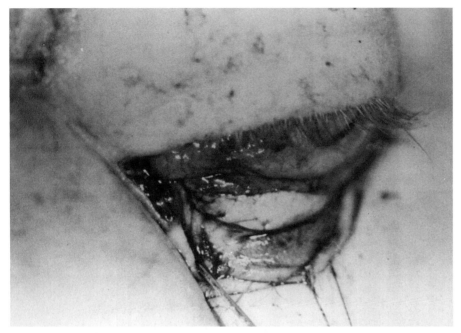

Figure 11-24. Tarsus from the contralateral upper eyelid is sutured into the lower eyelid to correct unilateral retraction.

has a curvature after it is removed, and it can be sutured to the lower eyelid with appropriate placement to incorporate that curvature, or vertical partial thickness cuts in the cartilage can be used to straighten it. We suture the dermis of the ear closed and have observed no ill effects. The ear cartilage is placed into the lower eyelid in the same manner as a scleral graft. Data on auricular cartilage spacers are too limited to adequately evaluate the results.[17,18,20]

Several groups have used autologous, hard-palate, free grafts for lower eyelid spacers.[45–47] These grafts are somewhat thicker than other tissue sources with resultant shrinkage in the range of 30%.[45] The graft should be obtained with local or general anesthesia from the posterior hard palate between the alveolar ridge and the midline. A major artery enters at about the third molar, and the graft should be taken anterior to this point to avoid bleeding, as shown in Figure 11-26. Most authors have advocated a 2 to 1 height of graft versus amount of eyelid retraction.[45–47] The results have been quite good, although I prefer a tarsal-conjunctival graft if possible. As has been demonstrated for eyelid cancer surgery, hard-palate grafts are contraindicated for the upper eyelid.[48]

Other options for spacers include fascia lata or synthetic materials, such as polytetrafluoroethylene.[49,50] In a report of seven eyelids of four patients, good results were observed with a polytetrafluoroethylene spacer; however, the postoperative lower eyelid position routinely was 0.5–1.0 mm lower than that noted at surgery.[49]

Several authors have devised procedures to lessen the lower eyelid alterations that occur with surgery on the inferior rectus. Most have included wide dissection around the inferior rectus muscle and advancement of the capsulopalpebral head.[51]

As mentioned above, we prefer not to use spacers for repair of upper eyelid retraction since levator recession and Müller's muscle surgery are effective and cosmetically more acceptable. If scleral grafts are used in the upper eyelid, the surgical

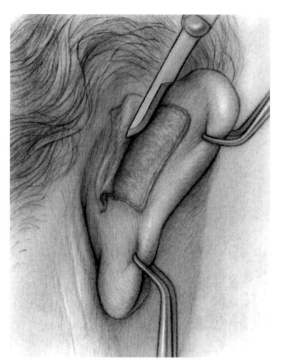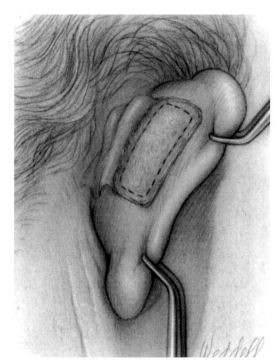

Figure 11-25. Schematic diagram of harvesting ear cartilage for use as a spacer for eyelid surgery (see text).

procedure is analogous to that described for the lower lid, with two exceptions: Müller's muscle is extirpated and the lacrimal ductules avoided laterally. Some reports have noted relatively poor results with this approach in the correction of upper eyelid retraction.[21] The graft shape is shown in Figure 11-21.

Waller demonstrated that the amount of upper eyelid surgery correlated with the amount of reduction of eyelid retraction; however, this was not the case in lower eyelid repair.[27] We would concur; while surgery for upper eyelid retraction is usually quite successful, lower eyelid retraction has been less effective. Small has emphasized the need in lower eyelid repair to perform a lateral canthoplasty to help support the lower eyelid.[52] Severe lower eyelid retraction is less common than upper eye lid malpositions.

TARSORRHAPHY

Before the use of decompression, radiation, steroids, and more sophisticated eyelid surgical techniques, tarsorrhaphy was the most common means of protecting an exposed cornea. Now it is used generally in association with one of the eyelid retraction procedures discussed above or in patients with severe lid retraction if it is unclear how long horizontal shortenings of the lid will be necessary (i.e., patients before decompression or radiation). If lateral lid shortening is to be permanent, a canthoplasty is performed.[53] Slight shortening of the palpebral fissure, especially in a markedly proptotic patient who is not going to be treated with orbital decompression, improves the cosmesis. Before performing this surgery, pinching the lids together will help in estimating the length of tarsorrhaphy necessary.

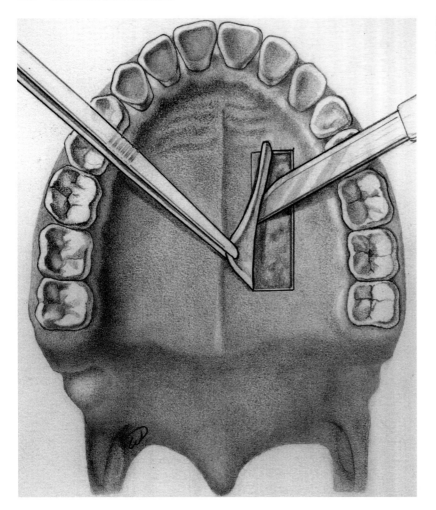

Figure 11-26. Harvesting of a hard palate graft for repair of lower eyelid retraction.

The techniques used in tarsorrhaphy and canthoplasty are similar (Figure 11-27), except that in canthoplasty the anterior lid margin, including the lash follicles, are excised. In tarsorrhaphy, the lashes are retained. A scalpel can be used to incise and remove a 1- to 2-mm strip at the gray line to the depth of the tarsus along the length of the proposed lid closure (see Figure 11-27). The lids can be brought together with running 5-0 Dermalon or interrupted 5-0 silk mattress sutures, which are tied over bolsters to decrease skin scarring.

CONCLUSION

Eyelid retraction with "scleral show" is one of the more cosmetically disfiguring aspects of thyroid ophthalmopathy. While proptosis can also alter facial appearance, a camouflage procedure that returns the lids to their correct position relative to the cornea can be quite successful in altering the patient's self image.

Figure 11-27. Schematic of the procedure for tarsorrhaphy. This procedure is often used as an adjunct to eyelid surgery and can be performed to temporarily or permanently horizontally shorten the eyelid.

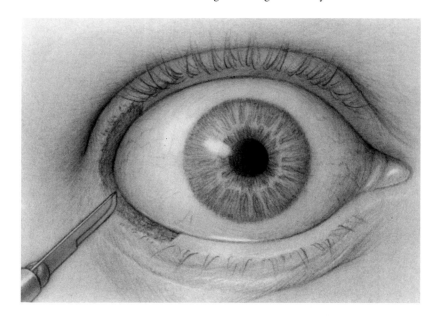

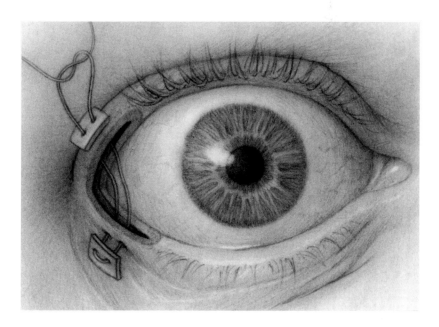

As discussed at the outset, many patients with eyelid retraction have apparent spontaneous resolution of this problem. Therefore, it seems wise to wait at least 6 months to 1 year from diagnosis of thyroid eye disease (unless the patient has corneal exposure) and until the eyelid position is stable before considering surgery. Similarly, since eye muscle surgery, radiation, steroids, and orbital decompression can all alter eyelid position, surgery on the lids should be deferred until these other therapeutic modalities are completed.

Figure 11-27. *(continued)*

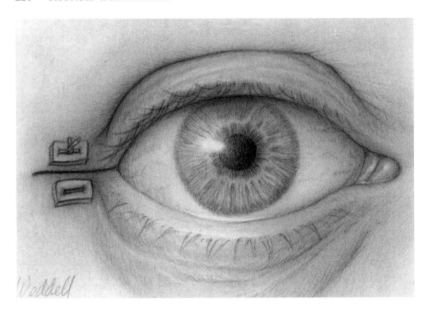

I routinely use eyelid retraction procedures alone on patients with minimal to moderate proptosis (generally <23 mm of exophthalmos) without optic neuropathy. Such patients often have excellent cosmetic results and appear to suffer significantly less ocular morbidity than with orbital decompression.

REFERENCES

1. Frueh BR. Graves' eye disease: orbital compliance and other physical measurements. Trans Am Ophthalmol Soc 1984;82:492.
2. Uldry AP, Regli F, Scazziga BR, Naegeli C. Palpebral asymmetry and hyperthyroidism. Two cases in connection with Graves' disease. J Neurol 1986;233:126.
3. Hales IB, Rundle FF. Ocular changes in Graves' disease. QJM 1960;29:113.
4. Hamilton HE, Schultz RO, DeGowin EL. The endocrine eye lesion in hyperthyroidism. Arch Intern Med 1960;105:675.
5. Goldstein I. Recession of the levator muscle for lagophthalmos in exophthalmic goiter. Arch Ophthalmol 1934;11:389.
6. Cusick PL, Sarrail J. Cited in JH King, JAC Wadsworth (eds), An Atlas of Ophthalmic Surgery (2nd ed). Philadelphia: Lippincott, 1970;186.
7. Blaskovics L. Cited in C Berans, JH King Jr. An Atlas of Ophthalmic Surgery. Philadelphia: Lippincott, 1961;76.
8. Dryden RM, Soll DB. The use of scleral transplantation in cicatricial entropion and eyelid retraction. Trans Am Acad Ophthalmol Otolaryngol 1977;83:669.
9. Putterman AM, Urist MJ. A simplified levator palpebrae superioris muscle recession to treat overcorrected blepharoptosis. Am J Ophthalmol 1974;77:358.
10. Grove AS Jr. Upper eyelid retraction and Graves' disease. Ophthalmology 1981;88:499.
11. Castanares S. Blepharoplasty in exophthalmos. Plast Reconstr Surg 1971;47:215.
12. Schimek RA. Surgical management of ocular complications of Graves' disease. Arch Ophthalmol 1972;87:655.
13. Moran RE. The correction of exophthalmos and levator spasm. Plast Reconstr Surg 1956;18:411.
14. Baylis HI, Cies WA, Kamin DF. Correction of upper eyelid retraction. Am J Ophthalmol 1976;82:790.

15. Henderson J. Relief of eyelid retraction: a surgical procedure. Arch Ophthalmol 1965;74:205.

16. Callahan A. Reconstruction of the eyelids with cartilage and mucosa from the nasal septum. Trans Ophthalmol Soc U K 1976;96:39.

17. Mehrotra ON. Repairing defects of the lower eyelid with a free chondromucosal graft. Plast Reconstr Surg 1977;59:689.

18. Zbylski JR, LaRossa DD, Rich JD. Correction of lower eyelid ptosis in the anophthalmic orbit with an autogenous ear cartilage graft. Plast Reconstr Surg 1978;61:220.

19. Crawford JS, Easterbrook M. The use of bank sclera to correct lid retraction. Can J Ophthalmol 1976;11:309.

20. Flanagan JC. Retraction of the eyelids secondary to thyroid ophthalmopathy: its surgical correction with sclera and the fate of the graft. Trans Am Ophthalmol Soc 1980;78:657.

21. Thaller VT, Kaden K, Lane CM, Collin JRO. Thyroid lid surgery. Eye 1987;1:609.

22. Beard C, Quickert MH. Anatomy of the Orbit: A Dissection Manual. Birmingham, AL: Aesculapius Publishing, 1969.

23. Berke RN. Cited in C Beard (ed), Ptosis. St. Louis: Mosby, 1969;211.

24. Tenzel RR. Treatment of Eyelid Retraction by Stretching of the Levator Aponeurosis. In JL Smith (ed), Neuro-Ophthalmology Update. New York: Masson, 1977;17.

25. Stephenson C. A review of the surgical treatment of the ophthalmopathy of Graves' disease with emphasis on newer techniques in lid surgery. Pacific Coast Otolaryngol-Ophthalmol Soc Trans 1975;56:203.

26. Beyer-Machule C-K. Surgical treatment of thyroid lid retractions. Int Ophthalmol Clin (in press).

27. Waller RR. Eyelid malpositions in Graves' ophthalmopathy. Trans Am Ophthalmol Soc 1982;80:855.

28. Putterman AM. Surgical treatment of thyroid-related upper eyelid retraction. Graded Müller's muscle excision and levator recession. Ophthalmology 1981;88:507.

29. Wesley RE, Bond JB. Upper eyelid retraction from inferior rectus restriction in dysthyroid orbit disease. Ann Ophthalmol 1987;19:34.

30. Putterman AM, Fett DR. Müller's muscle in the treatment of upper eyelid retraction: a 12-year study. Ophthalmic Surg 1986;17:361.

31. Harvey JT, Anderson RL. The aponeurotic approach to eyelid retraction. Ophthalmology 1981;88:513.

32. Uccello G, Vassallo P, Strianese D, Bonavolonta G. Free levator complex recession in Graves' ophthalmopathy. Orbit 1994;13:119.

33. Hurwitz JJ, Rodgers KJA. Prevention and management of postoperative lateral upper-lid retraction in Graves' disease. Can J Ophthalmol 1983;18:329.

34. Small RG. Upper eyelid retraction in Graves' ophthalmopathy: a new surgical technique and a study of the abnormal levator muscle. Trans Am Ophthal Soc 1988;86:725.

35. Small RG. Surgery for upper eyelid retraction: three techniques. Trans Am Ophthalmol Assoc 1995;93:353.

36. Hamed LM, Lessner AM. Fixation duress in the pathogenesis of upper eyelid retraction in thyroid orbitopathy: a prospective study. Ophthalmology 1994;101:1608.

37. Quickert MH, Dryden RM. Lower eyelid advancement. Presented at the meeting of the American Society of Ophthalmic Plastic and Reconstructive Surgery, Las Vegas, 1971.

38. Colvard DM, Waller RR, Campbell JR, Friedt R. Sterilization of scleral homografts with ionizing irradiation. Am J Ophthalmol 1979;87:494.

39. Soll DB. Scleral transplantation in ophthalmic plastic surgery. Trans Am Acad Ophthalmol Otolaryngol 1977;83:679.

40. Flanagan JC. Eyebank sclera in oculoplastic surgery. Ophthalmic Surg 1974;5:45.

41. Feldman KA, Puterman AM, Farber MD. Surgical treatment of thyroid-related lower eyelid retraction. A modified approach. Ophthal Plast Reconstr Surg 1992;8:278.

42. Hawes MJ, Jamell GA. Complications of tarsoconjunctival grafts. Ophthal Plast Reconstr Surg 1996;12:45.

43. Gardner TA, Kennerdell JS, Buerger GF. Treatment of dysthyroid lower lid retraction with autogenous tarsus transplants. Ophthal Plast Reconstr Surg 1992;8:26.

44. Baylis HI, Rosen N, Neuhaus RW. Obtaining auricular cartilage for reconstructive surgery. Am J Ophthalmol 1982;93:709.

45. Kersten RD, Kulwin DR, Levartovsky S, Tiradellis H. TSE DT: management of lower-lid retraction with hard-palate mucosa grafting. Arch Ophthalmol 1990;108:1339.

46. Cohen MS, Shorr N. Eyelid reconstruction with hard palate mucosa grafts. Ophthal Plast Reconstr Surg 1992;8:185.

47. Beatty RL, Harris GH, Bauman GR, Mills MP. Intraoral palatal mucosal graft harvest. Ophthal Plast Reconstr Surg 1993;9:120.

48. Char DH. Clinical Ocular Oncology. Philadelphia: Lippincott-Raven, 1997.

49. Karesh JW, Fabrega MA, Rodrigues MM, Glaros DS. Polytetrafluoroethylene as an intrapositional graft material for the correction of lower eyelid retraction. Ophthalmology 1989;96:410.

50. Morax S, Hurbli T. Choice of surgical treatment for Graves' disease. J Craniomaxillofac Surg 1987;15:174.

51. Meyer DR, Simon JW, Kansora M. Primary infratarsal lower eyelid retractor types to prevent eyelid retraction after inferior rectus muscle recession. Am J Ophthalmol 1996;122:331.

52. Small RG, Scott MM. The tight retracted lower eyelid. Arch Ophthalmol 1990;108:438.

53. Leone CR Jr. The management of ophthalmic Graves' disease. Ophthalmology 1984;91:770.

12

Surgical Orbital Decompression: History and Rationale

In 1911, Dollinger first reported a technique for surgical orbital decompression of thyroid ophthalmopathy patients using a modification of the Krönlein lateral orbitotomy.[1,2] Before that time, a number of authors had reported on patients with blindness (unilateral or bilateral) or enucleations resulting from thyroid eye disease.[3,4] Since Dollinger's time, five approaches to surgical decompression of the orbit have been set forth and modified (Figure 12-1). In 1933, Naffziger[5] described a successful orbital decompression using a neurosurgical transfrontal approach. Orbital contents were allowed to prolapse into the potential space created by removal of the orbital roof.[5] Welti and Offret used a pterional approach to orbital decompression in 1943.[6] Several authors proposed decompression into the sinuses. In the early 1930s, Hirsch and Urbanik reported a modified Caldwell-Luc procedure characterized by removal of the floor of the orbit through the maxillary antrum. Sewall proposed a fronto-ethmoidectomy in 1936.[7,8] In 1950, Hirsch recommended a transantral removal of the floor.[9] In 1947, Ogura first performed a combined transantral removal of the floor and medial orbital wall to decompress the orbit.[9,10]

Most of the more recent orbital decompression procedures are modifications of these basic approaches. Most clinicians now use a modification of the Ogura procedure for almost all orbital decompressions; these sinus-based orbital expansion procedures can be performed through the nose (endoscopy), orbit, or via a Caldwell-Luc transantral incision.[11] As Stabile and Trokel demonstrated in an osteologic study, removal of the lateral orbital wall increased intraorbital volume by only 2 ml, removal of the medial wall increased volume by 6 ml, and removal of ethmoid air cells and the orbital floor nasal to the infraorbital nerve increased available volume by 13–14 ml.[12]

Two other approaches based on a different mechanism of decompression or an apparent reduction of proptosis have been advocated. Both may be useful in highly selected patients as a secondary procedure if insufficient retroplacement of the globe was obtained with the standard decompression. Orbital fat can be removed with resultant mild decrease in proptosis—adipose tissue is mainly removed from the inferior orbit, since vessel damage in the superior orbit is more of a risk.[13–17] I have rarely used this defatting procedure to achieve some retroplacement of the globe and when apical decompression is not needed. As discussed below, many thyroid orbitopathy patients require apical decompression, and that is not optimally achieved

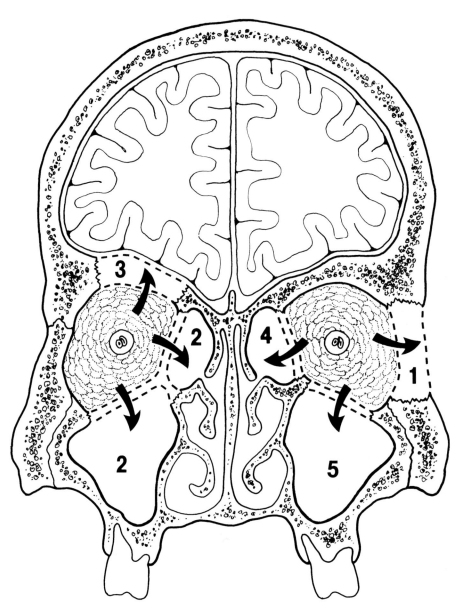

Figure 12-1. Schematic diagram of approaches for orbital decompression. 1. Lateral (Krönlein). 2. Transantral (Ogura). 3. Transfrontal (Naffziger). 4. Ethmoidal (Sewall). 5. Maxillary (Hirsch).

with this technique. As Trokel and colleagues noted, in most cases only 2–3 mm of globe retroplacement is achieved with orbital fat removal.[16] Olivari, however, has noted more success with this approach. In his experience there was transient diplopia in about 25% of cases.[17]

A second ancillary procedure is an outgrowth of Tessier's work on surgical repair for craniofaciostenosis. Wulc and colleagues have performed modified three-wall decompression (as described below) but also used titanium mini-plates to fasten the removed lateral rim forward and laterally, and smoothed the contour with methylmethacrylate.[18] The anterior displacement of the lateral orbital rim achieves a camouflage effect similar to a greater amount of globe retroplacement.

The original rationale for orbital decompression was to salvage the eye and its vision in cases of extreme proptosis with corneal exposure complications or optic nerve compression intractable to medical therapy. More surgeons now perform orbital decompression for non–vision threatening cosmetic defects. As examples of the degree of change, in a report from Warren and colleagues in 1989, 30% of orbital decompressions were performed for cosmetic reasons.[19] As many as 40% are now performed for cosmesis.[20]

LATERAL ORBITAL DECOMPRESSION

Early results with lateral orbitotomy were mixed. After Guyton reintroduced this approach in 1946, a few large trial series were reported in the American literature.[21] In 1966, Long and Ellis reported the results of 67 decompressions in 45 thyroid ophthalmopathy patients. They observed that patients with extreme proptosis had probably "autodecompressed" as a result of globe displacement and rarely experienced significant extraocular muscle dysfunction.[22]

Of the 45 patients treated with a modified Krönlein procedure (Figure 12-2), two were worse after surgery, four had no effect, and 38 had some benefit. Outstanding results were noted in two, great benefit in 14, moderate benefit in 18, and slight benefit in four cases.[22] Two cases in that series lost all vision after surgery. These authors surveyed 33 ophthalmic centers and discovered eight cases of total visual loss after lateral orbitotomy, including four after lateral decompression for thyroid ophthalmopathy.[23]

Kroll and Casten reported 32 lateral decompression operations in 18 thyroid eye disease patients.[24] Their indications for surgery were decreased vision (26 of 32), exposure, or severe discomfort. Improved vision was noted in 19 (73%) of 26 eyes after surgery; the vision in four eyes (15%) was unchanged, and in three eyes (12%) visual acuity diminished. They noted that patients with papilledema generally had slower improvement (11 eyes); usually visual acuity improved within the first few days after surgery.[24] Riley reported that approximately 50% of the 25 patients treated with lateral decompressions at the Mayo Clinic improved while the other patients' conditions remained stable or deteriorated.[25] Similar results have been reported by others.[26]

The major disadvantages of lateral orbitotomy as the sole procedure for orbital decompression are the small space it provides compared to procedures using the sinuses for orbital contents' prolapse and its minimally effective decompression of the apical portion of the orbit where optic nerve compression occurs (see below). The degree of globe retroplacement has been 2–4 mm in most reported series of lateral orbital decompression.

As discussed below, in certain cases, a lateral orbitotomy is an important adjunctive procedure in orbital decompression surgery. As Hurwitz and Birt showed, secondary strabismus is much less frequent after a lateral than an inferior-medial decompression.[27] In patients with marked proptosis, good motility, and no diplopia before surgery, use of a lateral orbitotomy and a smaller amount of sinus surgery probably results in a lower incidence of secondary muscle complications. As discussed under operative techniques, modifications in lateral orbitotomy as compared with a standard Wright-Stallard procedure for orbital tumor surgery are necessary to achieve optimal results.

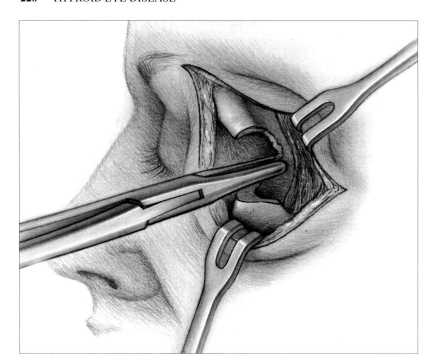

Figure 12-2. Schematic diagram demonstrating degree of lateral orbital bone removal in modified Krönlein procedure.

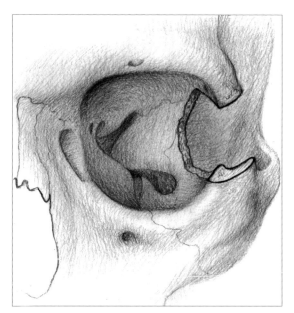

TRANSFRONTAL DECOMPRESSION

A neurosurgical approach to thyroid ophthalmopathy, transfrontal orbital decompression, proved more effective than lateral decompression but had significant real and potential morbidity, including increased length of hospitalization, frontal lobe signs (confusion, disorientation, etc.), rhinorrhea, pulsating globes, and possible meningitis.[28,29] Proptosis diminished 1–7 mm after surgery.

Two reports from the Mayo Clinic summarized results with transfrontal orbital decompression. In a series of 58 cases, Riley noted that the indications for surgery were optic nerve disease in 29 patients, progressive proptosis in 20, and corneal involvement in seven cases.[25] The average reduction of proptosis with surgery was 3 mm (range 1–9 mm). Optic nerve function partially improved in 10 cases and returned to normal in 11 patients. Usually, visual acuity improved in the first 2 weeks after surgery; however, papilledema often took months to resolve. Notably, 14 of 18 patients with optic neuropathy did not improve on corticosteroids before surgery. In 11 patients, extraocular muscle surgery was necessary, although muscle function improved in 20 cases and was stable in 18 after decompression.

McCarty and colleagues reported their results in 46 patients treated between 1951 and 1967 with transfrontal and lateral sphenoid ridge decompression. Vision was impaired in 31 patients. In nine patients, visual acuity returned to normal, 13 experienced some improvement, three were unchanged, and two deteriorated further.[30] Limited extraocular movement was present in 42 patients before surgery, 11 of whom reverted to normal function with treatment, 20 improved somewhat, three were unchanged, and eight were not measured.

While a number of investigators reported favorable results, hospitalization was longer and potential morbidity higher with transfrontal (as compared to transantral) surgery.[31] Gorman and coworkers compared the results in the same institution of combined lateral and transfrontal decompression versus transantral decompression and noted that both appeared to be equally effective. In transfrontal procedures, hospitalization was prolonged (10–12 days, compared to 5–6 days); however, none of the nine transfrontal cases developed the diplopia experienced by three of the 10 transantral decompression patients.[31]

The pterional approach has been used by some general plastic surgeons but appears to offer little advantage over transfrontal decompression. Algvere and colleagues reported 27 cases in which 20 of 22 with decreased vision improved after surgery.[32,33] Backlund, Hamby, and others have also used this approach with varying results.[34,35]

TRANSANTRAL DECOMPRESSION SURGERY

Most surgeons favor some form of orbital decompression into the maxillary antrum and ethmoid sinuses (medial-inferior decompression) or a combination of this approach with removal of other portions of the orbital bones. Decompression of orbital tissues into the sinuses can be accomplished via nasal endoscopy, through a transantral (Caldwell-Luc) approach, or through the orbit. There have been no randomized prospective series, and some of the larger series have come out of institutions with a strong bias against other forms of nonsurgical therapy, especially radiation. The two major advantages of a direct antral approach have been a greater degree of globe retroplacement and better exposure to the posterior ethmoid air cells—hence, a more reliable means of decompressing the apex than a direct orbital approach. While overall results have been good, significant complications have been reported (Table 12-1).

Ogura first reported on a large series of patients treated with transantral decompression by removing a portion of the orbital floor and medial wall.[36] Fifty-three of 76 patients before surgery had moderate to severe vision loss, and 16 had

Table 12-1. Complications of Orbital Decompression

Temporary lip numbness
Cerebrospinal fluid rhinorrhea
Sinusitis
Orbital cellulitis
Late enophthalmos
Diplopia
Blindness
Asymmetric correction of proptosis
Globe ptosis
Apparent increased upper eyelid retraction
Meningitis
Lower lid entropion
Epiphora (nasal lacrimal outflow obstruction)
Recurrent optic nerve compression

---

severe extraocular muscle problems. Most patients' vision improved after decompression; however, in four cases visual acuity diminished.[33] Other authors have reported good results with this technique.[19,37–44] In more than 90% of cases when visual acuities are better than 20/200 preoperatively and the patients are not diabetic, there is visual improvement.

DeSanto reported his results on transantral decompression in 200 thyroid ophthalmopathy patients treated between 1969 and 1976. Before surgery, vision was diminished in 87 patients (44%), 6% had papilledema, and 31% had normal extraocular muscle function. Four percent had corneal ulcers. Corticosteroids were used in 103 patients before surgery; 26 had some response, but medications were discontinued because of side effects or lack of continuing efficacy. The mean decrease in postsurgical exophthalmos was 5.5 mm (range 0–13 mm), although in 18 cases, proptosis increased immediately after surgery. Usually, final exophthalmos readings stabilized within 4–6 months. DeSanto observed that postoperatively, 79 of 87 patients with previously decreased visual acuity improved; most of those with visual field deficits of more than 1 year duration did not do as well. Vision usually improved within 1 week of surgery. Occasionally visual improvement continued for as long as 1 year after decompression.[45]

As discussed in Chapter 13, postoperative diplopia is a major complication of orbital decompression surgery. As many as 70% of patients had required some form of extraocular muscle surgery after an Ogura-type decompression.[19,40,42,45] This observation led to the recommendation of delaying extraocular muscle surgery in any patients who may require decompression since a number of patients may have increased diplopia after surgery (see below). Major complications of transantral decompression reported in DeSanto's series included postoperative diplopia (160 of 200 cases), cerebrospinal fluid rhinorrhea (2%), nasolacrimal duct obstruction (4.5%), fistulae (3.5%), temporary lip numbness (100%), and blindness in two patients.[45,46]

The results from several other series have been similar. Garrity summarized later results from the Mayo Clinic in 453 eyes.[43] Overall in that latter series, almost one-half of the patients required additional eye surgeries, and only 29% had no diplopia.

Incidence of secondary strabismus appears to be higher when this procedure is performed by an otorhinolaryngologist; new diplopia occurred in 74 of 116 who did not have this problem before decompression. In my experience, about 15% of patients will develop diplopia after a three-wall decompression; however, there are rare series with no diplopia following these procedures.[44] Usually the surgeon can achieve a symmetric result; Warren and colleagues found 89% of eyes were less than or equal to 2 mm of each other.[19] Sessions and colleagues noted a similar 5 mm mean decrease in proptosis (range 0–7 mm) and reported orbital cellulitis as an additional complication of surgery.[37] In a small series reported by Stell, the mean proptosis decrease was 3 mm.[38]

Review of all published series report a mean retroplacement of the globe of approximately 4–6 mm with a two-wall decompression, and up to 8 mm if a three-wall procedure is done. I have been able to tailor these results with reasonable accuracy at surgery. In some patients with mild proptosis and optic nerve compression, we deliberately just decompress the apex and do not attempt to achieve marked retroplacement of the globe. In other cases with extreme proptosis, we can and do achieve 10 mm of retroplacement by slightly altering the technique of three-wall decompression. Thus, the above figures for globe replacement probably reflect a tailored approach from most experienced surgeons' results. Generally, if greater than 5 mm of retroplacement is needed, a third wall should be decompressed. Calcaterra and Hepler reported on a series of 38 patients treated with transantral decompression between 1970 and 1975. Optic neuropathy was present in 21 cases (55%); 11 had preoperative diplopia. Corticosteroids were given to 34 patients; however, despite initial relief with medication, most patients had a recurrence or treatment side effects while on systemic steroids.[47]

A major, but uncommon, complication of decompression surgery is continued or recurrent visual loss. In some patients this has been due to continued or recurrent enlargement of the apical recti muscles.[48] In several series, the mechanism of recurrent visual loss is uncertain; however, as many as 20% of these patients have required radiation, corticosteroids, or both to control visual symptoms after surgery.[40,49] In my experience, less than 3% have recurrent visual loss, but I suspect that is a question of referral pattern. Certainly in patients who present with severe inflammation and optic nerve compression, surgery may alleviate the apical swelling, but continued optic nerve damage as a result of continued inflammation may require further therapy.

In any patient with recurrent or continued optic neuropathy after decompression, reimaging is mandatory. As shown in Figure 12-3, in this patient I thought I had obliterated the posterior ethmoid air cells but had failed to do so. Vision improved when those posterior air cells were exenterated.

OPHTHALMIC INFERIOR-MEDIAL-LATERAL DECOMPRESSION PROCEDURES

Ophthalmic surgeons have modified Ogura's procedure using a direct orbital approach with three intents: (1) to attempt to decrease ocular morbidity by direct visualization of orbital structures during decompression, (2) to decrease proptosis more completely when necessary by removal of more of the bony orbital walls, and (3) to improve cosmetic results.

In performing inferior-medial decompression surgery, ophthalmologists have used three incision placements: (1) through the conjunctival fornix, (2) through the subcilial lower lid (blepharoplasty-type), or (3) at the inferior orbital rim (Figure 12-

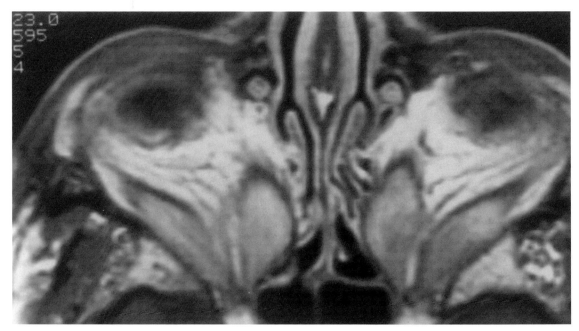

Figure 12-3. Posterior ethmoid air cells remain intact after orbital decompression. This was a surgical error I made in which I thought I had exenterated those structures and I had to do a second procedure to achieve excellent visual return.

4).[50–52] Most ophthalmic surgeons have noted approximately 4–6 mm reduction of proptosis with a two-wall removal (medial and inferior), and slightly more with a three-wall (medial, inferior, and lateral) decompression.

An increased number of orbital decompression surgeries have been reported. There are three important conclusions from this increased experience with decompression surgery. First, the type of incision and approach affect the incidence of strabismus. An antral approach, especially with a Caldwell-Luc incision, has a higher incidence of secondary strabismus than when surgery is performed through an ophthalmic incision (eyelid or conjunctiva). Second, there is a significant learning curve associated with these procedures and surgical experience is a major factor in success rate. Third, in a minority of patients, orbital decompression surgery does not successfully ameliorate cosmetic or compressive optic neuropathy deficits.

McCord surveyed American oculoplastic surgeons on orbital decompression experience.[53] An antral (75%) or a three-wall (20%) decompression was used in approximately 95% of cases; less than 4% of patients had only a lateral orbitotomy. Proptosis (60%) and visual loss (39%) were the major indications for surgery. Only 39% of questionnaires were returned and no visual acuities before or after decompression were reported.[53] Similarly, it is unclear what percentage of patients had surgery for cosmesis versus exposure or visual problems.[53,54] It appears that the indications for orbital decompression vary widely. In some reports, cosmesis was the indication for decompression in as many as 40% of cases.[55] In other series, cosmesis was the primary indication for orbital decompression in less than 5% of cases.[27,56,57]

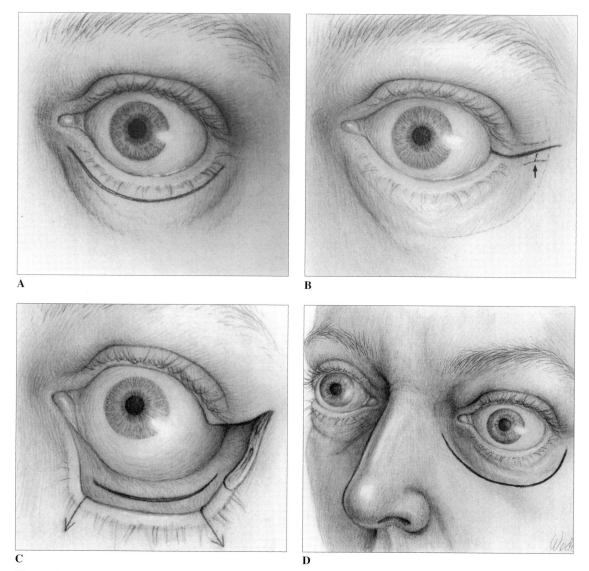

Figure 12-4. Schematic diagrams demonstrating: skin incisions for ophthalmic inferior-medial decompression approaches (A); swinging lower lid to expose the orbital floor so that an inferior fornix incision can be used to reach the roof of the maxillary antrum (B,C); and alternatively, an incision can be made directly over the floor of the orbit (D).

Secondary strabismus remains a major complication of orbital decompression.[32,42–45] Most reports have shown that this complication occurred more frequently with a transantral as compared with a lid or conjunctival approach to the sinuses.[27,53–54] In the University of California at Los Angeles experience, five of 10 patients with no strabismus before surgery developed it after transantral surgery, versus one of 11 after an ophthalmic approach.[55] Similarly, McCord reported that 5.6% of cases performed through a conjunctival or lid approach had motility complications, versus 41% when a transantral approach was used.[53] As would be expected, strabismus occurs much less frequently with lateral decompression. Hurwitz and Birt did not note it after a lateral approach; in contrast, motility disorders developed in 16 of 19 transantral decompressions they performed.[19] Fells noted that 11 of 14 patients developed ocular motility disorders after transantral or ethmoidal surgeries, and an A-pattern esotropia occurred in eight.[58] Torsional diplopias have also been described.[59] As discussed below, these data have led me to modify my surgical approach depending on the indications for decompression and the preoperative presence or absence of strabismus. In thyroid orbitopathy patients with good motility and sufficient proptosis to require decompression, I now prefer a modified three-wall procedure to minimize the amount of sinus surgery and hopefully decrease the incidence of secondary strabismus.

Approximately 2–4 mm of proptosis can be eliminated with a lateral orbital procedure alone, and this adjunct to medial-inferior decompression diminishes the amount of orbital contents that must be displaced into the sinuses. As Fells and others have noted, displacement of structures into the ethmoid sinuses probably results in a higher incidence of strabismus than antral surgery, although this remains to be proved.[58,60]

Indications for the cosmetic use of orbital decompression are still unclear. As discussed above, there is significant morbidity with this procedure; Table 12-1 lists some surgical complications.[53,57] Generally cosmetic decompression, as part of a staged reconstruction, is a reasonable approach in patients with Hertel exophthalmometry readings greater than 25 mm, especially if they already have strabismus. In patients with readings less than 22 mm on exophthalmometry, the risk/benefit ratio for cosmetic improvement versus complications is uncertain. Experienced oculoplastic surgeons, such as Crowell Beard, believe that eyelid camouflage procedures are safer and provide acceptable cosmetic results in patients with mild to moderate proptosis (personal communication, Crowell Beard, San Francisco, 1996). I agree with that concept, and unless the patient already has a significant motility disturbance, I tend not to advocate decompression in cases of mild proptosis. Obviously this decision is also predicated on a patient's cosmetic appearance, especially the appearance of the proptosis relative to their facial bones. Some patients remain attractive with a reasonable amount of proptosis while in others Hertel readings of more than 21 are cosmetically unacceptable.

If decompression is considered in any thyroid patient, it is important to advise the patient that a staged reconstruction will probably be required (decompression followed by muscle surgery followed by eyelid surgery) and that decompression surgery can exacerbate some cosmetic defects.[55–60] In addition to diplopia, a Caldwell-Luc decompression may often produce globe ptosis with an apparent, increased retraction of the upper eyelid (Figure 12-5). As Goldberg and colleagues showed, leaving a medial strut can diminish this former complication.[61] It is useful to give the patient a preoperative estimate of the time frame for the entire surgical reconstruction. I have examined a few patients where strabismus and eyelid surgery were performed too soon after decompression with less than optimal results. Maximum retroplacement of the eye following surgery is often delayed; in one series Lamberg and coworkers noted a mean retroplacement of the globe of 3.6 mm at 4 months and 5.3 mm at 6–12 months after decompression.[62,63]

The visual results after orbital decompression surgery are not uniformly excellent. As discussed above, while rare, loss of vision from surgical trauma can occur.[64,65] There are a number of etiologies of optic nerve damage in thyroid orbitopathy. In most cases, optic neuropathy is due to compression of the nerve by enlarged muscles at the apex, but in some instances this does not seem to be the case.[40,48,49,60,63] In some of these latter cases, optic nerve inflammation is probably a major cause of visual

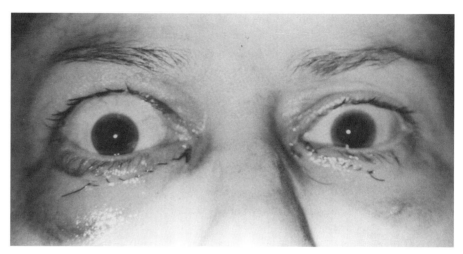

Figure 12-5. Globe ptosis and increased appearance of upper eyelid retraction after maximal antral/orbital floor decompression.

loss and orbital decompression is probably not effective. This problem is probably why some patients have required radiation, steroids, or cyclosporine after decompression to decrease optic nerve inflammation. Twenty-seven percent of cases cited by McCord required ancillary therapies after decompression.[53] Otto and colleagues noted that generalized increased intraorbital pressure could be another factor in thyroid optic neuropathy.[53a] In eight orbital decompression cases, they noted the mean retrobulbar pressure decreased from 28.7 mm Hg to 18.7 mm Hg.[53a] While failure of orbital decompression surgery to relieve visual loss is multifactorial, other causes include far advanced optic nerve damage and atrophy, surgical trauma, and decreased vision due to nonthyroid eye disease such as cataract, glaucoma, or macular degeneration. In some of the latter cases, magnetic resonance imaging (MRI) or computed tomography (CT) will show an absence of compression by the apical muscles. Those cases are probably better managed with an initial trial of high-dose systemic steroids, cyclosporine, or 20-gray photon irradiation. In my experience, patients with an insidious, chronic history of limited visual loss (i.e., better than 20/100 vision) can be managed nonemergently. We initially try nonsurgical techniques since rapid intervention is not necessary to prevent permanent visual sequelae. In contrast, when patients present with a rapid (less than 1 week) course of visual loss, relatively rapid progression of vision loss to below 20/100, or marked visual loss secondary to rapid proptosis, emergent decompression, with simultaneous high-dose systemic steroid therapy is indicated. The prognosis for visual return in patients with chronic poor (<20/200) vision is guarded after any form of therapy.

Three other factors are important in orbital decompression surgery for the visual loss associated with thyroid optic neuropathy. First, there is a long learning curve for this type of ophthalmic surgery. Often it is hard to divorce the effects of increased experience from changes in technique in a surgeon's series. McCord believed he obtained better visual results in compressive optic neuropathy patients when he changed from an ophthalmic (conjunctival or lid) to an otorhinolaryngologic (Caldwell-Luc) approach.[53] Probably the improved results were at least partially due to increased surgical experience.[53] In my experience, I have not had problems reaching the sphenoid sinuses and decompressing the orbital apex with an ophthalmic approach, but the technique took time to evolve. Second, as a corollary to the first, iatrogenic visual loss can also occur as posterior decompression surgery is being learned. Third, as discussed above, visual results after surgery are partially a function of preoperative visual acuities. Most eyes with visual acuities of 20/100 or better have excellent results.[66] In those cases that are 20/400 or worse, the return of vision is less assured; similarly, a patient with insulin-dependent diabetes has a worse visual prognosis.[40,67] It is often not possible to predict those patients with initially poor vision who will or will not have visual improvement after surgery.[66,67]

The overall reported incidence of most complications has appeared to remain stable over the last decade; however, some problems have been reported more frequently. Nasolacrimal duct obstruction associated with orbital decompression surgery was initially described more than 10 years ago.[68] Seiff and Shorr have noted that this complication occurred in 14 of 90 (16%) of transantral decompressions.[69] I am not aware of having produced this complication through an ophthalmic (lid or conjunctival) approach. Migliori has observed it and recommended that the nasolacrimal system be routinely probed at the time of orbital decompression.[70]

DeSanto pointed out the need to assess the sinus status before decompression surgery to avoid acute sinusitis or problems in surgical outcome.[45] CT or MRI studies of the orbit and sinuses are an important component of the preoperative evaluation of these patients. Lamberg and coworkers have described a patient with insufficient retroplacement of the globe, because of a small maxillary antrum that provided insufficient room to decompress orbital contents.[62]

Usually, strabismus surgery is performed several months after orbital decompression. In a few cases with less than 20 prism diopters of hypotropia, we have used an ipsilateral adjustable inferior rectus recession at the time of decompression with good results; however, I always warn the patient that it may not be sufficient.

In patients with greater than 30 mm of proptosis, two groups have described a combined ophthalmic-neurosurgical four-wall resection.[71,72] This surgical approach is not usually necessary, is quite tedious, and often has a poor cosmetic outcome.[61]

OPHTHALMIC OPERATIVE TECHNIQUE

I have continued to modify techniques for two and three-wall orbital decompression. The basic instrument set used for these procedures is shown in Figure 12-6. Figure 12-7 shows a fiber-optic headlight that is useful during some parts of the case. I have tried subciliary, conjunctival, rim, and Caldwell-Luc incisions (see Figure 12-4). Scarring with the rim incision seems acceptable; it apparently has a lower incidence of secondary lower lid entropion deformity (Figure 12-8) than the other two incisions.

Depending on whether a two-wall or three-wall decompression is planned, I start with a lateral orbitotomy (for three-wall) or a lower lid incision (two-wall). If a three-wall decompression is indicated in a patient with moderate proptosis and good motility, or in a patient with extreme proptosis to obtain near maximum retroplacement of the globe, the lateral orbitotomy is performed first to allow more space inferior-medially with less pressure and manipulation of the globe.

In a three-wall decompression, a modified Wright-Stallard lateral orbitotomy is performed (see Figure 12-2). After I remove the lateral orbital rim, I use the

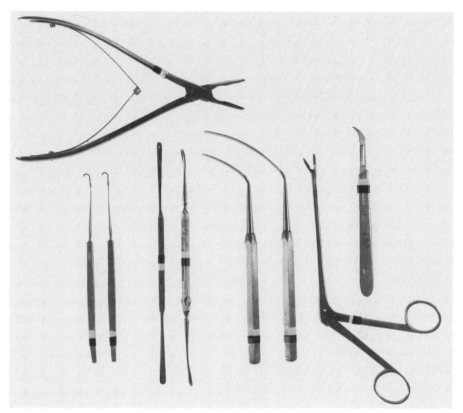

Figure 12-6. Orbital decompression surgical instruments.

minidriver saw and a burr to maximally reduce the size of the rim strut that I eventually replace at the end of the case (Figure 12-9). This reduction shaping of the lateral orbit rim allows more space for lateral tissue prolapse. If a strut is not placed back, especially in patients with a marked inflammatory component to their orbitopathy, significant cosmetic deficit can result (Figure 12-10). A Lempert rongeur is used to remove cancellous bone posteriorly, and periorbita in this area is obliterated. The lateral orbital rim is not replaced until after surgery on the inferior and medial walls of the orbit is completed.

I generally will try to minimize ethmoid surgery in those cases that have less than 25 mm of proptosis and good motility. Instead, a lateral orbitotomy combined with removal of the medial portion of the antral roof, and a minimal ethmoidectomy is performed. If there is greater than 27 mm of proptosis, a standard three-wall procedure is usually necessary, since I cannot routinely achieve more than 6–7 mm of retroplacement of the globe unless I decompress through the medial and inferior walls in addition to the lateral orbit. In patients with more than 31 mm of proptosis, a four-wall decompression may be indicated.[71,72] I have not personally had to resort to that procedure since a three-wall with removal of the entire orbital floor, save for the neurovascular strut, usually allows the globe to be retroplaced about 10 mm (Figure 12-11).[40–44,50–53]

In surgery through the lower lid it seems helpful to routinely inject 1% lidocaine (Xylocaine) with 1:100,000 epinephrine at the time of general anesthesia

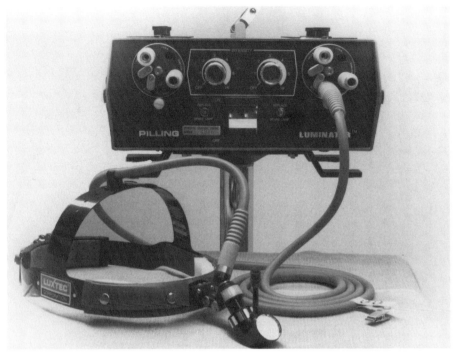

Figure 12-7. Fiber-optic light pipe is useful in posterior orbital decompression to ensure that all the bone fragments have been removed and to visualize areas where periorbital slits are to be made.

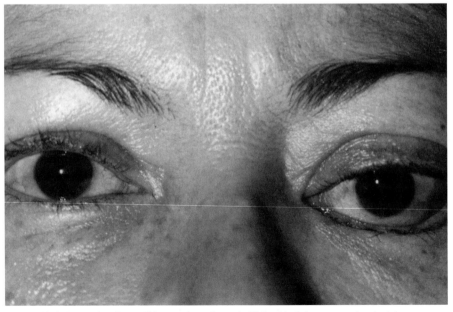

Figure 12-8. Secondary lower lid entropion after subcilial orbital decompression incision.

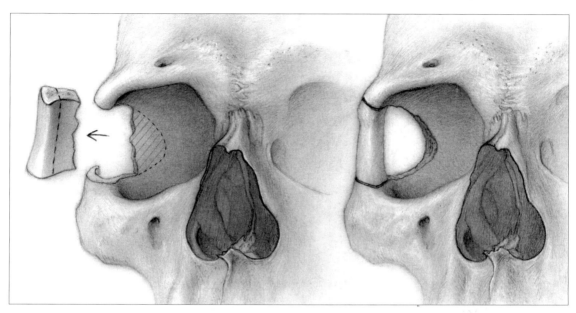

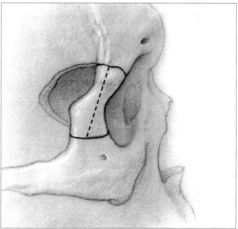

Figure 12-9. Schematic drawing shows sculpting of the orbital rim to decrease its bulk and allow more orbital contents to extrude laterally. After lateral rim is removed, it is sculpted (inset). Cancellous bone posterior to the rim is removed and the smaller rim is replaced.

induction, before surgical scrub, for improved hemostasis. After a skin incision with the scalpel, I use blunt and sharp dissection to reach the orbital rim (Figure 12-12). Periosteum is incised with a scalpel, and a Freer elevator is used to raise the periosteum on the inferior and medial walls of the orbit (Figure 12-13). A schematic diagram (Figure 12-14) demonstrates the extent of orbital wall removal in a standard two wall-decompression. A curved hemostat can be used to break into the medial portion of the roof of the maxillary antrum (Figure 12-15). In cases with an abnormally thick orbital floor, a pineapple-shaped drill bit can be used to sculpt out this bone. A front-biting Takahashi instrument is then used to remove

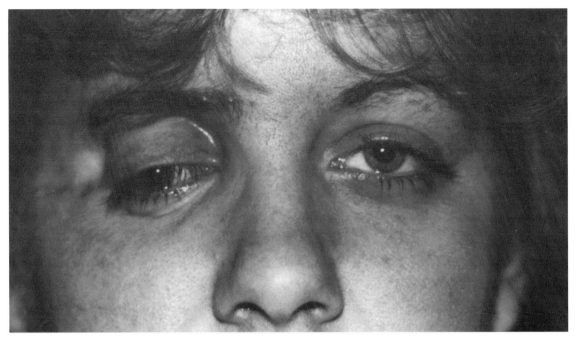

Figure 12-10. If the lateral orbital rim is not replaced after decompression, especially in patients that have a fibrotic/inflammatory component in their thyroid orbitopathy, a cosmetic defect can occur.

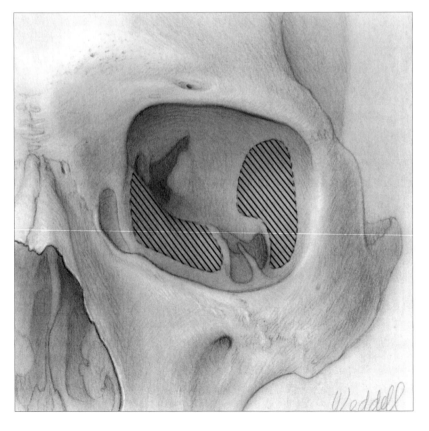

Figure 12-11. In patients with Hertel exophthalmometry readings greater than 30 mm, in conjunction with a standard three-wall decompression, the entire orbital floor, except for a central neurovascular strut, is removed, as shown in this schematic drawing.

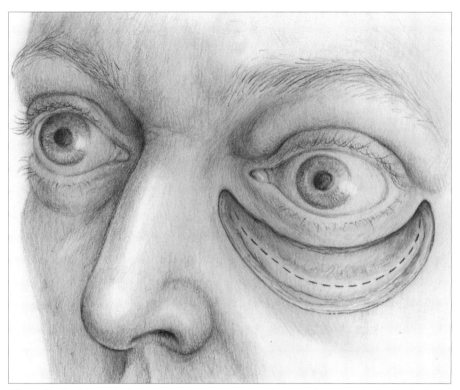

Figure 12-12. Schematic drawing showing exposed orbital rim; periosteum is incised and raised so that bone may be removed.

bone and the ethmoid sinus contents back to the apex of the orbit (Figures 12-16 and 12-17). Limiting anterior bone removal is advised to avoid the lacrimal fossa (nasal-lacrimal drainage system) and the orbital rim. Inferiorly, bone is removed laterally to the infraorbital groove, and superomedially, to the ethmoidal-frontal suture. Posteriorly, the orbital floor is removed and we routinely break into the sphenoid sinus. Often it is helpful to palpate posteriorly with an instrument, since a shelf of bone may be left inadvertently in the posterior orbital floor.

I routinely perform my initial inferior and medial bone removal without a headlight. Usually there is adequate visualization, and I tend to remove what I think will be an adequate amount of bone, pack the area with thrombin-soaked sponges, and if performing a bilateral decompression, then perform the same maneuver on the other side. Switching sides allows time for hemostasis to occur. I then put on a headlight with loupes (see Figure 12-7) and remove any additional bone necessary. I then repack the area, and go to the contralateral side (or wait for hemostasis). A microscimitar blade is then used to incise periorbita (see Figure 12-17).

The amount of globe retroplacement with surgery is mainly a function of the number and size of cuts made in the periorbita and the presence—and subsequent free prolapse—of normal fat. After bone is removed, there is virtually no retroplacement of the eye nor decompression of orbital contents. Lockwood's ligament, a thickened Tenon's capsule that blends with the capsulopalpebral fascia, forms a facial sling. A scimitar-shaped knife is useful for making anterior-posterior slits in the periorbita. This allows fat to freely prolapse into the maxillary and ethmoid cavities

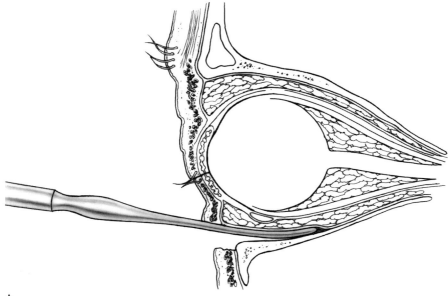

A

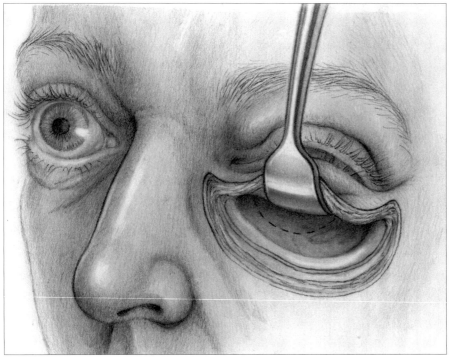

B

Figure 12-13. A. Schematic drawing demonstrating use of Freer elevator to elevate periosteum from floor of orbit. B. A soule retractor is used to elevate orbital contents and periosteum to the maxillary antral roof.

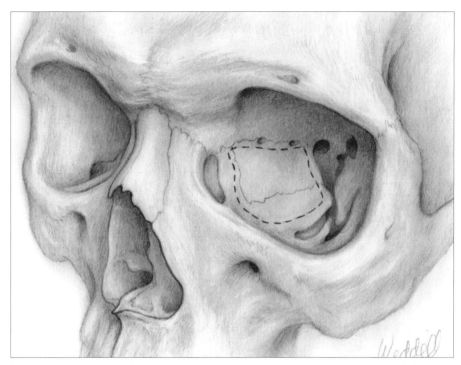

Figure 12-14. Schematic drawing demonstrating amount of bone removal in a two-wall decompression.

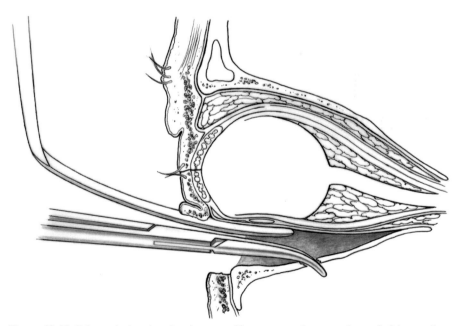

Figure 12-15. Schematic drawing showing curved hemostat used to enter the roof of the maxillary sinus.

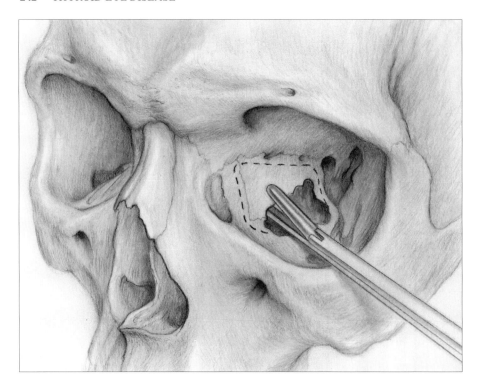

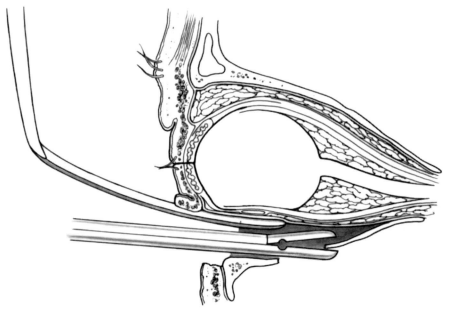

Figure 12-16. Schematic drawing showing front biting Takahashi instrument used to remove medial bony portion of orbital floor and inferior portion of the medial wall.

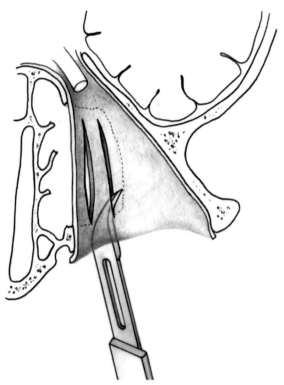

Figure 12-17. Schematic drawing showing scimitar blade used to make slits in periorbita.

to decompress the orbital contents (see Figure 12-17). The amount of manipulation necessary to achieve an acceptable degree of fat prolapse varies; with minimal fibrosis, fat lobules will ooze through the surgical slits. If significant fibrosis is present, orbital fat must be gently teased through the periorbital slits. In rare cases with marked orbital fibrosis, the fibrotic connective tissue that replaces normal orbital fat must be surgically excised to decompress the optic nerve. If bilateral decompressions are performed, the retroplacement should be symmetric at the time of surgery. I have not routinely made an antral window at the completion of surgery and have not observed a significantly higher incidence of postsurgical sinus disease.

Postoperative CT of a typical bone removal is shown in Figures 12-18 and 12-19.[73] This patient did not require apical decompression. In a two-wall decompression only the roof of the maxillary antrum is removed; however, I perform a complete ethmoidectomy.

Most of my experience has been in cases of compressive optic neuropathy not responsive to steroids or radiation, patients with marked proptosis with diplopia, or those with massive proptosis and exposure. If less than 7 mm of proptosis reduction is sought and the patient has preoperative diplopia, two-wall decompression, removing only the floor medial to the infraorbital nerve and the medial wall and ethmoid sinus contents is sufficient. In patients with no preoperative strabismus and only moderate proptosis, we use a three-wall decompression with minimal medial wall surgery.

In many patients with optic neuropathy, proptosis is minimal (Figures 12-20 and 12-21). In these cases, slits seem best placed only medially above and below the medial rectus muscle to avoid muscle prolapse. Where the object of surgery is decompression of the nerve and not retroplacement of the globe, this approach carries minimal risk of

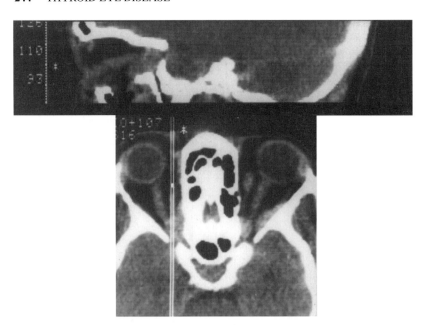

Figure 12-18. Axial computed tomography with parasagittal reconstruction after inferior-medial decompression.

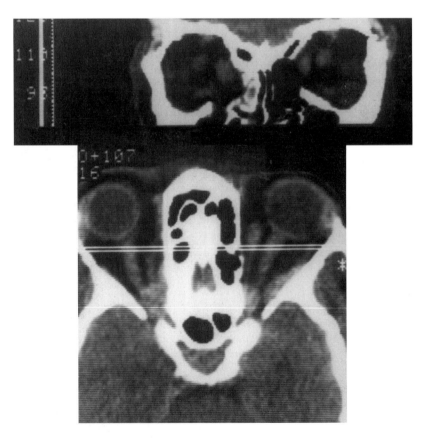

Figure 12-19. Axial computed tomography with coronal reconstruction after inferior-medial decompression. Note herniation of orbital structures into ethmoid area.

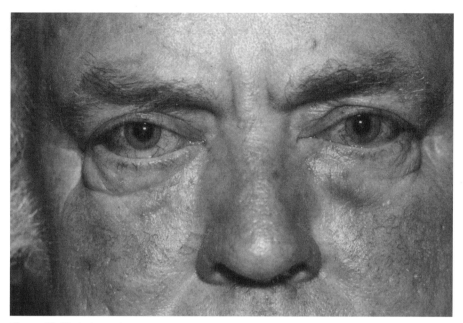

Figure 12-20. Patient with severe optic neuropathy, but minimal exophthalmos.

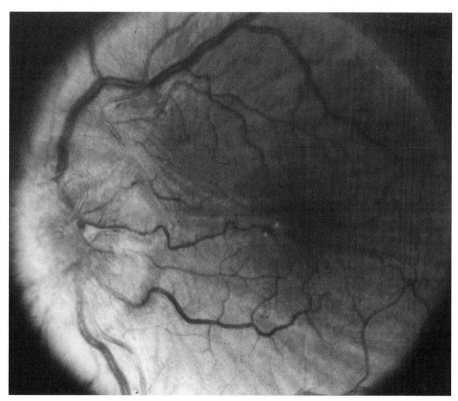

Figure 12-21. Fundus showing optic nerve changes in patient shown in Figure 12-20.

secondary diplopia or worsening of preoperative muscle status. When decompression is performed to diminish proptosis, slits of sufficient number and size must be made to allow the orbital contents, often including the extraocular muscles, to prolapse into sinus spaces with a resultant increase in extraocular muscle palsies. As previously noted, almost 70% of cases reported by DeSanto required muscle surgery. Shorr and coworkers noted that 30% of their patients developed consecutive diplopia in primary position after decompression, and 45% required some form of strabismus surgery.[74]

In those patients who are having surgery for extreme proptosis, and where the goal of surgery is to reduce proptosis by greater than 7 mm, a standard three-wall decompression is indicated. This can be performed using a two-incision approach or a conjunctival incision to reach all three walls.[51,53,56] The two-skin incision approach may be easier technically. I have had no experience with a four-wall decompression; this approach requires a combined ophthalmic-neurosurgical procedure and has significant potential morbidity.[71,72] In our experience, three-wall decompression coupled with camouflage eyelid surgery is effective and has less morbidity.

Many of the potential complications associated with orbital decompression can be minimized with alterations in surgical technique. One contraindication for this type of surgery is active sinusitis. As discussed above, if optic nerve decompression is the sole indication for surgical intervention, then care taken to avoid muscle prolapse into sinus space decreases the likelihood of secondary strabismus. Similarly, we prefer a lid approach in these cases since it has a lower incidence of secondary strabismus. In my experience, lower lid deformities occur less frequently (but are not eliminated) with a rim rather than subciliary skin incision. Medial bone removal should be below the ethmoidal-frontal suture and posterior to the lacrimal fossa.[68] The anterior and posterior ethmoidal arteries emerge from bone just superior to this suture line and bleed profusely when cut. If this occurs, a needle tip Bovie placed into the bony ostium controls bleeding; a suction Bovie is helpful for occasional profuse bleeding encountered deep in the orbit. I routinely have two independent suction lines set up in all orbital cases where bleeding may be likely. Bone incisions behind the lacrimal fossa seem unlikely to cause nasolacrimal duct obstruction. Bleeding is decreased if fat is allowed to freely prolapse and is not manipulated with forceps. In approximately 5–10% of severe thyroid ophthalmopathy cases, significant orbital fibrosis occurs; in rare instances, patients have been encountered in which Graves' disease and an "orbital wipe out" syndrome resulted in total replacement of fat by fibrosis (see Chapter 5, Figure 5-47). In such cases, after periorbital slits are made, the fibrotic tissue compressing the optic nerve must be surgically removed.

In patients with chronic, severe orbital proptosis, acute proptosis with exposure not amenable to nonsurgical management, or proptosis with rapid, severe visual loss, decompression is reasonable. Figures 12-22 and 12-23 show a patient who presented with a 1-week history of dramatic vision loss in her only functional eye with 30 mm of proptosis. The other eye was phthisical after multiple retinal procedures. Figure 12-24 shows 10 mm of retroplacement of the globe 2 days after a three-wall decompression. Vision returned from 20/400 to 20/25. The patients shown in Figures 12-24 through 12-27 similarly had orbital decompressions with good retroplacement noted within the first few days after surgery.

It is important for the patient to realize that orbital decompression may only be the first step in a multiple procedure surgical reconstruction, especially if they have eyelid malpositions and strabismus. Most of these patients require additional surgery and can develop worse diplopia that may only be correctable in the primary position of gaze after decompression surgery (Table 12-2; see also Chapter 13). Figures 12-28, 12-29, and 12-30 show a patient with unilateral exposure and diplopia treated with a three-

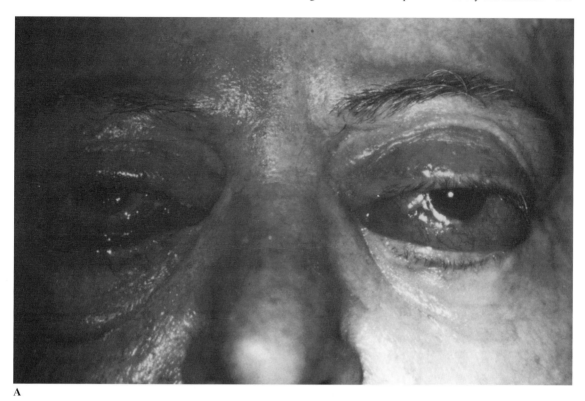

A

Figure 12-22. A. Preoperative photograph of patient with a 1-week history of severe visual loss in only functional eye; opposite eye is phthisical. Best visual acuity is 20/400. B. Axial computed tomography scan (right eye is phthisical).

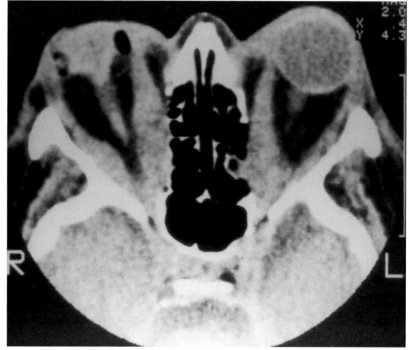

B

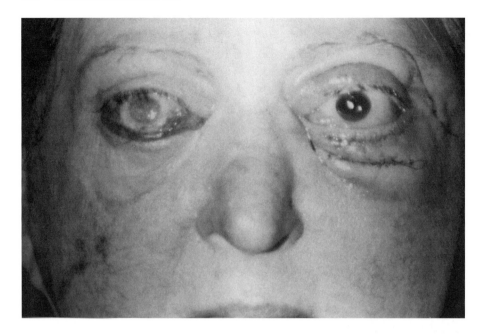

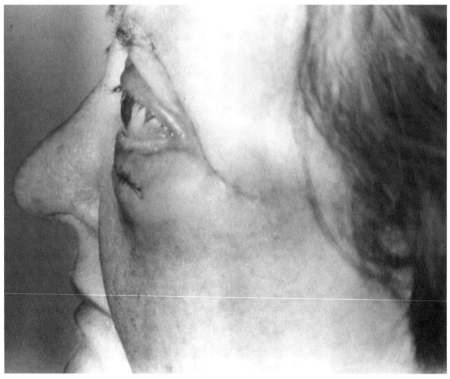

Figure 12-23. Patient shown in Figure 12-22, 2 days after three-wall decompression. Eye has been retroplaced 10 mm and vision has returned to 20/25.

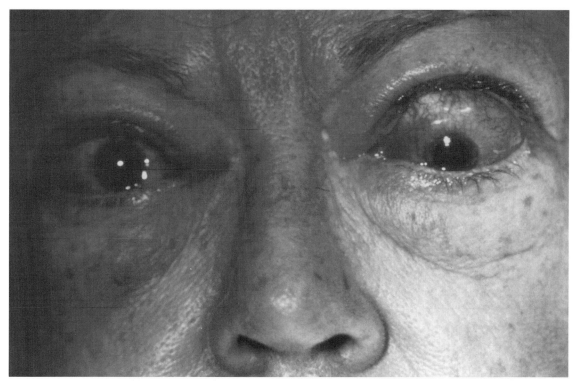

Figure 12-24. Preoperative photograph of a patient with severe inflammatory thyroid eye disease and compression optic neuropathy.

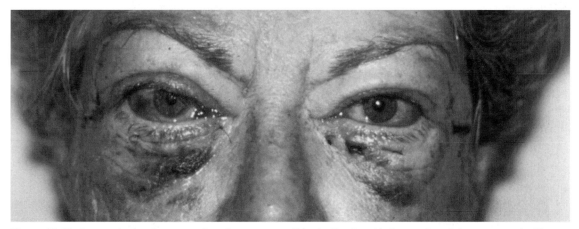

Figure 12-25. One week after decompression, the eyes are well back. Continued inflammation of the nerve required long-term anti-inflammatory therapy.

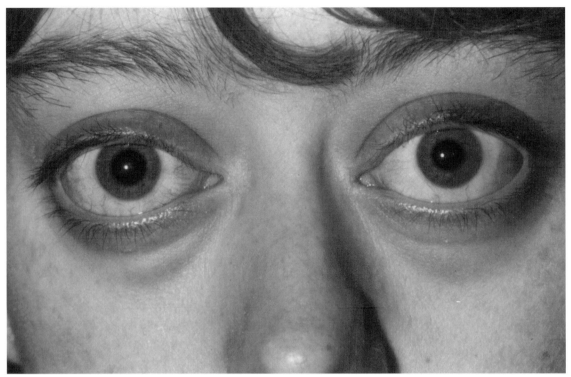

Figure 12-26. Preoperative photograph of a young patient with severe thyroid orbitopathy.

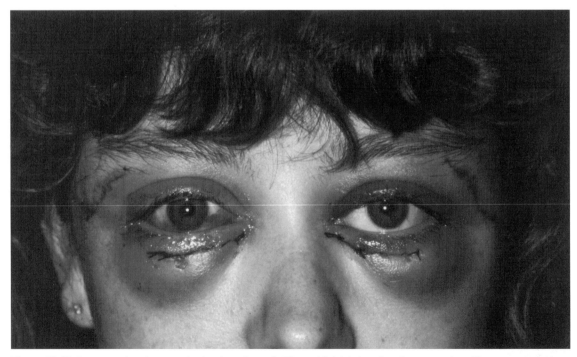

Figure 12-27. Postoperative photograph of patient shown in Figure 12-26 1 day after decompression. The eyes are nicely retroplaced.

Table 12-2. Surgical Approach to Severe Exophthalmos

1. Orbital decompression surgery
2. Repair of lid deformities
3. Extraocular muscle surgery

wall decompression. As a second stage the muscle was moved, and later he had placement of an autologous tarsal graft to correct the lower eyelid deformity.

Cosmetically, with minimal proptosis (Hertel exophthalmometry <23 mm) often camouflage eyelid surgery is acceptable. If there are 23- to 27-mm readings with preoperative diplopia, a standard two-wall procedure is indicated. In patients with 23–27 mm of exophthalmos with good motility, we use a modified three-wall decompression. Figures 12-31 and 12-32 show such a patient with good vision, no diplopia, and cosmetically unacceptable unilateral proptosis. She had a modified three-wall decompression without secondary strabismus. The lower eyelid deformity was corrected with an autologous tarsal graft from the opposite eyelid. In patients with more than 27 mm of proptosis, an expanded three-wall procedure is performed with removal of the entire floor, except for the neurovascular strut (see Figure 12-11), and medial and lateral walls. Tailoring the decompression approach based on optic nerve status, motility status, and the amount of proptosis can lessen the surgical morbidity associated with this procedure.

As discussed in Chapter 13, strabismus surgery is usually performed several months after orbital decompression. In a few cases of hypotropia alone, good results have been obtained with adjustable inferior rectus recession performed at the time of decompression. Often the inferior rectus malfunction can simulate a medial rectus disturbance (Figure 12-33).

New or increased strabismus is probably the most frequent major ocular problem associated with decompression surgery. In a retrospective review, Rosenbaum

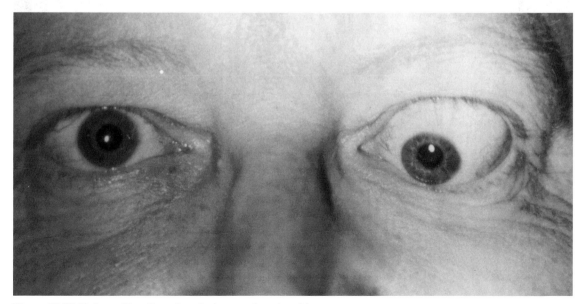

Figure 12-28. Patient with unilateral marked proptosis and strabismus.

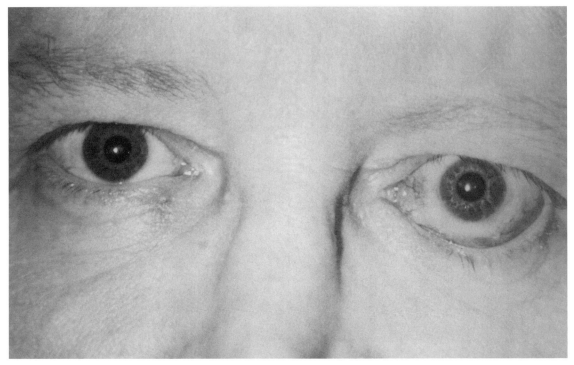

Figure 12-29. Three-wall orbital decompression of patient shown in Figure 12-28 has produced symmetric eye position. Patient has had surgery on the inferior rectus muscle but has lower eyelid malposition.

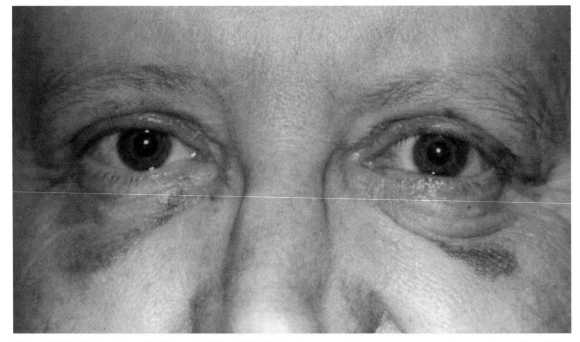

Figure 12-30. Patient shown in Figures 12-28 and 12-29 after decompression surgery, eye muscle surgeries, and eyelid repair (free graft of contralateral upper eyelid tarsus).

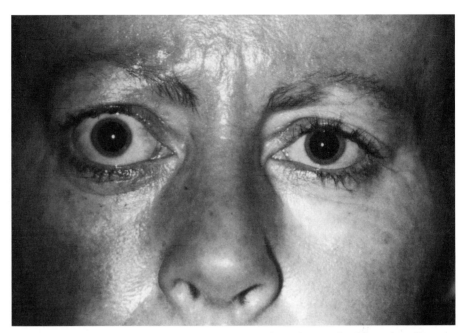

Figure 12-31. Patient with cosmetically unacceptable unilateral proptosis with good motility.

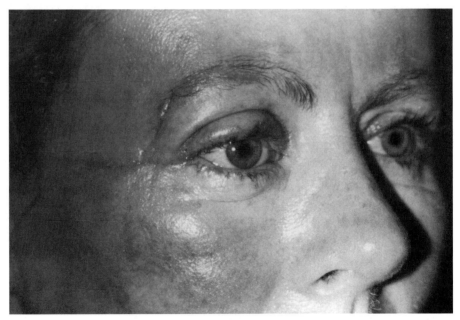

Figure 12-32. Repair with modified three-wall decompression of patient shown in Figure 12-31, and transplantation of contralateral upper eyelid tarsus to repair lower eyelid defect.

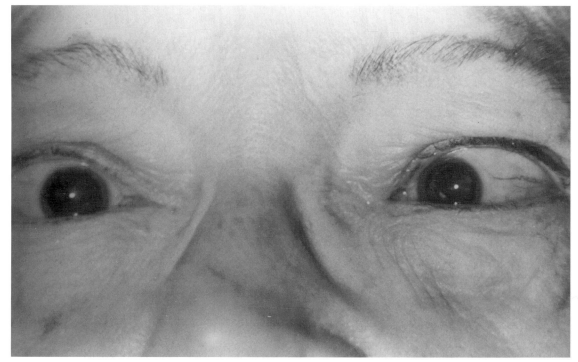

Figure 12-33. Inferior rectus fibrosis simulates medial rectus abnormality and produces esotropia.

observed that secondary diplopia occurred in approximately 26% of patients after decompression surgery; 9–69% of patients (mean 45%) required strabismus surgery after decompression.[75,76] Chapter 13 discusses why, while most of these patients' problems can be corrected sufficiently to produce single vision in the primary position, only a very small minority have return of full versions. This complication is a major reason for avoiding cosmetic decompression surgery in equivocal cases, especially if extraocular movement is acceptable.

Rarely, other complications can occur with an orbital decompression. Figure 12-34 shows the one case in which I have produced a rent in the superior orbital roof that occurred when we were exenterating the ethmoid sinuses inferior to the penetrating arteries. We did not actually manipulate the bony orbital roof, but it developed a posterior rent and had a cerebrospinal fluid leak.

OTOLARYNGOLOGIC APPROACHES FOR DECOMPRESSION

Some authors believe that a transantral approach gives better access to posterior ethmoidal air cells than an orbital approach. I have not found this to be the case. In a study by Mourits and coworkers, no difference in visual results was found when they compared surgical decompression via an orbital versus a coronal approach.[69] While I have used this approach extensively to reach small apical intraconal tumors just below the optic nerve, the transantral approach has a higher complication rate.[36,38,45,53,69]

A Caldwell-Luc procedure is the most commonly used approach for a sinus decompression procedure.

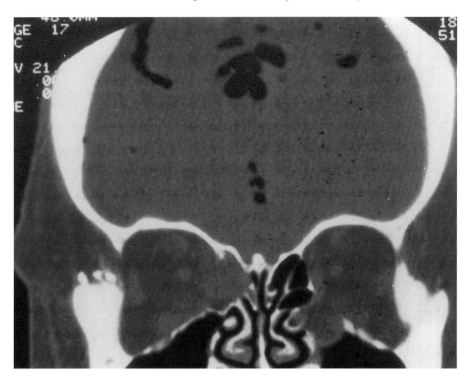

Figure 12-34. Postdecompression coronal reformatted computed tomography scan demonstrates air in the central nervous system secondary to a leak that occurred as a result of decompression surgery.

Caldwell-Luc Procedure

The Caldwell-Luc procedure was first described in the late nineteenth century.[77,78] The anatomy and inter-relationships of sinuses and orbit may confuse the ophthalmic surgeon not accustomed to viewing the orbit from medially and below. It is important to realize that the ethmoidal bulla is immediately superior to the natural ostium of the maxillary antrum. The nasolacrimal duct is just anterior to the natural ostium in the posterior superior wall. The medial wall of the maxillary antrum is directly under the lamina papyracea. Finally, the posterior limit of the ethmoid air cells are at approximately the posterior end of the maxillary sinus.

The canine fossa, an area of mucoperiosteum superior to the upper teeth on the face of the maxilla, is infiltrated with a combination of 2% lidocaine and 1:100,000 epinephrine. A scalpel is used to make a horizontal incision that is carried down to the bone in this tissue, not tightly adherent to bone, so that it is easier to close at the end of the procedure. This tissue is elevated superiorly off the maxillary face until the maxillary nerve, which exits the infraorbital foramen in the midpupillary line, is identified and avoided. Instruments placed for traction to visualize the surgical field should be positioned to minimize trauma to the nerve and lessen postoperative hypesthesia (Figure 12-35). The face of the maxillary antrum is then entered and an anterior antrostomy is carried out with chisel and Kerasin rongeurs.

A schematic (Figure 12-36) shows the surgical pathway. The natural ostium of the maxillary antrum is identified and enlarged. An exenteration of the ethmoidal air cells is performed through this opening. The medial half of the orbital floor is re-

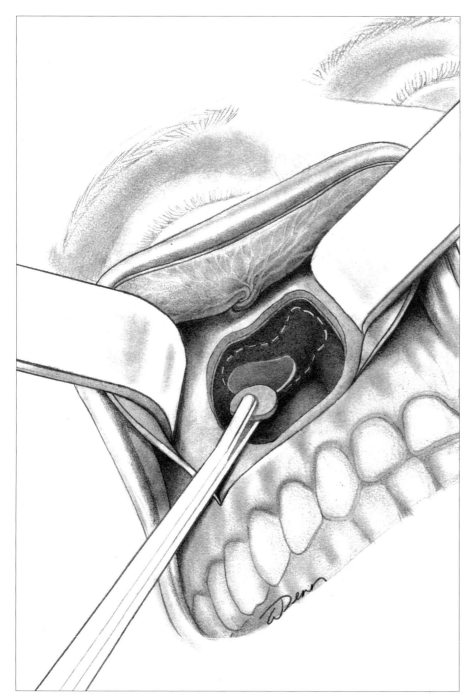

Figure 12-35. Schematic drawing showing bony landmarks for antrostomy for Caldwell-Luc approach to orbital decompression. The retractors should be placed to provide exposure, but avoid traction on the nerve. The incision should be in the relatively lax gingival tissue that is easier to close than mucosa closer to the teeth.

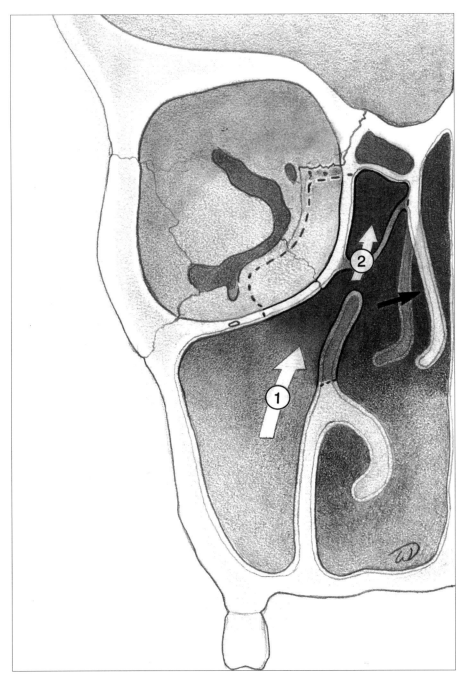

Figure 12-36. Schematic drawing showing a mid-orbital coronal section demonstrates the surgical pathway used for a Caldwell-Luc transantral decompression. Labels 1 and 2 refer to the order of the surgical approach through the sinuses (see text).

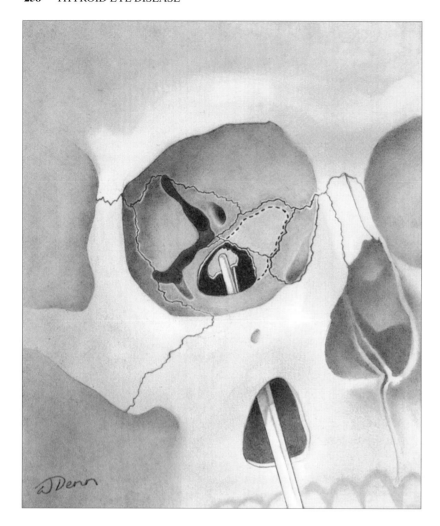

Figure 12-37. Schematic drawing showing how the roof of the medial portion of the maxillary antrum is removed, along with an ethmoidectomy to provide orbital decompression.

moved with rongeurs, in a manner analogous to that used in other approaches (Figure 12-37). After ethmoid exenteration and removal of the maxillary floor, the periorbita is incised to complete the orbital portion of the procedure.

An inferior nasal antrostomy is performed for drainage. A trocar is placed through the nose in the area of the inferior meatus. A window is created with chisel and rongeur. The nose is packed and the patient is placed on systemic antibiotics. Many surgeons have converted from a Caldwell-Luc to a nasal endoscopic approach.

Intranasal Endoscopic Approaches for Orbital Decompression

Two major advantages of an endoscopic approach are the lack of an external cutaneous scar and the ability to directly visualize the apical area and possibly decompress it better. There are a number of contraindications to endoscopic decompression; these include active sinusitis, polyps, or other processes that increase intranasal hemorrhage, a thick orbital floor, and a contracted maxillary antrum. An endoscopic approach does not allow as much anterior orbital floor to be removed as with other procedures.

Figure 12-38. A transnasal endoscopic decompression is initiated, as shown in this schematic drawing, after the nasal mucosa is treated with a topical decongestant, by placement of the nasal endoscope under the elevated middle turbinate. Some surgeons infracture the inferior turbinate. An incision in the ethmoidal bullae is then made.

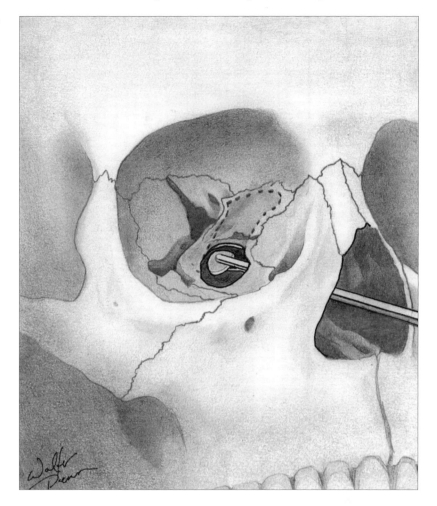

The most important parameter in the decision paradigm for the choice of operation is the relative expertise of the surgeon with a given procedure. Endoscopic surgery has an especially steep learning curve, and major complications are more common in less experienced hands, including bilateral vision loss, brain damage, or death.[79–81] In most centers, these endoscopic procedures are done jointly by ophthalmologists and otolaryngologists; several of the pioneering endoscopists have also advocated using their approach in conjunction with a lateral orbitotomy.[82,83]

A preoperative CT or MRI is mandatory to minimize complications.[84] It is important to assess sinus clarity, the relative height and slope of the roof of the ethmoid sinuses, the orbital floor thickness, and the relationship of the ethmoidal air cells to the walls of the maxillary antrum.

Every effort must be made to obtain hemostasis and decrease bleeding, which obstructs endoscopic visualization.[85,86] The nasal mucosa is treated with oxymetazoline hydrochloride (Afrin) nasal spray or a similar drug. The area of surgery around the middle turbinate is injected with lidocaine with 1:100,000 epinephrine. The initial incision for nasal endoscopic approach is made in the area of the uncinate process, opening the mucosa with a sickle knife followed by a Cottle elevator (Figure 12-38).

An uncinectomy is performed and then the lower limit of the ethmoid system is identified and the ethmoid bulla is entered and removed. Using various types of rongeurs, care is taken to remove the bone without damaging the orbital periosteum. The natural ostium of the maxillary sinus is entered just above the inferior turbinate; this structure is immediately below the ethmoidal bulla. The ground lamella posterior to the bullae is opened and the posterior as well as anterior ethmoidal air cells are exenterated (Figure 12-39). The medial half of the orbital floor, up to but not including the infraorbital neurovascular bundle, is then removed. After bony removal, the orbital periosteum is incised in a manner similar to other procedures.

Several investigators reported on about 30 patients operated on with only nasal endoscopy to decompress thyroid orbitopathy.[82,87,88] There is, on average, approximately 3–4 mm of retroplacement of the globe. In 18–50% of cases, there is worsening of strabismus after this surgical approach.[89,90]

Finally, orbital decompression has been done for a number of other non-Graves' conditions. These include proptosis due to sphenoid ridge meningioma, enlarged globe, and congenital orbital malformation.[89,90,91]

CONCLUSION

The role of decompression surgery in the management of thyroid ophthalmopathy continues to evolve. In experienced treatment centers, morbidity with the transantral or maxillary-ethmoidal decompression is usually limited to increased strabismus when maximum retroplacement of the globe is sought. The cosmetic effect of lid procedures without decompression in patients with exophthalmometry measurements of less than 23 mm seems satisfactory, even excellent, and morbidity is significantly less than with decompression.

Thyroid ophthalmopathy patients with relatively acute onset and severe proptosis with good vision should probably be given a trial of short-term, high-dose systemic steroids; if a partial effect or relapse occurs after medical therapy is withdrawn, orbital radiation is often effective. Many of these patients have a satisfactory response with nonsurgical procedures and do not require orbital decompression.

Decompression is indicated for patients who have severe compressive optic neuropathy, unacceptable proptosis, or corneal exposure from the anterior displacement of the globe, or those who have borderline corneal exposure but strabismus that will require repair with recessions.

It is important to emphasize that orbital decompression surgery does not affect the course of the inflammatory or fibrotic components of thyroid orbitopathy. Some patients may require continued or further medical treatment; rarely, optic compression can recur even after successful surgery. Since surgery does not affect the disease course, some patients may later require further medical treatment.

Many thyroid optic neuropathy cases can be adequately controlled with short-term steroids or steroids followed by orbital irradiation (see Chapter 10). Morbidity associated with these nonsurgical procedures seems sufficiently low as to obviate the use of surgical decompression unless the patient has acute, marked visual loss or fails medical therapy. In my experience, as many as 33% of radiated thyroid optic neuropathy patients have achieved only temporary remission, so these patients must be closely followed; some irradiated patients eventually require surgical decompression.

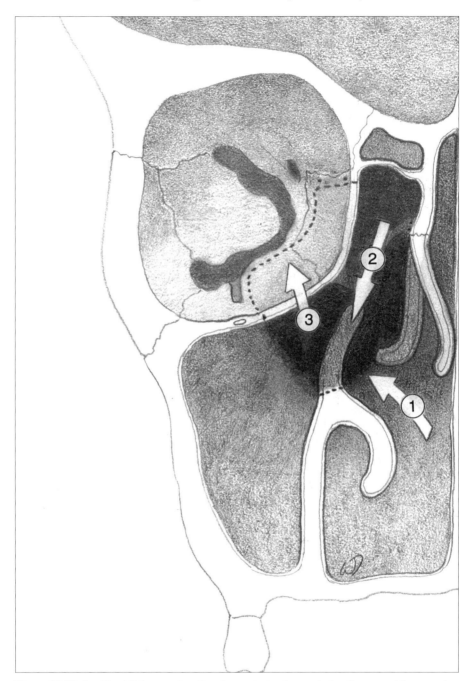

Figure 12-39. A mid-orbital coronal section demonstrates the surgical pathway used for a nasal endoscopic decompression. The ethmoidectomy is performed first, followed by removal of the medial portion of the maxillary roof. Labels 1, 2, and 3 refer to the order of the surgical approach through the sinuses (see text).

Often, in patients who undergo orbital decompression, if strabismus or eyelid retraction is present preoperatively, other procedures will have to be performed and the patient must be aware of this.

Since there is a long learning curve, complications are probably minimized if orbital decompression surgery is performed by a team with extensive experience. I do not believe that there are absolute indications or contraindications (other than listed above) to any one of the three commonly used approaches. In my experience, most problems arise when an inexperienced surgeon attempts to do these procedures, although some disasters have occurred around the country even with superb, highly experienced surgeons. If the beginning surgeon wishes to use a Caldwell-Luc or a nasal endoscopic approach, the first several procedures should be performed jointly with an experienced ear, nose, and throat surgeon.

REFERENCES

1. Dollinger J. Die druckentlastung der augenhoehle durch entfernung der aeusseren orbitalwand bei hochgradigem exophthalmus (morbis basedoweii) und konsecutiver hornhauterkrankung. Dtsch Med Wochenschr 1911;37:1888.
2. Krönlein RU. Die Traumatische Meningitis. In Handbuch der Praktischen Chirurgie (Vol 4). 1913–1914.
3. Jessop L. Three cases of exophthalmic goiter with severe ocular lesions. Trans Ophthalmol Soc U K 1896;16:187.
4. Juler FA. Acute purulent keratitis in exophthalmic goiter treated by repeated tarsorrhaphy resection of cervical sympathetic and x-rays: retention of vision in one eye. Trans Ophthalmol Soc U K 1913;33:58.
5. Naffziger HC. Pathologic changes in the orbit in progressive exophthalmos with special reference to alterations in extra-ocular muscles and optic disks. Arch Ophthalmol 1933;9:1.
6. Welti H, Offet G. Indications et technique de la trépanation decompressive de l'orbite dans le traitement des exophtalmies malignes basedowiennes. Lyon Chir 1943;38:542.
7. Hirsch VO, Urbanek AG. Behandlung eines exzessiven exophthalmus (Basedow) durch entfernung von orbitalfett vonder kieferhöhle aus. Monatschr Ohrenh-Laryngorhinol 1930;64:212.
8. Sewall EC. Operative control of progressive exophthalmos. Arch Otolaryngol 1936;24:621.
9. Hirsch VO. Surgical decompression of malignant exophthalmos. Arch Otolaryngol 1950;51:325.
10. Walsh TE, Ogura JH. Transantral orbital decompression for malignant exophthalmos. Laryngoscope 1957;67:544.
11. Ogura JH, Pratt LL. Transantral decompression for malignant exophthalmos. Otolaryngol Clin North Am 1971;4:193.
12. Stabile JR, Trokel SM. Increase in orbital volume obtained by decompression in dried skulls. Am J Ophthalmol 1983;95:327.
13. Hecht SD, Guibor P, Wolfley D, Wiggs EO. Orbital dissection defatting technique for Graves' disease. Ann Ophthalmol 1984;16:314.
14. Haddad HM. Pathogenesis and treatment of endocrine exophthalmos. Int Surg 1973;58:482.
15. Roncevic R, Jackson IT. Surgical treatment of thyrotoxic exophthalmos. Plast Reconstr Surg 1989;84:754.
16. Trokel S, Kazim M, Moore S. Orbital fat removal. Decompression for Graves' ophthalmopathy. Ophthalmology 1993;100:674.
17. Olivari N. Transpalpebral decompression of endocrine ophthalmopathy (Graves' disease) by removal of intraorbital fat: experience with 147 operations over 5 years. Plast Reconstr Surg 1991;87:627.
18. Wulc AE, Popp JC, Bartlett SP. Lateral wall advancement in orbital decompression. Ophthalmology 1990;97:1358.
19. Warren JD, Spector JG, Burde R. Long-term follow-up and recent observations on 305 cases of orbital decompression for dysthyroid orbitopathy. Laryngoscope 1989;99:35.

20. Lyons CJ, Rootman J. Orbital decompression for disfiguring exophthalmos in thyroid orbitopathy. Ophthalmology 1994;101:223.

21. Guyton JS. Decompression of the orbit. Surgery 1946;19:790.

22. Long JC, Ellis GD. Temporal decompression of the orbit for thyroid exophthalmos. Am J Ophthalmol 1966;62:1089.

23. Long JC, Ellis PP. Total unilateral visual loss following orbital surgery. Am J Ophthalmol 1971;71:218.

24. Kroll AJ, Casten VG. Dysthyroid exophthalmos. Palliation by lateral orbital decompression. Arch Ophthalmol 1966;76:205.

25. Riley FC. Surgical management of ophthalmopathy in Graves' disease. Transfrontal orbital decompression. Mayo Clin Proc 1972;47:986.

26. Moran RE. The correction of exophthalmos and levator spasm. Plast Reconstr Surg 1956;18:411.

27. Hurwitz JJ, Birt D. An individualized approach to orbital decompression in Graves' orbitopathy. Arch Ophthalmol 1985;103:660.

28. Naffziger HC. Exophthalmos. Some principles of surgical management from the neurosurgical aspect. Am J Surg 1948;75:25.

29. Poppen JL. The surgical treatment of progressive exophthalmos. J Clin Endocrinol 1950;10:1231.

30. MacCarty CS, Kenefick TP, McConahay WM, Kearns TP. Ophthalmopathy in Graves' disease treated by removal of roof, lateral walls and lateral sphenoid ridge: review of 46 cases. Mayo Clin Proc 1970;45:488.

31. Gorman CA, DeSanto LW, MacCarty CS, Riley FC. Optic neuropathy of Graves' disease. Treatment by transantral or transfrontal orbital decompression. N Engl J Med 1974;290:70.

32. Algvere P, Almqvist S, Backlund EO. Pterional orbital decompression in progressive ophthalmopathy of Graves' disease. I. Acta Ophthalmologica 1973;51:461.

33. Wende S, Aulich A, Nover A, et al. Computed tomography of orbital lesions. Neuroradiology 1977;13:123.

34. Backlund EO. Pterional approach for orbital decompression. Acta Ophthalmol (Copenh) 1968;46:535.

35. Hamby WB. Pterional approach to the orbits for decompression or tumor removal. J Neurosurg 1964;21:15.

36. Ogura JH, Walsh TE. The transantral orbital decompression operation for progressive exophthalmos. Laryngoscope 1962;72:1078.

37. Sessions RB, Wilkins RB, Weycer JS. Endocrine exophthalmos. Arch Otolaryngol 1972;95:46.

38. Stell PM. Transmaxillary orbital decompression for malignant exophthalmos. Proc R Soc Med 1969;62:23.

39. Golding-Wood PH. Trans-antral ethmoid decompression in malignant exophthalmos. J Laryngol Otol 1969;83:683.

40. Carter KD, Frueh BR, Hessburg TP, Musch DC. Long-term efficacy of orbital decompression for compressive optic neuropathy of Graves' disease. Ophthalmology 1991;98:1435.

41. Girod DA, Orcutt JC, Cummings CW. Orbital decompression for preservation of vision in Graves' ophthalmopathy. Arch Otolaryngol Head Neck Surg 1993;119:229.

42. Fatourechi V, Garrity JA, Bartley GB, et al. Graves' ophthalmopathy. The results of transantral orbital decompression performed primarily for cosmetic indications. Ophthalmology 1994;101:938.

43. Garrity JA, Fatourechi V, Bergstralh EJ, et al. Results of transantral orbital decompression in 428 patients with severe Graves' ophthalmopathy. Am J Ophthalmol 1993;116:533.

44. Leone CR Jr, Piest KL, Newman RJ. Medial and lateral wall decompression for thyroid ophthalmopathy. Am J Ophthalmol 1989;108:160.

45. DeSanto LW. The total rehabilitation of Graves' ophthalmopathy. Laryngoscope 1980;90:1652.

46. Maniglia AJ, Chandler JR, Goodwin WJ Jr, Flynn J. Rare complications following ethmoidectomies: a report of eleven cases. Laryngoscope 1981;91:1234.

47. Calcaterra TC, Hepler RS. Antral-ethmoidal decompression in Graves' disease. Five-year experience. West J Med 1976;124:87.

48. Wendz R, Levine MR, Putterman A, et al. Extraocular muscle enlargement after orbital decompression for Graves' ophthalmopathy. Ophthal Plast Reconstr Surg 1994;10:34.

49. Hurwitz JJ, Freeman JL, Eplett CJ, et al. Ethmoidectomy decompression for the treatment of Graves' optic neuropathy. Can J Ophthalmol 1992;27:283.

50. Anderson RL, Linberg JB. Transorbital approach to decompression in Graves' disease. Arch Ophthalmol 1981;99:120.

51. McCord CD Jr. Orbital decompression for Graves' disease. Exposure through lateral canthal and inferior fornix incision. Ophthalmology 1981;88:533.

52. Leone CR Jr, Bajandas FJ. Inferior orbital decompression for thyroid ophthalmopathy. Arch Ophthalmol 1980;98:890.

53. McCord CD Jr. Current trends in orbital decompression. Ophthalmology 1985;92:21.

53a. Otto AJ, Koornneef L, Mourits MP, deen-van Leeuwen L. Retrobulbar pressures measured during surgical decompression of the orbit. Br J Ophthalmol 1996;80:1042.

54. Antoszyk JH, Tucker N, Codere F. Orbital decompression for Graves' disease: exposure through a modified blepharoplasty incision. Ophthalmic Surg 1992;23:516.

55. Shorr N, Seiff SR. The four stages of surgical rehabilitation of the patient with dysthyroid ophthalmopathy. Ophthalmology 1986;93:476.

56. McCormick MS, Stell PM. Orbital decompression for progressive exophthalmos. J R Coll Surg Edinb 1986;31:18.

57. Trokel SL, Cooper WC. Orbital decompression: effect on motility and globe position. Ophthalmology 1979;86:2064.

58. Fells P. Orbital decompression for severe dysthyroid eye disease. Br J Ophthalmol 1987;71:107.

59. Garrity JA, Saggau DD, Gorman CA, et al. Torsional diplopia after transantral orbital decompression and extraocular muscle surgery associated with Graves' orbitopathy. Am J Ophthalmol 1992;113:363.

60. Garrity J, Gorman C. Pitfalls associated with orbital decompression for thyroid-related orbitopathy. Exp Clin Endocrinol 1991;97:338.

61. Goldberg RA, Shorr N, Cohen MA. The medial orbital strut in the prevention of postdecompression dystropia in dysthyroid ophthalmopathy. Ophthal Plast Reconstr Surg 1992;8:32.

62. Lamberg BA, Grahne B, Tommila V, et al. Orbital decompression in endocrine exophthalmos of Graves' disease. Acta Endocrinol 1985;109:335.

63. Grahne B, Lamberg B-A, Rinne J, et al. Transantral orbital decompression in the treatment of Graves' disease. J Laryngol Otol 1985;99:865.

64. Neigel JM, Rootman J, Belkin RI, et al. Dysthyroid optic neuropathy. Ophthalmology 1988;95:1515.

65. Barrett L, Glatt HJ, Burde RM, Gado MH. Optic nerve dysfunction in thyroid eye disease: CT. Radiology 1988;167:503.

66. Hallin ES, Feldon SE. Graves' ophthalmopathy: III. Effect of transantral orbital decompression on optic neuropathy. Br J Ophthalmol 1988;72:683.

67. Mourits MP, Koornneef L, Wiersinga WM, et al. Orbital decompression for Graves' ophthalmopathy by inferomedial, by inferomedial plus lateral, and by coronal approach. Ophthalmology 1990;97:636.

68. Colvard DM, Waller RR, Neault RW, DeSanto LW. Nasolacrimal duct obstruction following transantral ethmoidal orbital decompression ophthalmus. Ophthalmic Surg 1979;10:25.

69. Seiff SR, Shorr N. Nasolacrimal drainage system obstruction after orbital decompression. Am J Ophthalmol 1988;106:204.

70. Migiori ME. Nasolacrimal drainage system obstruction after orbital decompression. Am J Ophthalmol 1989;107:91.

71. Stranc M, West M. A four-wall orbital decompression for dysthyroid orbitopathy. J Neurosurg 1988;68:671.

72. Kennerdell JS, Maroon JC. An orbital decompression for severe dysthyroid exophthalmos. Ophthalmology 1982;89:467.

73. Lanzieri CF, Sacher M, Biller HF, Som PM. Orbital decompression: postoperative computed tomography. J Comput Assist Tomogr 1984;8:957.

74. Shorr N, Neuhaus RW, Baylis HI. Ocular motility problems after orbital decompression for dysthyroid ophthalmopathy. Ophthalmology 1982;9:323.

75. Small RG, Meiring NL. A combined orbital and antral approach to surgical decompression of the orbit. Ophthalmopathy 1981;88:542.

76. Rosenbaum AL. Discussion. Ophthalmology 1982;89:327.
77. Caldwell GW. Diseases of the accessory sinuses of the nose, and an improved method of treatment for suppuration of the maxillary antrum. N Y Med J 1893;58:526.
78. Luc H. Nouvelle method opératoire pour la cure radicale et rapide de l'empyème chronique du sinus maxillaire. Bull Med Soc Fr 1897;3:457.
79. Stankiewicz JA. Complications of endoscopic intranasal ethmoidectomy. Laryngoscope 1987;97:1270.
80. Vanden Abeele D, Clemens A, Tassignon MJ, Van de Heyning PH. Blindness due to electro-coagulation following functional endoscopic sinus surgery. Acta Otorhinolaryngol Belg 1994;48:11.
81. Jorissen M, Heulens H, Feenstra L. Functional endoscopic sinus surgery under local anesthesia. Acta Otorhinolaryng Belg 1996;50:1.
82. Buess G. Review: transantral endoscopic microsurgery (TEM). J R Coll Surg Edinb 1993;38:239.
83. Sacks EH, Anand VK, Lisman RD. Orbital Decompression: Endoscopic Perspective. In VK Anand, WR Panje (eds), Practical Endoscopic Sinus Surgery. New York: McGraw-Hill 1993;138.
84. Henick DH, Kennedy DW. Endoscopic Orbital Decompression—Graves' Disease. In JA Stankiewicz (ed), Advanced Endoscopic Sinus Surgery. St. Louis: Mosby 1995;103.
85. Ritter FN, Fritsch MH. Atlas of Paranasal Sinus Surgery. New York: Igaku-Shoin Medical Publishers 1992;110.
86. Rice DH, Schaefer SD. Endoscopic Paranasal Sinus Surgery (2nd ed). New York: Raven 1993;215.
87. Michel O, Bresgen K, Russmann W, et al. Endoskopish kontrollierts endonasale orbitadekompression beim malignan ophthalmus. Klaryngorhinootologie 1991;70:656.
88. Metson R, Dallow RL, Shore JW. Endoscopic orbital decompression. Laryngoscope 1994;104:950.
89. Neugebauer A, Nishino K, Neugebauer P, et al. Effects of bilateral orbital decompression by an endoscopic endonasal approach by dysthyroid orbitopathy. Br J Ophthalmol 1996;80:58.
90. Gum KB, Frueh BR. Transantral orbital decompression for compressive optic neuropathy due to sphenoid ridge meningioma. Ophthal Plast Reconstr Surg 1989;5:196.
91. Goldberg RA, Hwang MM, Garbutt MN, Shorr N. Orbital decompression for non-Graves' orbitopathy. A consideration of extended indications for decompression. Ophthal Plast Reconstr Surg 1995;11:245.

13

Therapy of Thyroid Myopathy

Thyroid ophthalmopathy is the most common cause of acute-onset diplopia in middle-aged or older individuals; restrictive myopathy secondary to thyroid eye disease is probably the most frequent serious ocular complication of Graves' disease.[1,2] The differential diagnosis of enlarged extraocular muscles (see Table 5-1) is discussed in detail in Chapter 5. The forced duction test (see Figure 5-52) is helpful in differentiating a restrictive thyroid myopathy from a nonrestrictive ophthalmoplegia associated with myasthenia gravis, skew deviation, or a form of paralytic or nonparalytic strabismus. It does not, however, differentiate thyroid myopathy from such other causes of restrictive extraocular muscle disorders as entrapment in a sinus or idiopathic myositis. Occasionally, thyroid eye disease can coexist with myasthenia gravis, multiple sclerosis, or other endocrine or neurologic diseases.[3–8]

As discussed in Chapters 1 and 6, there are no satisfying hypotheses to explain why the inferior rectus appears to be preferentially involved in thyroid ocular myopathy.[9–11] The nature of mechanical disorders responsible for thyroid-related esotropia or hypotropia has not been well delineated. As discussed in Chapter 6, histologic studies are not correlative with clinical patterns of restrictive thyroid extraocular myopathies. The extraocular muscles in thyroid eye disease are usually inflamed, enlarged, and, late in the disease, fibrotic. Some of the propensity to develop problems in the field of the inferior rectus muscle may be due to the importance of downgaze for modern literate life, although data supporting this hypothesis is tenuous.

Most commonly, these patients present with unilateral or bilateral apparent elevator palsies with diplopia in upgaze. While almost all extraocular muscles may appear enlarged on computed tomography or ultrasonography, clinically detectable involvement is most frequent in the inferior and medial recti; the superior and lateral recti are much less commonly involved.[12–15] The oblique muscles are rarely affected, although cyclodeviations or inflammatory Brown's syndrome can occur in thyroid myopathy.[16,17]

Extraocular muscle involvement in thyroid eye disease was first reported in 1853.[18] Most early investigators observed an apparent paralysis of upgaze,[19–21] which, although it was not appreciated at that time, was due to the restrictive, rather than paralytic, nature of the myopathy. Dunnington and Berke's 1943 work with the forced duction test (see Chapter 5) demonstrated the restrictive nature of most thyroid eye muscle disease.[22]

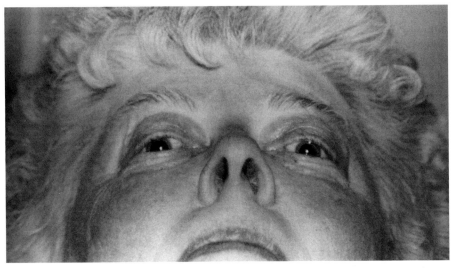

Figure 13-1. Adaptive head position to minimize diplopia secondary to fibrotic inferior recti.

Most thyroid ophthalmopathy patients have simple hypotropia or hypotropia with esotropia. Diplopia may be intermittent or constant and become manifest as an acute or slowly discernible process. Usually patients initially develop transient diplopia on awakening, and develop recurrent symptoms when they are tired or use alcohol or drugs.[23] Patients may assume a compensatory head position; the patient in Figure 13-1 has a bilateral restrictive inferior rectus myopathy with single vision when she has her chin markedly elevated. Unlike many other acquired adult extraocular muscle problems, some thyroid eye patients are able to ignore the second image and do not complain of diplopia.[24]

The vast majority of patients with symptomatic thyroid myopathy complain of vertical diplopia. Evans and Kennerdell noted that 96% of their patients had involvement of the inferior or medial rectus muscle, and 32 of 45 patients (71%) had pure hypotropia.[25] Scott and Thalacker observed that 80% of thyroid ophthalmopathy patients had some inferior rectus involvement, 44% had medial rectus involvement, and much less frequently the superior rectus contributed to the strabismus.[26] Similarly, Sterk and coworkers noted that 76% of 50 patients had vertical diplopia while 22% had a purely horizontal diplopia.[27] In this latter study, limitation of upgaze or lateral gaze was noted in 90% of cases, whereas diffuse limitation or downgaze restriction was noted in the other cases. Mourits and colleagues noted 47% of their thyroid myopathy patients presented with hypotropia, 21% with esotropia, and 32% with both findings.[28]

Six general caveats are important in the discussion of thyroid myopathy management:

1. Surgery on the involved muscles is always a recession procedure and, as described below, better results occur when adjustable sutures are used.

2. Patients who present with exotropia in thyroid eye disease should be evaluated for the possibility of myasthenia gravis. As discussed elsewhere, up to 8% of thyroid eye disease patients have other endocrine and immunologic abnormalities.

3. It has been appreciated for some time that the eye muscle findings in thyroid orbitopathy are variable and often abate as the systemic hyperthyroidism is controlled or as the eye disease spontaneously remits.[27,29] Most experienced clinicians do not operate on a thyroid patient with myopathy unless the systemic disease is in remission and the eye muscle findings have been stable for at least 3–6 months. When this dictum is not obeyed, second or third surgeries are generally necessary to repair over- or undercorrection. Even when surgery is delayed until the strabismus is stable, it is not uncommon to note further changes months later. We and others have shown in animal models and thyroid myopathy patients that magnetic resonance spectroscopy (MRS) can be used to delineate active inflammation versus fibrosis of the extraocular muscles.[30–32] These noninvasive test data have not yet been sufficiently verified in clinical trials to determine if earlier surgery can be performed on the basis of MRS data with acceptable morbidity.

4. It has been known for many years that patients with severe proptosis and ophthalmoplegia without corneal exposure can develop exposure keratitis if muscle surgery is performed before decompression. In these patients, restrictive myopathy prevents further forward placement of the globe, and recession of extraocular muscles allows more proptosis to develop with secondary exposure keratopathy. We therefore will perform an orbital decompression first if the patient has had previous episodes of corneal damage from proptosis, or requires muscle surgery and has readings greater than 25 mm on Hertel exophthalmometry.

5. As discussed in Chapter 12, as many as 79% of patients who have surgical decompression of the orbit require eye muscle surgery, and secondary diplopia develops in 3–80% (mean 26%).[33,34] Decompression surgery often causes or exacerbates pre-existing esotropia or hypotropia; if orbital decompression is likely to be necessary, it should be performed before any extraocular muscle procedures. While repair of strabismus after orbital decompression is not entirely satisfactory, the alterations in muscle alignment after orbital structures are decompressed into the sinuses results in secondary diplopia, even if the muscle was repaired before decompression.

6. Reading position (downgaze) is crucial for older patients. It is important not to cripple the inferior rectus in a strabismus procedure so that downgaze is not possible. Usually that is not a problem if the inferior rectus is not recessed more than 8 mm and an A-pattern (esotropia greater in upward gaze than downward) is not present. Most thyroid myopathy patients do better with separate reading and distance glasses. If a bifocal is prescribed, a large add segment should be used.

There are six options in the management of symptomatic thyroid myopathies: (1) observation, (2) medical treatment (corticosteroids or cyclosporine), (3) prisms, (4) radiation, (5) botulinum toxin injection, or (6) surgery. As discussed previously, neither medical treatment nor radiation is usually effective in the therapy of chronic diplopia, although some patients with acute or subacute symptoms who are treated with these modalities early in the disease course do well (see Chapters 7, 9, and 10). Some patients have transient diplopia during the acute phase of hyperthyroidism, and while this is less likely to spontaneously resolve than eyelid malpositions, it can do so. In patients with newly diagnosed hyperthyroidism or those with acute symptoms, treatment with systemic steroids is a reasonable option. In one report of 50 thyroid myopathy patients, 11 appeared to improve spontaneously or after systemic steroids.[27] Medical therapy is not effective in the fibrotic stage of the disease.

BOTULINUM TOXIN INJECTION

There are limited data on the use of botulinum toxin for thyroid myopathy. Its use has been advocated as a possible interim measure in patients with diplopia of less than 6 months. Dunn and coworkers studied the use of botulinum toxin in eight patients with a mean deviation of 20 prism diopters (PD). They performed the botulinum injections under electromyographic control using between 1.25 and 5 units. Results were generally good, although some complications occurred, including ptosis and prolonged overcorrection.[35,36] These authors believed indications for this therapy in thyroid myopathy were patients with subacute disease that did not respond to medical treatment. Lyons and colleagues summarized their results with intramuscular botulinum injections in 38 thyroid myopathy patients.[37] In only six cases (16%) was botulinum alone effective. Approximately 75% of injections had some effect, with a mean duration of 2 months. This medical approach has also been used in some patients with idiopathic myositis.[38] Alan Scott (San Francisco, personal communication, 1996) has found that botulinum has very limited indications, and data supporting its efficacy are limited. Scott believes that botulinum may be useful in three specific instances: (1) the patient with an acute-onset deviation not responsive to oral corticosteroids who is incapacitated by the strabismus; (2) the subacute patient with a small-angle (<6 PD) hypotropia who may benefit from injection; (3) the patient with a small-angle esotropia and hypotropia where the vertical or horizontal deviation is dealt with surgically but the other component is managed with botulinum.

PRISMS

Prisms are useful in some patients; most often they are helpful in cases with small-angle, relatively concomitant deviations. Generally patients with less than 12 PD of concomitant strabismus with good fusional amplitudes are reasonable candidates for prisms. In one series, up to 30% were treated with prisms and success was noted in 10 of 15 cases. Success probably should be defined in most patients as single vision in primary and reading positions of gaze. Usually prismatic correction of more than 5 PD is not accepted; however, a few patients with up to 15 PD have had good results, especially if separate distance and reading glasses are used.[39] Blur is associated with large-angle prisms. Inconcomitant strabismus is the major limiting factor in prism use in most cases. Lueder and associates tried prisms as primary treatment in 24 thyroidopathy patients, and prisms were not acceptable in 16.[40] They also used prisms as an adjuvant for residual small-angle strabismus after muscle surgery and found that they were helpful in nine of 43 patients.[40] In addition to prisms, occasionally convergence exercises are helpful, and this was found to be of benefit for the small number of patients with that problem.[41]

SURGERY

A number of surgical approaches have been tried to improve the accuracy of muscle recessions and decrease scarring associated with this type of strabismus. Most of these procedures, including the use of Supramid sleeves and allogeneic scleral grafts, have been discontinued because they were no more effective than conventional techniques.[42–45] The inflammatory and fibrotic nature of thyroid myopathy has resulted in diminished use of marginal myotomies or muscle restriction procedures in thyroid myopathy. Some authors pretreat patients with steroids or radiation, although there have been no controlled trials, and it is doubtful that these agents are efficacious except during the inflammatory portion of the disease.[46] Similarly, in a small number of patients, we have used mitomycin-C topically at the time of muscle surgery in an attempt to prevent progressive fibrosis, but we were not impressed with the efficacy of this adjunctive approach.

Jampolsky noted that deficient elevation and abduction can be caused solely by a tight inferior rectus muscle.[47] The inferior rectus plays a secondary role in adduction; its tightness at the time of surgery can cause esotropia. The inferior rectus contraction is probably the major cause of strabismus in patients with an A-pattern esotropia. Until the inferior rectus is recessed, it may be impossible to determine the contribution of the medial rectus development of esotropia in this restrictive strabismus.[47] After inferior rectus recession, forced duction tests on the medial rectus can help to elucidate its role in muscle imbalance. Forced duction tests on the medial rectus muscle should be done, intraoperatively, in primary as well as downgaze.

Results of extraocular muscle surgery for thyroid eye disease in the era before the use of adjustable sutures were less effective than now.[48,49] Dyer reported that 55% of patients operated on for thyroid myopathy had the condition corrected with only one procedure, 27% required two, and 18% required additional surgeries.[50] Similarly, Evans and Kennerdell noted a 29% incidence of two or more surgeries in patients operated on without adjustable sutures.[22] Kraus and Bullock reviewed pooled data from their and other centers' experience and noted a 77% success rate with adjustable sutures as compared with 46% when nonadjustable sutures were used.[51] Lueder and colleagues noted good or excellent results in 73% of 47 cases using an adjustable suture technique.[40] In 40 of their cases, a single surgical procedure achieved binocular vision in primary and reading positions; most failures were due to progressive fibrosis in other extraocular muscles.[40] In some patients, hypertropia develops when the superior rectus muscle becomes fibrotic and contracts.

Operations on extraocular muscles are complicated by their enlarged, sometimes inflamed, and fibrotic nature that hinders visualization and surgery. In some reports, the amount of surgical manipulation of inferior and medial recti muscles has not been too large; often recessions for thyroid myopathies need to be significantly larger than for most other strabismus procedures.[28] Inferior medial recessions of 7–8 mm are not infrequent. As discussed, recession of the inferior rectus muscle often alters the position of the lower eyelid either in a beneficial or adverse manner. It is surprising that even when attempts are made to lyse all adhesions between the inferior rectus and eyelid retractors, deformities can result (see Chapter 11). In the experience from Iowa, in 28% of their thyroid strabismus cases, eyelid retraction increased.[40] However, as shown in Figures 13-2 and 13-3, recession of an inferior rectus muscle alone can sometimes improve the lower eyelid position; this case illustrates one of several reasons why eyelid surgery should be delayed until after extraocular muscle surgery is performed. Inferior rectus fibrosis can also affect the upper eyelid position, and recession of the rectus can sometimes correct upper eyelid retraction.[52]

Several different approaches have been used to decrease the incidence and severity of secondary lower eyelid malpositions after inferior rectus muscle recessions.[52a–c] In our experience, none of these modifications is completely satisfactory, but exquisite care to dissect the rectus from the lower eyelid retractors and to reposition the latter if moved as a result of muscle manipulation does decrease the magnitude of the problem.

In 1975, Jampolsky first reported on the use of an adjustable suture for reoperations in strabismus surgery.[53] He noted that traction tests were important in all cases

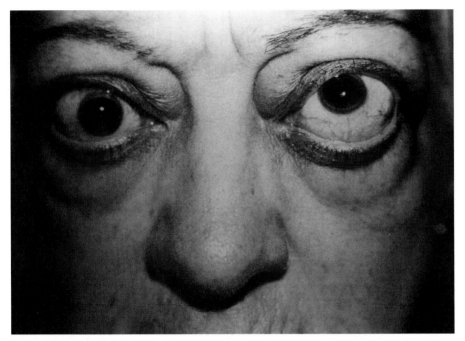

Figure 13-2. Patient with fibrotic inferior rectus and diplopia before recession.

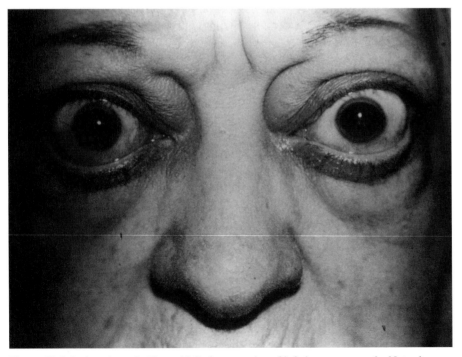

Figure 13-3. Patient shown in Figure 13-2 after recession of inferior rectus muscle. Note alteration of lower eyelid position after only rectus muscle surgery.

and that adjustable sutures allowed further refinement of muscle position after surgery. A number of clinicians have modified this approach for thyroid restrictive myopathy; most strabismologists now use an adjustable suture in all thyroid myopathy cases. This technique is excellent in a cooperative patient; generally patients more than 15 years old can be treated with an adjustable suture to recess recti muscles. The results obtained at adjustment the morning after surgery usually correlate with those several months later.[53,54] There are very few factors that predict outcome, and the major problem that resulted in an unacceptable strabismus surgery outcome was progressive restriction of other muscles.[40] Progressive overcorrection or undercorrection can occur months after inferior rectus recession. In one series, nine of 18 thyroid myopathy patients developed this problem after surgery, and the authors queried whether this late complication was more common in a group that had adjustable sutures.[55] My interpretation would be that it could also be explained by the fact that the group treated with adjustable sutures probably had a worse prognosis.

Four general guidelines are paramount for effective surgical management of thyroid myopathy. First, use recessions for all strabismus surgery; resections are almost never performed. Second, conserve sufficient inferior rectus function to avoid impairment of downgaze. It is unusual to obtain single vision and complete duction in all fields of gaze. Therefore, it is better to slightly undercorrect a tight inferior rectus than to cripple this muscle's function and severely limit the downgaze necessary for normal reading. Rarely, a Faden approach may be used; Buckley and Meekins noted good results in six patients with thyroid myopathy in whom the rectus belly was sutured to the sclera 10 mm posterior to its normal insertion to allow it to retain ocular alignment in the better eye.[56] Third, for inferior rectus problems, recess the muscle approximately 1 mm for every 2.5 PD of squint. Intraoperative repeated forced duction tests are critical to establish that the amount of muscle recession is adequate. If more than 30 PD of hypotropia is present, recessions on adjustable sutures of the inferior rectus and the superior rectus in the opposite eye are usually necessary. Fourth, in many cases of restrictive disease the conjunctiva and Tenon's capsule are pathophysiologically involved and must be recessed sufficiently to minimize hypotropia. In addition to these structures, other orbital tissue may also produce constriction, and again, intraoperative forced duction tests are helpful to delineate the relative contribution of these structures.

I prefer to recess the muscle by severing it from the globe after it has been imbricated with suture, and then attempting to place it in an appropriately correct recessed position (Figures 13-4A and 13-4B). The suture is brought through a long scleral tunnel starting posterior to the original muscle insertion and ending just anterior to it (Figure 13-4C). The sutures are grasped on each side of the tunnel and pulled back and forth through the tunnel in a "sawing" fashion to improve sliding for later adjustment. The muscle is placed in an apparently appropriate position and temporarily tied down with a single throw of a knot. Forced ductions are performed to try to establish restrictive parity in both eyes, particularly when there is bilateral involvement. The recession is then remeasured and, if it is satisfactory, tied with an adjustable suture in a double throw single knot followed by a bow knot (Figure 13-4D). Conjunctiva is recessed to eliminate any restrictive effect it may have and to allow sufficient visualization of the muscle's original insertion. The eye is then patched without an antibiotic ointment; inclusion of a salve makes it more difficult to adjust sutures the next morning.

There are a few necessary modifications to standard strabismus surgical procedures if an adjustable suture technique is used. We try to eliminate any unnecessary preoperative or anesthetic medications that may alter perception or muscle tone (i.e., diazepam [Valium], phenobarbitol, succinylcholine, etc.). A double-armed 6-0 Vicryl

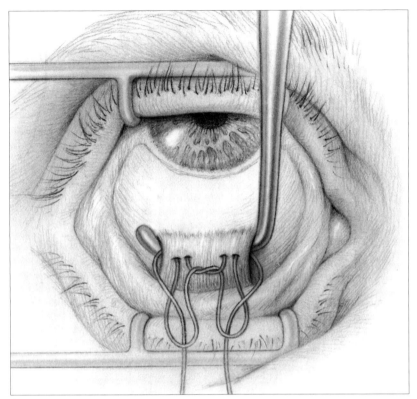

A

Figure 13-4. Schematic diagrams showing adjustable suture technique (see text for specifics).

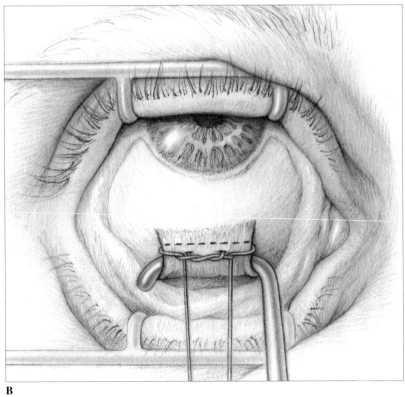

B

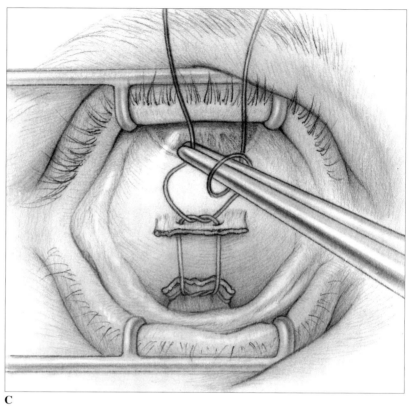

C

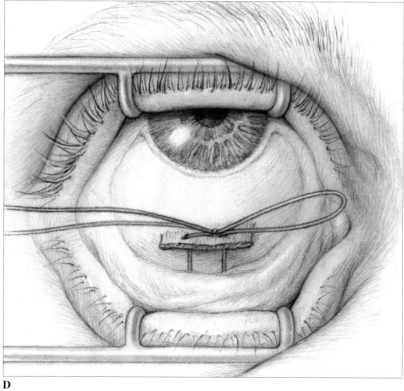

D

suture works well. In pure hypotropia, the inferior rectus muscle is isolated and carefully dissected free from adhesions to the inferior oblique caudad and retractors of the inferior lid. Even with extreme care in isolating the muscle from the lower eyelid retractors, lower lid deformity or entropion can occur in large recessions.[52a–c] Generally for less than 10–20 PD of hypotropia, one can recess the inferior rectus 5–9 mm; for 20–30 PD of hypotropia, 9–12 mm of recession may be necessary. The muscle is imbricated with the 6-0 Vicryl suture and locked at the medial and lateral edges. This locking bite is slightly larger, to collapse some horizontal muscle width and make it slightly easier to slide forward or aft at the time of adjustment. The muscle is severed from its insertion and allowed to retract. We usually adjust the suture the following morning, although some surgeons do this on the afternoon of surgery. Cooperative patients will accept the use of topical anesthesia and placement of a small wire speculum in the palpebral fissure for a cover-uncover test. If the muscle position is correct, the bow knot is tightened and the suture cut. If adjustment is required, a cotton-tip applicator soaked with 4% lidocaine (Xylocaine) can be placed over the muscle insertion for 1 minute, then the suture adjusted. Most discomfort is due to conjunctival manipulation, which should be minimized. As is obvious to experienced strabismologists, it is much easier to tighten a suture that is too loose than to further recess the muscle on the first postoperative day. If this is necessary and the suture must be loosened; the patient is asked to look superiorly. Additional recession can be achieved by actually pulling the muscle inferiorly. If too great a recession was performed at surgery, the sutures are pulled tighter. In either event, the bow knot is retied, and a cover-uncover test is again performed. Once the adjustment is satisfactory, the suture is tied and cut and the eye redressed; the patient is re-examined the next day. While there have been some algorithms for nonthyroid adjustable suture manipulations, there are limited data for thyroid cases.[57] Rarely, an oculocardiac reflex can occur during manipulation of an adjustable suture, and this procedure should be performed in an area of the hospital where resuscitation can be readily performed.[58] In one series, the authors observed that those patients who had alterations in heart rate at the time of surgery were more likely to have a problem at the time of postoperative suture adjustment.[59]

I support Jampolsky's recommendation to operate first on the inferior rectus, even if there is some esotropia in addition to hypotropia.[60] Especially after orbital decompression, when the inferior rectus may be moved inferiorly and nasally, the adduction effect may be heightened. Many patients with significant esotropia have required inferior rectus surgery only. After the inferior rectus is positioned, a medial rectus forced duction test will indicate whether medial rectus surgery will be required. In vertical or horizontal rectus surgery, recessions are used to align the eyes; very large deviations require bilateral surgery.

A major component in the surgical decision process is the degree of restriction noted before surgery, and in many cases after a single inferior rectus muscle is recessed. Forced duction tests performed before and after movement of each muscle at surgery are necessary to monitor and decide on the appropriate number of muscles to operate on and the amount of recession to do. Even large vertical deviations can usually be managed with only ipsilateral inferior rectus recession. The risk of performing a contralateral superior rectus recession is overcorrection, since the opposite eye may have a subclinical inferior rectus restriction. Recession of the superior rectus in such a case will produce contralateral hypotropia. If it is likely that contralateral surgery on the superior rectus muscle will be necessary, that muscle should be recessed on an adjustable suture to minimize the likelihood of this complication. Similarly, when inferior rectus recession alone does not appear sufficient to correct a hypotropia-esotropia, then adjustable sutures are used to recess inferior and medial recti muscles; however, exotropia in downgaze can result in poor reading vision. If a marked A-pattern is present in downgaze, weakening of the superior oblique muscles should be done when the inferior recti are recessed. Excision of most of the posterior superior oblique tendon has been described for torsion problems.[57]

In 1981, Scott and Thalacker reported on the largest series of thyroid myopathy patients to date. [26] They evaluated 175 patients with thyroid eye disease; 25 had diplopia. Thyroid myopathy patients have limited fusional amplitudes and inconcomitant deviations, which limit the use of prisms. In that series, prisms were only effective in three of 12 cases in which they were tried; however, as previously discussed, efficacy is markedly influenced by definition of success.

Scott and Thalacker attempted to achieve binocular vision in primary position and as far from it as possible. Eighteen of 22 patients had fusion in primary position; however, only four had full versions and normal motility. Many had limitation of adduction, downgaze, or upgaze. In patients with combined medial and inferior rectus surgeries, an A-pattern in downgaze was found postoperatively.[26]

Sterk and coworkers noted that nine of 13 patients who had primary strabismus surgery (without previous decompression) had a good result with one operation, while the success rate in those operated on after other thyroid orbitopathy reconstruction procedures had poorer results (two of seven).[27] In a series of postdecompression cases, 26 of 355 (7.3%) had persistent diplopia despite multiple surgical procedures.[61] In contrast, the Iowa experience did not note an adverse effect of orbital decompression in the 17 patients for which that procedure had been performed.[40] An update of the Iowa experience reported that 73% had a good or excellent result from surgery.[40] In 56 strabismus procedures reported, 22 involved one muscle, 13 involved two muscles, 14 involved three muscles, and seven had four muscles operated on.[40] In 37 of 47 patients, postoperative adjustment of sutures was performed. Sterk and colleagues noted that three of 20 successfully operated cases developed late motility limitations (15%), sometimes alleviated with prednisone.[27] In another Dutch series, smaller amounts of recession were used with good results.[46] In 23 patients, nine had surgery on only one muscle, 11 on two muscles, and three on three muscles. Usually, less than 5 mm of recession was performed on the horizontal recti and less than 6 mm on the vertical recti.[39] As mentioned above, the time course to obtain an optimal result after strabismus surgery is variable. In a recent series, 74% of patients stabilized within 1 month of surgery; however, in 26% of cases it took up to 3 months to obtain final ocular position.[28]

Numerous complications are observed following strabismus surgery for thyroid myopathy. In the series reported by Scott and Thalacker, only four of 22 patients followed for more than 6 months had full versions and normal motility. As noted above, 28% of patients develop secondary abnormalities of the lower eyelid.[36] While anterior segment ischemia is a rare problem,[33,40] a case report was published of necrotizing scleritis in a patient who had bilateral medial and inferior recti.[62] The most common eye muscle problem is limited motion in the recessed muscle's field of action. A second common problem is the occurrence of a secondary A-pattern in downgaze when medial and inferior recti require recession. A slight undercorrection with better function in downgaze can help avoid this development. A third ocular muscle problem is occasional instability due to secondary to progressive disease or (possibly) due to the unmasking of previously hidden superior rectus myositis revealed by recession of the inferior rectus muscle. While increased intraocular pressure has been noted during strabismus surgery on thyroid orbitopathy patients, its effect on the optic nerve is uncertain.[63]

CONCLUSION

Myopathy is a common component of thyroid eye disease; however, some acute and subacute cases resolve spontaneously as part of the natural history of Graves' disease. Management may be difficult, especially after surgical decompression. Patients who request orbital decompression for cosmesis are likely to be bothered most by new-onset diplopia that may occur as a consequence of that procedure. Myopathy can resolve and then recur, apparently spontaneously, so that surgery, even that performed when eye muscle measurements appear to have stabilized, can result in latent under- or overcorrection. Muscular problems can be corrected surgically, but full postsurgical return of normal extraocular motility and single vision in all fields of gaze is uncommon, especially in patients who have undergone orbital decompression.[64] Adjustable sutures have improved operative success rates; however, even this surgical modification cannot produce totally acceptable results.

REFERENCES

1. Brain WR, Turnbull HM. Exophthalmic ophthalmoplegia. QJM 1938;7:293.
2. Mulvaney JH. The exophthalmos of hyperthyroidism. Am J Ophthalmol 1944;27:589.
3. Morgan DC, Mason AS. Exophthalmos in Cushing's syndrome. Br Med J 1958;2:481.
4. Weidler WB. Acromegaly with extreme degree of exophthalmos. Boston MSJ 1916;174:506.
5. Zondek H, Ticho A. Myasthenia gravis and malignant exophthalmos. Report of case. Lancet 1951;2:1018.
6. Cushing H. Basophil adenomas of pituitary body and their clinical manifestations (pituitary basophilism). Bull Johns Hopkins Hosp 1932;50:137.
7. Vail D. Exophthalmos. Postgrad Med 1949;5:439.
8. Hermann JS. Paretic thyroid myopathy. Ophthalmology 1982;89:473.
9. Hodes BL, Frazee L, Szmyd S. Thyroid orbitopathy: an update. Ophthalmic Surg 1979;10:25.
10. Havard CWH. Endocrine exophthalmos. Br J Med 1972;1:1360.
11. Kriss JP, Konishi J, Herman MM. Studies on the pathogenesis of Graves' ophthalmopathy. Recent Prog Horm Res 1975;31:533.
12. Inoue Y, Inoue T, Ichikizaki K. The role of extraocular muscle in the development of dysthyroid ophthalmopathy. Jpn J Clin Ophthalmol 1978;32:901.
13. Forrester JV, Sutherland JR, McDougall IR. Dysthyroid ophthalmopathy: orbital evaluation with B-scan ultrasonography. J Clin Endocrinol Metab 1977;45:221.
14. McNutt LC, Kaefring SL, Ossoinig KC. Echographic measurement of extraocular muscles. In D White, R Brown (eds), Ultrasound in Medicine (Vol 3). New York: Plenum, 1977;927.
15. Enzmann D, Donaldson SS, Kriss JP. Appearance of Graves' disease on orbital computed tomography. J Comput Assist Tomogr 1979;3:815.
16. Caygill WM. Excyclotropia in dysthyroid ophthalmopathy. Am J Ophthalmol 1972;73:437.
17. Trobe JD. Cyclodeviation in acquired vertical strabismus. Arch Ophthalmol 1984;102:717.
18. Naumann M. Herzleiden mit anschwellung der schilddruese und exophthalmos. Dtsch Klinik 1853;5:269.
19. Goldstein JE. Paresis of superior rectus muscle. Arch Ophthalmol 1964;72:5.
20. Moore RF. Exophthalmos and limitation of eye movements of Graves' disease. Lancet 1920;2:701.
21. Schultz RO, Van Allen MW, Blodi FC. Endocrine ophthalmoplegia. With an electromyographic study of paretic extraocular muscles. Arch Ophthalmol 1960;63:217.

22. Dunnington JH, Berke RN. Exophthalmos due to chronic orbital myositis. Arch Ophthalmol 1943;30:446.
23. Fells P, Lawton NF, Shine B, McCarry B. Management of dysthyroid eye disease. Aust N Z J Ophthalmol 1988;16:37.
24. Fells P, McCarry B. Diplopia in thyroid eye disease. Trans Ophthalmol Soc U K 1986;105:413.
25. Evans D, Kennerdell JS. Extraocular muscle surgery for dysthyroid myopathy. Am J Ophthalmol 1983;95:767.
26. Scott WE, Thalacker JA. Diagnosis and treatment of thyroid myopathy. Ophthalmology 1981;88:493.
27. Sterk CC, Bierlaagh JJM, De Keizer RJW. Motility disorders in endocrine ophthalmopathy. Doc Ophthalmol 1985;59:71.
28. Mourits MP, Koorneef L, Mourik-Noordenbos AM, et al. Extraocular muscle surgery for Graves' ophthalmopathy: does prior treatment influence surgical outcome? Br J Ophthalmol 1990;74:481.
29. Hamilton HE, Schultz RO, DeGowin EL. The endocrine eye lesion in hyperthyroidism. Arch Intern Med 1960;105:675.
30. Winguth S, Kurhanewicz J, Wang ML, et al. ^{31}P magnetic resonance spectroscopy (MRS) of orbital myositis. Invest Ophthalmol Vis Sci 1991;32:2417.
31. Laitt RD, Hoh B, Wakeley C, et al. The value of the short tau inversion recovery sequence in magnetic resonance imaging of thyroid eye disease. Br J Radiol 1994;67:244.
32. Hoh HB, Laitt RD, Wakeley C, et al. The STIR sequence MRI in the assessment of extraocular muscles in thyroid eye disease. Eye 1994;8:506.
33. Rosenbaum AL. Discussion. Ophthalmology 1982;89:327.
34. Fells P. Orbital decompression for severe dysthyroid eye disease. Br J Ophthalmol 1987;71:107.
35. Dunn WJ, Arnold AC, O'Connor PS. Botulinum toxin for the treatment of dysthyroid ocular myopathy. Ophthalmology 1986;93:470.
36. Fells P. Thyroid-associated eye disease: clinical management. Lancet 1991;338:29.
37. Lyons CJ, Vickers SF, Lee JP. Botulinum toxin therapy in dysthyroid strabismus. Eye 1990;4:538.
38. Bessant DAR, Lee JP. Management of strabismus due to orbital myositis. Eye 1995;9:558.
39. Kulla S, Moore S. Orthoptics in Graves' disease. Trans Am Acad Ophthalmol Otolaryngol 1979;86:2053.
40. Lueder GT, Scott WE, Kutschke PJ, Keech RV. Long-terms results of adjustable suture surgery for strabismus secondary to thyroid ophthalmopathy. Ophthalmopathy 1994;99:993.
41. Burke JP, Shipman TC, Watts MT. Convergence insufficiency in thyroid eye disease. J Pediatr Ophthalmol Strabismus 1993;30:127.
42. Long JC. Surgical management of tropias of thyroid exophthalmos. Arch Ophthalmol 1966;75:634.
43. Swan KC. Fascia in relation to extraocular muscle surgery. Arch Ophthalmol 1970;83:134.
44. Dunlap EA. Plastic implants in muscle surgery: plastic materials in the management of extraocular motility restrictions. Arch Ophthalmol 1968;80:249.
45. Beisner DH. Extraocular muscle recessions utilizing silicone tendon prostheses. Arch Ophthalmol 1970;83:195.
46. Mailette LJJM, Wenniger-Prick DB, Van Mourik-Noordenbos AM, Koorneef L. Squint surgery in patients with Graves' ophthalmopathy. Doc Ophthalmol 1986;61:219.
47. Jampolsky A. Surgical Leashes and Reverse Leashes in Strabismus Surgical Management. In Symposium on Strabismus: Transactions of the New Orleans Academy of Ophthalmology. St. Louis: Mosby, 1978;244.
48. Pratt-Johnson JA, Drance SM. Surgical treatment of dysthyroid restriction syndromes. Can J Ophthalmol 1972;7:405.
49. Sugar HS. Management of eye movement restriction (particularly vertical) in dysthyroid myopathy. Ann Ophthalmol 1979;11:1305.
50. Dyer HAA. The oculorotary muscles in Graves' disease. Trans Am Ophthalmol Soc 1976;74:425.
51. Kraus DJ, Bullock JD. Treatment of thyroid ocular myopathy with adjustable and nonadjustable suture strabismus surgery. Trans Am Ophthalmol Soc 1993;91:67.

52. Wesley RE, Bond JB. Upper eyelid retraction from inferior rectus restriction in dysthyroid orbit disease. Ann Ophthalmol 1987;19:34.

52a. Pachecco EM, Guyton DL, Reyka MX. Changes in eyelid position accompanying vertical rectus muscle surgery and prevention of lower eyelid retraction with adjustable surgery. J Ped Ophthal Strab 1992;29:265.

52b. Kushner BJ. A surgical procedure to minimize lower-eyelid retraction with inferior rectus recession. Arch Ophthalmol 1992;110:1011.

52c. Meyer DR, Simon JW, Kansora M. Primary infratarsal lower eyelid retractor lysis to prevent eyelid retraction after inferior rectus recession. Am J Ophthalmol 1996;122:331.

53. Jampolsky A. Strabismus reoperation techniques. Trans Am Acad Ophthalmol Otolaryngol 1975;79:704.

54. Rosenbaum AL, Metz HS, Carlson M, Jampolsky AJ. Adjustable rectus muscle recession surgery. A followup study. Arch Ophthalmol 1977;95:817.

55. Sprunger DT, Helveston EM. Progressive overcorrection after inferior rectus recession. J Pediatr Ophthalmol Strabismus 1993;30:145.

56. Buckley EG, Meekins BB. Faden operation for the management of complicated inconcomitant vertical strabismus. Am J Ophthalmol 1988;105:304.

57. Clorfeine GS, Parker WT. Adjustment sensitivity of horizontal rectus muscles and adjustable strabismus surgery. Arch Ophthalmol 1987;105:1664.

58. Vrabec MP, Presian MW, Kushner BJ. Oculocardiac reflex during manipulation of adjustable sutures after strabismus surgery. Am J Ophthalmol 1987;104:61.

59. Hertle RW, Granet DB, Zylan S. The intraoperative oculocardiac reflex as a predictor of postoperative vaso-vagal responses during adjustable suture surgery. J Pediatr Ophthalmol Strabismus 1993;30:306.

60. Jampolsky A. Strategies in Strabismus Surgery. Trans New Orleans Acad Ophthalmol 1986;363.

61. Bartley GB, Fatourechi V, Kadrmas EF, et al. Long-term follow-up of Graves ophthalmopathy in an incidence cohort. Ophthalmology 1996;103:958.

62. Kaufman LM, Folk ER, Miller MT, Tessler HH. Necrotizing scleritis following strabismus surgery for thyroid ophthalmopathy. J Pediatr Ophthalmol Strabismus 1989;26:236.

63. Raizman MB, Beck RW. Sustained increase in intraocular pressure during strabismus surgery. Am J Ophthalmol 1986;101:308.

64. Shorr N, Neuhaus RW, Baylis HI. Ocular motility problems after orbital decompression for dysthyroid ophthalmopathy. Ophthalmology 1982;89:323.

14

Conclusion

It is difficult to be concise and inclusive in a relatively short book on thyroid eye disease. Investigators from many disciplines have studied various aspects of this problem: endocrinology, ophthalmology, ocular plastic surgery, radiation oncology, and immunology. It is somewhat difficult to try to incorporate ideas that are sometimes contradictory and often in a state of evolution into a lucid framework.

This book covers general principles and ideas regarding the pathogenesis, pathophysiology, diagnosis, and treatment of thyroid ophthalmopathy. It is appropriate to end the discussion with a short survey of what we do not know and with some comment on the direction further research into the pathogenesis and management of thyroid eye disease may take.

As discussed in Chapter 2, it appears that immunologic alterations are central to the development of autoimmune thyroid syndromes, including Graves' disease. The nature of these immunologic abnormalities is still poorly delineated. More data suggest that an antireceptor antibody is a central component of the pathophysiology of Graves' disease; however, the trigger for this disorder is poorly understood. I think it is unlikely to be a systemic immunologic disorder, but why local thyroid immunity develops is unclear. While it is somewhat discouraging to have seen a number of immunologic theories developed and refuted in less than 20 years, it appears that we are getting closer to understanding the immunologic perturbations that occur, but we cannot yet delineate the pathogenesis of thyroid eye disease.

In the last 10 years, since the first edition of this book, improvements in laboratory tests, most notably the development of a sensitive test for serum thyrotropin, and routine availability of antithyrotropin antibodies plus the routine use of magnetic resonance imaging have made diagnosis of thyroid eye disease easier. These assays improve our ability to differentiate thyroid orbitopathy from most other simulating lesions. The sensitivity and specificity of these diagnostic tools in the detection of euthyroid ophthalmopathy and the differentiation of thyroid eye disease from idiopathic orbital inflammations (orbital pseudotumors) is still uncertain. Use of modern imaging techniques, laboratory studies, and, when necessary, fine-needle aspiration biopsy under computed tomography control has made differential diagnosis straightforward. Probably some euthyroid ophthalmopathy patients who do not display evidence of systemic thyroid disease have idiopathic orbital myositis of a different etiology, although we have a few patients who initially had normal serum thyrotropin and an absence of antibodies when they first presented with eye disease, then developed systemic thyroid disease in the subsequent years. More sequential follow-up data on such patients is necessary.

Over the last 10 years, neither clinical nor basic research work has greatly increased our understanding of the nature of some peculiarities of thyroid eye disease. For example, it remains unclear why the inferior rectus is the predominant extraocular muscle involved in this disease. Is this because modern humans use vision in downgaze (and hence the inferior rectus) more than in other gaze angles? This explanation seems adumbrated. What differentiates Graves' disease patients who develop ophthalmopathy from those who do not? Some have slightly different systemic immunologic abnormalities, but these are not consistent. Similarly, why are elderly male patients who develop hyperthyroidism more likely to develop severe ophthalmopathy? Finally, why do approximately 5–10% of thyroid eye disease patients develop visually threatening optic neuropathy?

Therapeutically, increased understanding of immunologic circuits has resulted in the gradual introduction of less toxic, more specific immunomodulatory drugs, the first generation typified by cyclosporine. The relative indications of steroids, immunomodulatory agents, and radiation are still uncertain, although as discussed in Chapters 8–10, sufficient clinical data have become available to allow us to develop rational treatment protocols. Current surgical therapies have significant side effects and do not affect the underlying disease process. In the future, it is hoped that we can prevent development of thyroid eye disease, or with newer gene therapies, diminish the incidence of fibrotic disease and thus reduce the need for ocular surgery. These treatments still remain more of a hope than a reality.

Index

Note: Page numbers in italic indicate figures; page numbers followed by t indicate tables.